Cancer and the LGBT Community

Ulrike Boehmer • Ronit Elk
Editors

Cancer and the LGBT Community

Unique Perspectives from Risk to Survivorship

Springer

Editors
Ulrike Boehmer
Department of Community Health Sciences
Boston University School of Public Health
Boston
USA

Ronit Elk
College of Nursing
University of South Carolina
Columbia
USA

ISBN 978-3-319-15056-7 ISBN 978-3-319-15057-4 (eBook)
DOI 10.1007/978-3-319-15057-4

Library of Congress Control Number: 2015941732

Springer Cham Heidelberg New York Dordrecht London

Printed on acid-free paper

Springer International Publishing is part of Springer Science+Business Media (www.springer.com)

We dedicate this book to the innumerable LGBT patients with cancer and their families of choice, who have so willingly and courageously shared their cancer experience; and to the dedicated cancer researchers, clinicians, and policy makers who have paved the way for future generations.

Foreword

In 1999, a group of us worked on a white paper that was to provide background information to Health and Human Services (HHS) investigators who were considering the inclusion of LGBT populations in Healthy People 2010 (1). Research on cancer in LGBT populations was limited—mostly addressing HIV/AIDS -related cancers in men and breast cancer in women. The section of the white paper that reviewed knowledge then available about cancer started and ended with notes on the need for further research to help in understanding cancer in LGBT populations. Fifteen years later, this book, which comprises 19 chapters edited by Boehmer and Elk, is an important response to the call for knowledge on cancer in LGBT populations. This book provides an indispensable resource for information about the many aspects of cancer.

The chapters assembled for this book cover impressively broad areas of research and practice, with authors providing diligent analysis and integration of research conducted on the epidemiology, clinical care, and policy of LGBT cancer. Part I discusses risks for cancer, with careful analysis addressing women and men, including transgender individuals, separately. Chapters address risk related to infection in LGBT men and women and lifestyle risks, related to obesity and nutrition, substance use and smoking, and physical activity. Part II addresses cancer prevention by focusing on issues related to early screening. Again the authors avoid generalizations by carefully covering issues of concern to GBT men (e.g., HPV) and LBT women (e.g., breast, reproductive organs) separately. Part III provides a review of the epidemiology of cancer in LGBT populations and addresses clinical issues, treatment and survivorship. The unique issues of LGBT people in cancer are made especially clear here as authors discuss issues such as disclosure of one's sexual orientation to care providers, sensitivity to special concerns of LGBT individuals (e.g., sexual performance after prostate cancer treatment, Chap. 10), and social support and, specifically, the inclusion of expanded definition of family that is so important to LGBT people (e.g., inclusion in care-giving of ex-lovers of a lesbian entering hospice, Chap. 12). Of course, cultural competence in providing cancer care, including in support groups, is crucial for providers to be able to address these issues sensitively (Chap. 13).

Although authors of all the chapters are sensitive to including concerns of transgender individuals and to address, as possible, issues affecting diverse LGBT populations, Part IV takes a special look at concerns of transgender populations and LGBT people of color. For example, authors highlight the combined impact of social, economic, and cultural factors that place barriers to screening, health care services, and engagement in risk behaviors (Chap. 16). Also addressed in all chapters are implications of the research findings and observations to healthcare policy but the editors address this important issue specifically in Part V where authors review implications of new U.S. policies and how they have impacted healthcare for LGBT populations, as well as discuss challenges, and suggest a roadmap for LGBT cancer health.

One question that emerges from the pages of the book, sometimes implicitly, is whether LGBT disparity in cancer outcomes is the main reason for studying LGBT populations in cancer. Authors review data to try to understand cisgender/heterosexual vs. LGBT cancer disparities. The focus on health disparities is an important topic for the U.S. Health and Human Services, as described in Healthy People 2010 and Healthy People 2020. It is a key motivation for studying social epidemiology because health disparities reveal important structural inequities that ought to be addressed. But as Boehmer notes in the context of breast cancer (Chap. 9), the "absence of a disparity must not be interpreted as lack of need for programs for and interventions with sexual minority women who live with breast cancer" (p. 155). Although understanding health disparities is important, it is not the only reason to study LGBT people and cancer and should not be the only topic of study. As many chapters demonstrate, even where there are no differences in rates of disease or screening, special attention ought to be paid to LGBT issues. For example, Blank, Descartes, and Asencio (Chap. 7) ask not only whether screening rates in gay and bisexual men and transgender people differ from screening rates of cisgender heterosexual men, but also whether there are specific factors related to these populations that may merit screening guidelines being different. These authors, like most of the book's authors, explore these and other distinctions among LGBT and cisgender heterosexual populations and reveal important areas for research and intervention.

Indeed, the book is impressive in the broad perspectives taken by the authors in discussing cancer in LGBT populations. For example, although risks for cancer are often discussed at the individual genetic and behavioral levels, authors in this volume have incorporated a broader health equity perspective that identifies larger structural factors (e.g., Chaps. 4, 16). Indeed, by the very act of focusing on LGBT populations in cancer, all authors adopt a social-cultural view of medicine, where one's identity and position in society are as important determinants of health as are biological and behavioral factors. In weaving these social-cultural factors together with individual lifestyle risks and vulnerabilities, the book enlightens us not only about cancer in LGBT populations but also about the many ways that cancer is affected by seemingly non-medical factors. One of the research respondents in Margolies and Kamen's chapter noted this connection when he talked about the importance of support: "My partner IS MY FAMILY and when [health care providers] treat him as such my [health] outcomes are much better. He is my advocate and can remember everything I can't. Good [health] outcomes depend on his involvement as does my emotional well being" (p. 208). Behind this observation is a profound realization, explicated by authors throughout the book, that LGBT identity matters because it is connected with a host of structural factors related to stigma, prejudice, and access to resources, which determine health outcomes.

Despite the great progress in knowledge about LGBT cancer since the 2000 white paper, as chronicled here in the book reveals important continuing challenges for researchers, clinicians, and policy makers. For example, several authors have noted that cancer registries still do not include information about sexual orientation or gender identity, making vast invaluable information about cancer unusable with regard to issues that may be specific to LGBT populations (Chap. 3, Chap. 8). As Tracy noted: "If we are to enhance our understanding of basic epidemiology of STI-associated cancers in LBT women, we must start by integrating data collection of sexual identity and gender identity into our national surveillance systems as crucial demographic variables, and we must urge members of the scientific community to adopt standards for collecting demographic variables related to sexual identity, sexual behavior and gender identity so that results can be compared meaningfully across studies" (p. 32). Several authors noted that the recent decision by HHS to include sexual orientation questions in the National Health Interview Survey, like the inclusion of sexual orientation questions in other state-based surveys, is an important first step in improving knowledge on LGB health. Still, as Fredriksen-Goldsen, Hoy-Ellis, and Brown (Chap. 4) remind us, to date only one survey—the Massachusetts Behavioral Risk Factor Surveillance System—includes information about gender identity.

Another challenge for cancer in LGBT population is the paucity of specialized targeted programs and culturally competent care in general. As several authors noted, there are too few evaluations of both primary interventions to reduce risk for cancer and secondary and tertiary interventions with LGBT people with cancer (Chaps. 4, 13). It may not be apparent to service providers, but even when the information provided to a cancer survivor is the same regardless of sexual orientation and gender identity, an LGBT person can be alienated when services are not tailored and culturally sensitive to the him or her. As Margolies and Kamen (Chap. 13) said: "LGBT survivors … may feel most comfortable and most supported when talking to another LGBT survivor who shares their concerns and experiences." The authors report on one of their research participants, who said "Without knowing other lesbians who had had breast cancer who helped me through the process, I am not sure how I would have fared" (p. 215). Fredriksen-Goldsen, Hoy-Ellis, and Brown concluded "it is imperative that tailored community-based prevention efforts and interventions be designed and tested to improve health and promote health equity in these communities" (Chap. 4., p. 54).

Thanks to the editors, this book goes a long way toward providing knowledge, ideas, and resources that can help researchers, clinicians, and policy makers achieve the goal of improving health and promoting health equity in LGBT communities. It also points to challenges ahead which, hopefully, will encourage researchers to study the topics covered in the book and bring about more progress in the study of LGBT cancer.

Ilan H. Meyer

References

Dean L, Meyer IH, Robinson K, Sell RL, Sember R, Silenzio VMB, et al. Lesbian, Gay, Bisexual, and Transgender Health: Findings and Concerns. J Gay Lesbian Med Assoc. 2000;4(3):101–51.

Book Note

The following individuals have contributed to this book by reviewing chapters and assisting with other tasks: Bryn Austin (Children's Hospital, Boston, MA), Kellan Baker (Center for American Progress www.americanprogress.org), Jose Bauermeister (University of Michigan School of Public Health, Ann Arbor, MI), Thomas Blank (University of Connecticut, Storrs CT), Jack Burkhalter (Memorial Sloan-Kettering Cancer Center, New York, NY), Rachel M. Ceballos (Fred Hutchinson Cancer Research Center, Seattle, WA), Brian Chen (University of South Carolina, Columbia, SC), Julie Fish (De Montfort University, Leicester, United Kingdom), Danielle Gentile (University of South Carolina, Columbia, SC), Ayad Hamdan (Harvard Medical School, Boston, MA), Michael Hoyt (City University of New York, New York, NY), Tonda Hughes (University of Illinois at Chicago, Chicago, IL), David Latini (Baylor College of Medicine and Michael E. DeBakey VA Medical Center, Houston, TX), Jeanne Marrazzo (University of Washington, Seattle, WA), Nick Mule (York University Toronto, Ontario, Canada), Henry Ng (GLMA: Health Professionals Advancing LGBT Equality), Nancy Orel (Bowling Green State University, Bowling Green, OH), Julie Palmer (Boston University, Boston, MA), Jennifer Potter (Harvard Medical School, Boston, MA), Paul Reiter (The Ohio State University, Columbus, OH), Gary Stein (Yeshiva University, New York, NY).

Contents

Contributors

Madina Agénor Department of Social and Behavioral Sciences, Harvard School of Public Health, Boston, MA, USA

Gilad E. Amiel Scott Department of Urology, Baylor College of Medicine, Houston, TX, USA

Frances Aranda College of Nursing, University of Illinois at Chicago, Chicago, IL, USA

Marysol Asencio University of Connecticut, Storrs, CT, USA

Swagata Banik Baldwin Wallace University, Berea, OH, USA

Thomas O. Blank University of Connecticut, Storrs, CT, USA

Ulrike Boehmer Department of Community Health Sciences, Boston University School of Public Health, Boston, MA, USA

Maria Brown Syracuse University, NY, USA

Jack E. Burkhalter Memorial Sloan Kettering Cancer Center, New York, NY, USA

Melissa A. Clark Department of Epidemiology and Obstetrics & Gynecology, School of Public Health and Warren Alpert Medical School, Brown University, Providence, RI, USA

Lara Descartes Brescia University College, London, ON, Canada

Suzanne L. Dibble Institute of Health and Aging, School of Nursing, University of California, San Francisco, CA, USA

Michele J. Eliason Department of Health Education, San Francisco State University, San Francisco, CA, USA

Ronit Elk College of Nursing, University of South Carolina, Columbia, SC, USA

Karen I. Fredriksen-Goldsen School of Social Work, University of Washington, Seattle, Washington, USA

Heather H. Goltz Social Work Program, University of Houston—Downtown, Houston, TX, USA

Section of Infectious Diseases, Department of Medicine, Baylor College of Medicine, Houston, TX, USA

Missak Haigentz Departments of Medicine (Oncology) and Otorhinolaryngology - Head and Neck Surgery, Albert Einstein College of Medicine, Montefiore Medical Center, Bronx, NY, USA

Tae L. Hart Department of Psychology, Ryerson University, Toronto, ON, Canada

Charles P. Hoy-Ellis School of Social Work, University of Washington, Seattle, Washington, USA

Charles Kamen Department of Surgery, University of Rochester Medical Center, Rochester, NY, USA

Michael R. Kauth VA South Central Mental Illness Research, Education and Clinical Center, Houston, TX, USA

Mental Health Care Line, Michael E. DeBakey VA Medical Center, Houston, TX, USA

Center for Innovations in Quality, Effectiveness and Safety, Michael E. DeBakey VA Medical Center, Houston, TX, USA

Department of Psychiatry & Behavioral Sciences, Baylor College of Medicine, Houston, TX, USA

Stewart Landers John Snow, Inc., Cambridge, MA, USA

David M. Latini Mental Health Care Line, Michael E. DeBakey VA Medical Center, Houston, TX, USA

Scott Department of Urology, Baylor College of Medicine, Houston, TX, USA

Meenhye Lee College of Nursing, University of Illinois at Chicago, Chicago, IL, USA

Emilia Lombardi Department of Public Health, Baldwin Wallace University, Berea, OH, USA

Liz Margolies National LGBT Cancer Network, New York, NY, USA

Alicia K. Matthews College of Nursing, University of Illinois, Chicago, IL, USA

I Mary Poynten The Kirby Institute, The University of New South Wales, Sydney, Australia

Samantha Rosenthal Department of Epidemiology, School of Public Health, Brown University, Providence, RI, USA

Natalie Ross Howard Brown Health Center, Chicago, IL, USA

Scout LGBT HealthLink at CenterLink: The Community of LGBT Centers, Fort Lauderdale, FL, USA

J. Kathleen Tracy Department of Epidemiology and Public Health, University of Maryland School of Medicine, Baltimore, MD, USA

Evan P. Wenker Scott Department of Urology, Baylor College of Medicine, Houston, TX, USA

Chapter 1
Introduction

Ulrike Boehmer and Ronit Elk

Abstract Cancer affects people globally, the numbers of cancer survivors are increasing, and cancer counts among the leading causes of death. Despite cancer's universal impact, this is the first book to focus on the cancer burden among the lesbian, gay, bisexual, and transgender (LGBT) community. Multiple challenges are discussed that have impeded research of the cancer burden in the LGBT community until this first publication brought together dedicated researchers, advocates, and scientists who are at the forefront of LGBT cancer research. The cancer control continuum is the underlying structure for the content of the book, ranging from cancer prevention, detection, diagnosis, and cancer survivorship to the end of life. Specific chapters are dedicated to transgender individuals, as well as racial or ethnic minority LGBT individuals to emphasize the diversity of the LGBT community. In addition, this book includes chapters on the impact of policy in the US and internationally and a final chapter that addresses the crosscutting themes and discusses the next steps for LGBT communities and cancer.

In the United States, cancer is the second leading cause of death, and increasing numbers of academic and clinical publications, alongside the popular media, discuss and bring awareness about the steadily increasing numbers of cancer survivors. Moreover, cancer has been recognized as a worldwide problem, given that in many low and middle-income countries more people die from cancer annually than from AIDS, malaria, and tuberculosis combined. Yet to date, this is the first book that focuses on cancer and the LGBT population. It's not that such a book could not have been written earlier, but rather, anyone dealing with this topic would have chosen a much shorter publication method, possibly an opinion piece or several articles to summarize what is known about LGBT populations and just a select few cancers. A great number of challenges stood in the way of compiling such a book until

U. Boehmer (✉)
Department of Community Health Sciences, Boston University School of Public Health, 801 Massachusetts Avenue, Crosstown Center, Boston, MA 02118, USA
e-mail: boehmer@bu.edu

R. Elk
College of Nursing, University of South Carolina, Columbia, SC, USA
e-mail: elk@mailbox.sc.edu

U. Boehmer, R. Elk (eds.), *Cancer and the LGBT Community*,
DOI 10.1007/978-3-319-15057-4_1

now. Unfortunately, many of these challenges continue to hinder greater knowledge about LGBT populations and cancer.

Possibly one of the most profound challenges that impede LGBT cancer research is the promotion of an exclusively biomedical and basic science perspective of cancer. Some funders, researchers, and members of the medical establishment call into question any focus on cancer in LGBT individuals, arguing that cancer cells grow in LGBT bodies the same as in heterosexual bodies. Without minimizing the contribution of the basic sciences, it nevertheless holds true that even if the proverbial "cure" for cancer was discovered in a lab today, social aspects would still come into play. It is likely that access to the cure would take longer or be more challenging for disenfranchised and underserved minorities, including LGBT individuals. In other words, cancer or health and well-being are not the outcome of cellular processes alone; there are social factors that contribute to cancer or health and well-being. Another challenge is the myth of sexual orientation being synonymous with sexual behavior; a perspective that holds that the only aspect that distinguishes lesbian, gay, and bisexuals' lives from heterosexuals' is their same-sex sexual activities. Such reductionist thinking of LGBT lives has been an impediment noted in a recent review of gay and bisexual men and cancer, which noted that most available information focuses on cancers that have infectious causes linked to sexual transmission [1]. Ironically, a number of medical journals, including oncology journals, even have a policy against the use of the terms gay and bisexual men, allowing exclusively the term men who have sex with men. The usage of the terms, "men who have sex with men" and "women who have sex with women" has long been identified as problematic; it erases lesbian, gay, or bisexual identity, cultural and political content, as well as the larger perspective of the LGBT community [2]. Another challenge for LGBT research is that the focus on sexual and gender minorities often minimizes the diversity that exists within the LGBT community, such as LGBT individuals who are poor or from racial or ethnic minorities. Transgender individuals are without question the most marginalized and neglected community members not only in terms of cancer, but also in terms of LGBT health in general. Often even the most well-intentioned efforts that focus on LGB***T*** fall short on the ***T***. Understanding LGBT populations and cancer has long been plagued by data challenges; most importantly, cancer registries do not collect information on sexual orientation and gender identity. Although increasing numbers of federal and state-level datasets are now available that include at least some measure of sexual orientation, a measure of gender identity is rarely included. The available datasets have been instrumental in providing a growing understanding of LGBT risk behaviors that are linked to cancers. Yet, to date, the datasets upon which research commonly relies to gather information about incidence, survivorship, and mortality, state and SEER cancer registries, have not followed suit and do not collect sexual orientation and gender identity data. This continues to be an obstacle for much of LGBT cancer survivorship and mortality research. However, it has not stopped such research from taking place. Moreover, there are important research questions about LGBT and cancer to be answered that do not require large population-based datasets. While this speaks to the vibrancy and emergence of research about LGBT and cancer, it has to be noted that possibly one of the most difficult challenges to overcome has to do with obtaining support and funding to conduct research that focuses on LGBT populations and cancer. A recent review of the National Institutes of Health funding portfolio for the years 1989–2011 showed that over these 22 years, only 35 funded studies focused on LGBT and cancer, further reduced to a mere 13 studies, once research conducted in the context of HIV/AIDS and sexual health had been excluded [3]. One of the major consequences of the lack of funding is a serious gap in research that can, in turn, inform evidence-based programs, services and interventions to improve risk, prevention, or suffering from cancer among LGBT communities. This list of challenges that have long hindered and still interfere with current endeavors of deepening our understanding of cancer in LGBT communities is brief and incomplete, yet it provides some context to the reader about the kind of milestone this book represents.

In 2011, the Institute of Medicine published *The Health of Lesbian, Gay, and Bisexual, and Transgender People*, currently the pivotal document for the National Institutes of Health, the research community, and all other individuals and agencies interested in understanding the health of lesbian, gay, bisexual, and transgender LGBT individuals [4]. Within this report cancer is discussed as one of the conditions that affect LGBT individuals. Around the same time, Elk and Landrine published their edited book, *Cancer Disparities: Causes and Evidence-Based Solutions,* which discussed cancer causes and evidence-based research programs aimed at reducing cancer health disparities in populations in which such disparities exist, including LGBT populations [5]. In each of these landmark publications, only a few of the hundreds of pages were devoted to LGBT populations and cancer. It is therefore a great honor to edit a book on LGBT and cancer, which is entirely devoted to cancer and LGBT communities. The time is ripe for such a publication; we feel fortunate to have brought together a group of dedicated researchers, advocates and scientists who are the forefront of this field, having spent many years and tremendous efforts in overcoming considerable challenges in their work in this field.

To organize our thinking and the content of the book, we relied on the cancer control continuum (http://cancercontrol.cancer.gov/od/continuum.html). While admittedly, this is an old concept with well-recognized shortcomings, we feel it is a useful concept to apply to LGBT communities and cancer, as it organizes the state of the current knowledge about LGBT communities and cancer and identifies the research gaps that remain. Applying this framework, the sequence of book chapters follows the trajectory from cancer risks and cancer detection to cancer survivorship. In a deliberate attempt to include transgender populations, so often neglected from health research, we encouraged chapter authors to address transgender individuals in their respective chapter whenever possible, but also decided to devote a chapter to transgender individuals and cancer to ensure that this book about LGB***T*** and cancer will be relevant to all members of the LGBT community. Similarly, to ensure that this book on LGBT populations and cancer is responsive to LGBT individuals of diverse race and ethnicity, we have included a chapter that deals with the intersection of race, ethnicity and sexual and gender minorities. Understanding the impact a country's policies have on health outcome is key to obtaining a broad perspective, hence we have included chapters on the impact of policy in the US and internationally. The final chapter addresses the crosscutting themes of this book and discusses the next steps for LGBT communities and cancer. This framework has been useful in organizing the available knowledge on cancer among LGBT communities.

In order to provide a comprehensive review of cancer in the LGBT community, we have addressed the most common cancer risks, cancer detection methods, and survivorship issues that cut across cancer types. Not all types of cancer are addressed in this book; LGBT individuals who wish to get information about their specific cancer type may need to consult other sources that answer questions about their specific cancer (e.g., ACS http://www.cancer.org/ and NCI http:// www.cancer.gov/).

References

1. Boehmer U, Cooley TP, Clark MA. Cancer and men who have sex with men: a systematic review. Lancet Oncol. 2012;13(12):E545–53.
2. Young RM, Meyer IH. The trouble with "MSM" and "WSW": erasure of the sexual-minority person in public health discourse. Am J Public Health. 2005;95(7):1144–9.
3. Coulter RWS, Kenst KS, Bowen DJ, Scout. Research funded by the national institutes of health on the health of lesbian, gay, bisexual, and transgender populations. Am J Public Health. 2014;104(2):e105–e12.
4. Institute of Medicine. The health of lesbian, gay, bisexual, and transgender people: building a foundation for better understanding. Washington, DC: The National Academies Press; 2011.
5. Elk R, Hope L, editors. Cancer disparities: causes and evidence-based solutions. New York: Springer; 2011.

Part I
Understanding and Reducing the Risk for Cancer

Chapter 2
Risk for Cancer in Gay, Bisexual and Transgender Men via Infection

Stewart Landers

Abstract A number of infections play a significant role in cancer risk for gay, bisexual and transgender (GBT) men. The association between Human Immunodeficiency Virus (HIV), the virus that attacks and degrades the immune system, frequently leading to Acquired Immune Deficiency Syndrome (AIDS) and cancer, has been studied extensively. In addition, human papillomavirus (several types), human herpes virus (also several types), and Hepatitis virus (primarily Hep B and Hep C), each contribute to additional cancer risk in the form of infection-related cancers. This chapter reviews these infections and associated cancers among GBT men including viral transmission and prevalence both independently and in comparison to other men. It further explores the risk of cancer associated with these infections and, given the wide varieties and potential cancer sites, where elevated cancer rates have been observed. In response to these elevated risks, efforts to improve screening, educate GBT men about the increased risk, and new treatment strategies have been implemented. This chapter explores how programs to address infection-related cancer in GBT men have fared to date, including efforts to reduce transmission of infectious agents, early intervention and screening, cost effectiveness of screening, advances in cancer treatment itself, and changes in knowledge, attitudes and behavior among GBT men. The chapter ends with unique challenges with respect to treatment of GBT men with infection related cancers.

1. Prevalence of Cancer-related STIs (HIV, HPV, Herpes, Hepatitis, Epstein-Barr)

a. Human Immunodeficiency Virus (HIV)

HIV has been associated with GBT men since the onset of the AIDS epidemic [1], as well as with cancer–Kaposi's sarcoma (KS). KS, along with Pneumocystis Carinii Pneumonia, was the presenting illness among one of the initial cohorts of AIDS patients, before the disease had a name or its cause was even known [2–3]. Gay and bisexual men, referred to as "men who have sex with men" or MSM by the federal Centers for Disease Control, are 42 times more likely to be living with HIV

S. Landers (✉)
John Snow, Inc., Cambridge, MA, USA
e-mail: stewart_landers@jsi.com

U. Boehmer, R. Elk (eds.), *Cancer and the LGBT Community*,
DOI 10.1007/978-3-319-15057-4_2

compared to other men [4]. Cancer risk is elevated among people living with HIV/AIDS (PLWH) for three AIDS-defining cancers (ADCs) including Kaposi's sarcoma, non-Hodgkin Lymphoma (NHL) and cervical cancer as well as for several non-AIDS-defining cancers (NADCs) including lung cancer, Hodgkin lymphoma, anal cancer, and liver cancer [5].

HIV risk for GBT men is well reported with risk related to anal intercourse and confounded by co- infection with other STIs including syphilis, gonnorhea, and human papillomavirus. A report based upon the CDC's National HIV Behavioral Surveillance system collected cross-sectional data in 21 U.S. cities in 2008 and found 19% of gay and bisexual men to be infected with HIV [6].

b. Human Papillomavirus (HPV)

HPV is the most common sexually transmitted infection and can be transmitted through oral, anal and vaginal sex [7]. Using DNA sequencing, more than 100 HPV types have been identified, of which 40 types infect the genital epithelia [8]. A person does not need to be symptomatic to transmit the virus [7]. Various health problems are associated with HPV including genital warts and cancers. However, most HPV infections do not cause symptoms or disease and are cleared by the body (Table 2.1).

HPV has been found to increase risk for oropharangeal, penile and anal cancers in men, including both HIV-negative and HIV-positive GBT men. Chin-Hong et al. [9] found anal HPV infection in 57% of a sample of urban HIV-negative men. Infection in this cohort was correlated with receptive anal intercourse and greater than five sex partners, both in the past 6 months. Rates of HPV among GBT men with HIV infection have been found to be as high as 93%–97.9% [10]. Two HPV types, HPV 16 and 18, are considered to carry the highest risk for cancer [11]. Reviewing

Table 2.1 List of common acronyms

ADC	AIDS Defining Cancers
EBV	Epstein-Barr Virus
HAART	Highly Active Antiretroviral Therapy
HBV	Hepatitis B Virus
HCV	Hepatitis C Virus
HHV	Human Herpes Virus
HL	Hodgkin Lymphoma
HPV	Human Papillomavirus
KS	Kaposi's sarcoma
NADC	Non-AIDS Defining Cancer
NHL	Non-Hodgkin Lymphoma
PLWH	People living with HIV/AIDS
SIR	Standardized Incidence Ratio

incident cases of anal cancer among men from 2004 to 2007, CDC attributed 93% to HPV infection and 87% specifically to HPV 16 and 18 [12].

c. Human Herpesvirus (HHV)

There are eight types of human herpesviruses including varicella/zoster (VZV/HH3), Epstein- Barr virus (EBV/HHV4), Cytomegalovirus (CMV/HHV-5) and Kaposi's sarcoma herpesvirus (KSHV/HHV-8) [13]. HHVs are transmitted both sexually and non-sexually with evidence of sexual transmission for HH2, EBV, CMV and KSHV [14].

In 1994, Chang [15] found that human herpesvirus 8 (HHV-8) was the cause of Kaposi's sarcoma. In one study, Del Mistro [16] compared rates of HHV-8 and HPV among three groups of PLWH–MSM, heterosexual men, and women, finding higher rates of both HHV-8 and HPV among gay and bisexual HIV+ men.

Epstein-Barr Virus (EBV) is another name for human herpesvirus 4 and one of the most common human viruses. Most people are infected in childhood and do not develop symptoms or have very minor symptoms [17]. EBV was identified over 40 years ago in a biopsy of Burkitt's lymphoma, becoming the first infectious agent to be directly associated with a human cancer 18].

While there is limited epidemiological data on rates of EBV infection in gay and bisexual men, one study found a higher prevalence of EBV type 2 among gay men compared to heterosexual men associated with HIV infection and a higher number of sexual partners [19]. Additional epidemiological research would be helpful to know more about prevalence rates of EBV among gay/bisexual/transgender and heterosexual men in a variety of geographic locations (unlike parts of Africa where EBV is endemic). EBV is associated with a diverse group of lymphomas and carcinomas including Burkitt's lymphoma, Hodgkin's disease, Post-transplant lymphoproliferative disease, AIDS- associated lymphoma, and nasopharyngeal and gastric carcinoma [17].

d. Hepatitis B (HBV) and Hepatitis C (HCV)

Hepatitis B and C are disproportionately found among gay and bisexual men [19]. Hepatitis B is spread in a manner similar to HIV, i.e. through blood or semen. Hepatitis B is considered to be 50–100 times more infectious than HIV [20]. Hepatitis C is primarily spread through sharing of needles and syringes. Over time, Hepatitis B and C attack the liver, causing a variety of liver diseases including liver cancer. It is estimated that 90% of liver cancers in less developed countries and 40% of liver cancers in more developed countries are attributable to HBV or HCV infection [22]. Approximately 20% of gay and bisexual men account for new Hepatitis B infections [20], disproportional to their 4% representation in the general population.

2. Reasons for different rates of cancer than in the heterosexual community

Why Higher Rates of Infection Lead to Higher Rates of Cancer

HIV can increase the risk of GBT men for rare cancers like non-Hodgkin Lymphoma, Kaposi sarcoma, and liver cancers. Additionally it has been shown that immunosuppression and infection with other viruses related to HIV/AIDS puts those infected at higher risk of anal, liver, lung cancer. HPV infection impacts disparate cancer rates in GBT men. HPV infection leads to penile cancer for men, cervical cancer for women, and cancers of the mouth, throat, and anus for people of both genders. Hep B and C can also put people at risk for liver cancer and lymphomas.

HIV-positive Patients Have Higher Risk for Some Cancers

The burden of cancer on PLWH has been well documented. However, the nature of this burden has shifted, specifically as a result of the introduction of highly active antiretroviral therapy (HAART) in 1996. For example, in a 2011 study, Shiels [23] found that during 1991–2005, an estimated 79,656 cancers occurred in the population of people living with AIDS in the United States. However, comparing the periods 1991–1995 and 2001–2005, the estimated number of AIDS-defining cancers decreased by greater than threefold from 34,587 to 10,325 cancers. In contrast, the number of non-AIDS-defining cancers increased by approximately threefold from 3193 to 10,059. An earlier meta-analysis by Shiels [24] found that the standardized incidence ratios (SIR) of NADC was approximately 2-fold higher risk for all NADC among PLWH compared with the general population. However, individual cancer types associated with infectious agents had different SIRs including anal cancer (SIR = 28), Hodgkin lymphoma (SIR = 11), and liver (SIR = 5.6).

Robbins [25], exploring data from 1996 to 2010, looked at cancer trends for three ADCs and seven NADCs to see if demographic changes for HIV positive individuals, changes in relative risks, and/or background incidence in the general population had an effect, and if so which. Table 2.2 includes a summary of changes identified by Robbins. Simard [26] had similar findings looking at data from 1980 to 2006.

Each of the ADCs has a viral cause suggesting that the advent of HAART in 1996 has had an effect on cancer reduction by improving the immune system's ability to manage the viral infection [25]. At the same time, demographic shifts were likely related to the increase in liver cancer and prostate cancer; specifically, the increase in liver cancer reflected additional years living with Hepatitis B and C viruses. Curtrell [27] explores several factors related to the increase in NADC including oncogenic effects of HIV, immunosuppression, chronic inflammation and immune activation, exposure to HAART, higher rates of oncogenic viral coinfections and traditional cancer risk factors. The same study found that when standard cancer therapy is given, PLWH have the same outcomes as the non-HIV population [27].

Other types of NADC have been identified among PLWH. Silverberg [28] compared a California cohort of HIV-infected persons, of whom 74 % were MSM, and compared them with a demographically similar group non-HIV-infected persons. He found adjusted rate ratios, coming HIV-infected with HIV-uninfected persons

Table 2.2 Trends in Cancer incidence among HIV infected persons [25]. (Source: Robbins et al. AIDS 2014 Mar 27)

Type of cancer	Trend 1996–2010 (unless otherwise indicated)		Summary
Kaposi's sarcoma (ADC)	1996–2000 2000–2010	−29.3% −7.8%	Decreasing
NHL (ADC)	1996–2003 2003–2010	−15.7% −5.5%	Decreasing
Cervical cancer (ADC)	−11.1%		Decreasing
Anal cancer (NADC)	3.8%		Increasing
Liver cancer (NADC)	8.5%		Increasing
Prostate cancer (NADC)	9.8%		Increasing
Hodgkin Lymphoma (NADC)	−4.0%		Decreasing
Lung cancer (NADC)	−2.8%		Decreasing

of 37.7 for ADC, 9.2 for infection-related NADC, and 1.3 for infection-unrelated NADC. The rates for individual NADC included anal squamous cell (rate ratio = 101.6), Hodgkin lymphoma (rate ratio = 19.4), penis (rate ratio = 5.8) liver (rate ratio = 2.7) and HPV-related oral squamous cell cancers (rate ratio = 2.0) [27]. Among infection- unrelated NADC there were increased rates for people with HIV infection for other anal (rate ratio = 35.3, nonmelanoma skin (rate ratio = 10.6), other head and neck (rate ration = 2.7), lung (rate ratio = 1.9) and melanoma (rate ratio = 1.5). HIV-infected persons also had a lower rate of prostate cancer (rate ratio = 0.7). HIV infection was not associated with higher rates of other infection-unrelated NADC [27]. Similarly, Grulich et al. [29] demonstrated that other cancers not known to be associated with an infection were also elevated in both immunosuppressed populations, that is, HIV-infected persons and transplant recipients, including lung and kidney cancers, multiple myeloma, and leukemia. Yanik [30] found decreasing rates from 2000 to 2011 of NHL among a cohort of HIV-infected individuals in North Carolina.

Silverberg [31] found that HIV-infected patients had a twofold higher incidence rate of non- melanoma skin cancers compared with non-HIV-infected subjects. Squamous cell cancers but not basal cell cancers were associated with immunodeficiency. Shebl [32] concluded that chronic pulmonary inflammation arising from infection contributes to recurrent pneumonia which puts PLWH at greater risk of lung cancer, independent of higher smoking rates. Similarly, Sigel [33] found HIV infection was an independent risk factor for lung cancer when controlling for potential confounders, including smoking and surveillance bias.

Persson [34] looked at data for 596,955 person with AIDS from 16 US population-based HIV/AIDS and cancer registries. Risk of stomach and esophageal malignancies in people with HIV/AIDS were compared with those of the general population using standardized incidence ratios (SIRs). People with HIV/AIDS had increased risk of carcinomas of the esophagus (SIR, 1.69) carcinoma of the stomach (SIR, 1.44), esophageal adenocarcinoma (SIR, 1.91), squamous cell carcinoma (SIR, 1.47), and carcinomas of the gastric cardia (SIR, 1.36) and noncardia (SIR, 1.53) compared with the general population. Rates of NHL decreased from 1980 to 2007 with HAART, but incidence of carcinomas remained consistent over time [34].

Thus while HAART has reduced the risk of cancer related to HIV and EBV i.e. NHL, other cancer risks continue to be elevated related to HIV infection and immunologic status, possibly unrelated to other infections.

Infection with HPV Raises Cancer Risk for GBT Men and Especially Those Co-infected with HIV

Beachler [35] found HIV infected gay and bisexual men to have higher rates of anal HPV infections compared to HIV-infected heterosexual men. In addition, anal HPV infection rates were higher than oral HPV infection rates, contributing to the higher burden of anal HPV associated cancer in HIV-infected individuals. Berry [36] described the progression from anal high-grade squamous intraepithelial lesions (HSIL) to anal squamous cell cancer.

Incident anal cancer has increased by 96 % in men and 39 % in women since the 1980 primarily due to the HIV epidemic [37]. Nearly all anal cancers in gay and bisexual men are associated with HPV [38]. The rate of abnormal anal cytology in a cohort of 60 young gay and bisexual men (mean age = 21.2 years) was found to be comparable to the rate among adult MSM [39]. Increased risk for developing anal cancer among PLWH was associated with prolonged survival and increasing immunosuppression [40].

The prevalence of cirrhosis and hepatocellular carcinoma in patients with human immunodeficiency virus infection. The Hepatitis C (HCV) epidemic has driven up the rate of cirrhosis and hepatocellular carcinoma (HCC) amongst HIV-infected persons. Among patients co-infected with HIV and HCV, there was a dramatic increase in the prevalence of cirrhosis (3.5–13.2 %), decompensated cirrhosis (1.9–5.8 %), and HCC (0.07–1.6 %). Little increase was observed among patients without HCV co-infection in the prevalence of cirrhosis [41].

However, HIV Infection Does Not Lead to Higher Risk or Different Types of Risk for all Kinds of Cancer

HIV does not appear to impact some of the most common cancer including colorectal and prostate cancer among GBT men. Shiels [42] found a reduced risk of prostate cancer among HIV-infected men, though attributed that primarily to lower rates of screening. There were no differences between rates of distant stage prostate cancer between people with AIDS and the general population, giving strength to this argument [42]. Incidence rates of head and neck squamous cell cancers were higher among HIV-infected patients, compared with other gay and bisexual men. However, the risk factors for head and neck cancer were similar for HIV-infected persons and the general population [43].

3. Interventions for risk reduction, include efforts to raise knowledge/awareness of how infections raise cancer risk, the role of vaccination in preventing infection and how screening and early treatment may reduce cancer incidence

a. Current Interventions and treatments for for STIs and HIV

Interventions to reduce STIs including HIV include behavioral interventions, use of highly active antiretroviral therapy (HAART), and both HPV and HBV vaccines, screening, and treatment, are frequently targeted to gay and bisexual men. In many situations, people with any STIs are recommended to undergo the same cancer screening and, if diagnosed, receive the same treatment regimens for both the infection and the cancer as those without infection. However this is not always the case, and there are many studies in progress to find more effective ways of treating these populations.

b. Interventions specific to infection and cancer risk

I. Knowledge, awareness and perceived risk

Gilbert [44] found there not to be much of a difference between HIV(+) and (−) men, but that overall there was acceptability for the vaccine, little understanding of how HIV increases risk for HPV-related diseases, and other misperceptions about the vaccines. This information can inform awareness/prevention efforts for gay men. Blackwell [45] conducted a descriptive study to assess knowledge of HPV, anorectal carcinoma, and anorectal screening in a sample of MSM in Orlando, FL. The 89 participants demonstrated low levels of knowledge with an average score on knowledge items of 38 % correct. Of the 49 participants who had heard of anal Papanicolau (Pap) smears, only five (10.2 %) discussed screening with a physician, while eight (16.3 %) had discussed it with a nurse, and 16 (32.7 %) with another health care professional.

Rosa-Cunha [46] found that only 54 % of men who have sex with men (MSM) reported discussing anal health with their HIV providers in the prior 12 months. Rates for MSM and heterosexual men were 5.56 times and 2.31 times more likely, respectively, than women to have to discuss anal health with their HIV provider. Interestingly, having reported unprotected sex with a partner who was HIV negative or whose HIV status was unknown was inversely related to having a discussion about anal health with their primary care provider [46].

Burkhalter [47] explored perceived risk of cancer in a large urban community center and found that men associated a higher number of sexual partners with a higher risk for cancer. Sanchez [48] found that a quarter of MSM attending a sexually transmitted disease clinic in New York City did not know that HPV is transmitted through anal sex and 77 % were unaware of the link between HPV and anal cancer.

II. Vaccinations

Vaccinations are available to reduce exposure to HPV and Hep B. In 2009, the FDA licensed the use of quadrivalent vaccine for the prevention of genital warts in males ages 9–26 and in 2010, its use was extended for prevention of anal cancer in the same group [49]. On October 25, 2011, the Advisory Committee on Immunization

Practices (ACIP) recommended routine use of quadrivalent HPV vaccine in males aged 11–12 and vaccination with HPV4 for males aged 13–21 who have not been previously vaccinated or did not complete the three dose series [50]. Males aged 22–26 may also be vaccinated [50]. To date, update of HPV vaccination among adolescent males generally has been limited. Reiter [51], looking at a nationally representative sample of adolescents, found that HPV vaccine initiation among males ages 13–17 increased from 1.4 % in 2010 to 8.3 % in 2011. Parents were more likely to get their sons vaccinated against HPV if they received a recommendation from their healthcare provider [51]. Gay and bisexual men have been found to have greater willingness to receive HPV vaccines as well as higher levels of concern about HPV-related diseases [52].

For GBT males, perceived benefits and barriers were the most proximate predictors of intention to be vaccinated against HPV, while knowledge and perceived threat exerted an indirect influence [53]. One study found 73 % of gay and bisexual men were willing to receive the HPV vaccine [52]. Another study of young gay and bisexual men found that 36 % were likely to be vaccinated based upon perceived stronger physical and psychological benefits [54]. Kim [55] found HPV vaccination to be cost effective using the standard measure of costs per QALY below $ 50,000. With respect to Hepatitis B vaccination, a study of 3,432 MSM age 15–22, found only 9 % immunization coverage and 11 % infection rates [56].

III. Screening innovations

Given the increasing rates of anal cancer, substantial effort has been placed on screening for anal intraephitelial neoplasia (AIN), primarily using high-resolution anoscopy. High resolution anoscopy (HRA) was developed in England in the 1980s and uses a colposcope to explore the anal mucosa. A swab, soaked in 5 % acetic acid, is inserted through the anoscope and applied topically for 1–2 min. Lesions reacting to the application are identified and biopsied [57]. Anal-rectal cytology collects non-gynecological specimens via exfoliative cytology tests which are then interpreted by a qualified pathologist. The smear is the same technique as a Pap test, whereby the exfoliated cells are quickly smeared and fixed onto a glass slide [58]. Cachay [59] found that despite the availability of several modalities for treatment of precursors of anal cancer, evidence that current treatment modalities favorably alter the natural history of human papillomavirus oncogenesis in the anal and perianal regions is still inconclusive. However, there is sufficient evidence to state that the accuracy of anal cancer screening procedures (cytology and high-resolution anoscopy directed biopsy) is comparable to the accuracy of those used in screening for cervical cancer precursors. More research is needed to assess the efficacy of anal cancer screening programs on reducing morbidity/mortality in the HIV-infect population [59].

Darragh [60] looked at inter-rater reliability in the reading of Papanicolaou-stained liquid based cytology cells being used for anal cancer screening among high risk populations of gay and bisexual men. Two observers had an overall agreement of 66 % and this increased to 86 % for dichotomized cytology results. Thus reviewers were able to detect which lesions were precancerous and which were not, similar to the methodology used for cervical cancer screening. A high rate of acceptability of screening was found at a Veteran's Affairs HIV Clinic [61]. When approached during a routine care visit to participate in the study by obtaining an anal Pap smear, 82% of HIV-patients agreed to do so. Another clinic was established at an HIV clinic in New York to comply with New York State AIDS Institute guidelines for anal cancer screening and treatment in HIV-positive persons. The intent is to reduce morbidity and mortality in young, HIV-infected persons [62].

However, a review of the literature found that screening for anal cancer in HIV-positive gay and bisexual men as well as HIV-positive women was not cost-effective [63]. Given the number of false-positives, results with treatment for high-grade AIN, there were no models that showed a 50% probability of cost-effectiveness to a quality-adjusted life year (QALY) gained reaching the value of 50,000 British pounds. This is contrary to earlier reports that found it to be cost effective to screen for anal squamous interepithelial lesions in gay and bisexual HIV-infected men [64].

Routine HIV testing, in the form of standard "opt-out" protocols is recommended by the CDC in all health care settings. This has not been widely implemented, but should be for cancer patients [65], in order to maximize effective HIV management during cancer treatment and improve clinical outcomes.

IV. Treatment innovation/cancer risk reduction

A review of recently published literature on the heightened risk for cancer in PLWH explored whether early HAART treatment can lower their risk [66]. The findings were that immunodeficiency still appears to be the key factor; however, there is emerging evidence that HIV may have direct oncogenic effects through inflammation and coagulation that HAART only partly normalizes. Analysis of studies comparing the impact of early versus delayed HAART was inconclusive [66]. Chiao [67] looked at a cohort of US veterans with HIV and in a multivariate analysis found that those with controlled (i.e. undetectable) viral load at 61–100% of follow-up time had significantly decreased risk of squamous cell anal cancer compared to those with undetectable viral load less than 20% of the time.

Compared to high-resolution anoscopy alone, it is more beneficial to health outcomes as well cost effective to use combined HRA and anal cytology at 6 and 12 months as a method of surveillance for HIV-positive MSM treated for high-grade anal intraepithelial neoplasia to prevent anal cancer and to maximize QALYs [68]. Use of HPV vaccine in HIV-infected children and adult men is safe and highly immunogenic [69]. More research is needed on the role of HPV vaccination for older adults living with HIV who have ongoing HPV infections [69].

A California-based study found an inverse association between statin use and risk of NHL in HIV(+) persons, and though there were limitations in the study design this may be an area for additional research [70].

4. Unique challenges

a. Effect of HAART

Although HAART has led to reductions in the incidence of Kaposi's sarcoma and non-Hodgkin lymphoma among HIV-infected individuals, it has not reduced the incidence of cervical cancer, which has essentially remained unchanged. Moreover, the incidence of several other cancers, particularly Hodgkin lymphoma and anal cancer, has been increasing among HIV-infected individuals since the introduction of HAART. The influence of HAART on the risk of these other cancer types is not well understood [71], [72], [40].

Research continues to show that in the post-HAART era, PLWH continue to be at increased risk for cancer late after AIDS onset [73] and that cancer-related mortality for PLWH is significant [74]. However, early treatment with HAART has been shown to lower cancer risk generally [28]. Overall, use of HAART was not associated with increased ADC or NADC risk, except for one NADC, anal cancer [75].

With respect to the leading cause of cancer-related death among HIV-infected individuals, Gopal [76] found that, over time, HIV-associated lymphoma is changing with less immunosuppression and greater HIV control at diagnosis. Both stable survival and increased mortality for lymphomas occurring on HAART need more research to improve outcomes [76].

b. Understanding mechanisms associated with infection and cancer

For some infections it is unclear exactly what the mechanism is that leads to cancer. For example, both HBV and HCV have been demonstrated to relate to increased risk, but the exact mechanisms are unknown and likely different for both viruses. Jiang [77] reports that while the integration of HBV into the host genome has been reported, the scale, impact and contribution to HCC development are not clear. With respect to HCV, there are a range of lympho-proliferative disorders that required clinical, pathological and molecular findings to establish diagnosis and treatment [78].

c. Special treatment concerns for management of cancer in HIV-infected individuals

Treatment of cancer in people with HIV needs to be cognizant of managing two complex treatment regimens simultaneously. Hadjuandreou [79] finds the key to controlling resistance is the optimal management of the frequency and magnitude of treatment interruptions. As we continue to learn about the interactions of multiple infections, clinicians need to ensure that innovations in treatment for HIV and other infections don't come with negative side effects. People with STIs or HIV may have not just higher risk, but also worse prognoses once diagnosed with cancer. For example, even when the stage of presentation and use of treatment was the same for HIV-infected and non-infected persons, HIV-infected person with non-small cell lung cancer (NSCLC) lived 6 months compared with 20 months for non- infected persons, suggesting this cancer might behave more aggressively in the presence of HIV [33]. Another study found people with HIV and NSCLC had more complications, rapid progression to disease recurrence and poorer post-op survival [80]. In the case of head and neck squamous cell carcinoma, chemotherapy appeared to be less effective in HIV-infected patient compared with non-HIV- infected patients [81].

5. Implications for the future: research, policy and practice

The risks of cancer are elevated in GBT men related to infection with HIV, HPV, human herpesvirus and hepatitis B and C. While there is much research regarding the impact of HIV on cancer in GBT men, there are challenges to deconstructing the impact on cancer incidence, progression and treatment of HIV infection itself, treatment with HAART, co-infections, as well as non-infection co-factors such as aging and behavioral risk factors. In addition, with rising rates of anal cancer among GBT men, more research is needed about the effectiveness of anoscopy and cytology screening and whether treatment of anal dysplasia truly affects long-term morbidity and mortality associated with anal cancer.

Despite extensive investigation into the current literature there is very little information available regarding the epidemiology, natural history, and treatment of infection-related cancers among transgender men. There is a substantial need to conduct and publish research related to cancer risk and outcomes among this population.

Educating GBT men about the cancer risks associated with HPV, HHV, Hep B and Hep C can help support a variety of prevention activities ranging from HPV vaccination to screening for anal dysplasia to initiation of Hepatitis C treatment. To date, efforts to educate GBT men about cancer risk, and especially the role of infections in cancer risk, are relatively limited. Such education, both for GBT men and those who provide health care and prevention services to them can lead to improved decision-making regarding strategies to reduce new infections and the sequelae of existing infections.

Acknowledgments Stewart Landers J.D., M.C.P. is a Senior Consultant and Director of the Health Services Division-Boston Office of John Snow Inc.
John Carper and Claire Perkins assisted in background research and organization of materials.

References

1. Gottlieb MA et al. Pneumocystis Pneumonia. Morbidity and Mortality Weekly Report. Los Angeles. June 5, 1981;30(21):1–3
2. Friedman-Kien AE. Disseminated Kaposi's sarcoma syndrome in young homosexual men. Am Acad Dermatol. 1981;5:468–71.
3. Centers for Disease Control and Prevention (CDC). Kaposi's sarcoma and Pneumocystis pneumonia among homosexual men—New York City and California. MMWR Morb Mortal Wkly Rep. 1981;30:305–8.
4. Purcell D, Johnson CH, Lansky A, et al. Estimating the population size of men who have sex with men in the United States to obtain HIV and syphilis rates. Open AIDS J. 2012;6(Suppl 1: M6):98–107.

5. Robbins HA, Shiels MS, Pfeiffer RM, Engels EA. Epidemiologic contributions to recent cancer trends among HIV-infected people in the United States. AIDS. 2014;28(6):881–90.
6. Morbidity and mortality report, prevalence and awareness of HIV infection among men who have sex with men—21 US Cities, United States, 2008, September 24, 2010/59(37);1201–7.
7. www.cdc.gov/std/HPV/STDFact-HPV.htm. Accessed 20 February 2014.
8. Canepa P, Orsi A, Martini M, Icardi G. HPV related diseases in males: a heavy vaccine- preventable burden. J Prev Med Hyg. 2013;54(2):61–70.
9. Chin-Hong PV, Vittinghoff E, Cranston RD, Buchbinder S, Cohen D, Colfax G, et al. Age-specific prevalence of anal human papillomavirus infection in HIV-negative sexually active men who have sex with men: the EXPLORE study. J Infect Dis. 2004;190:2070–6.
10. de Pokomandy A, Rouleau D, Ghattas G, Vezina S, Cote P, Macleod J, et al. Prevalence, clearance, and incidence of anal human papillomavirus infection in HIV-infected men: the HIP- VIRG cohort study. J Infect Dis. 2009;199:965–73.
11. Daling JR, Sherman KJ. Relationship between human papillomavirus infection and tumours of anogenital sites other than the cervix. IARC Sci Publ. 1992;(119):223–41.
12. www.cdc.gov/vaccines/pubs/surv-manual/chpt05-hpv.html. Accessed 3 March 2014.
13. Thomas H, Tidy C. www.patient.co.uk/doctor/human-herpes-viruses. Accessed 3 March 2014.
14. Pagano J. Is Epstein-Barr Virus Transmitted Sexually? J Infect Dis. 2007;195(4):469–70.
15. Chang Y, Cesarman E, Pessin MS, Lee F, Culpepper J, Knowles DM, Moore PS. Identification of herpesvirus-like DNA sequences in AIDS-associated Kaposi's sarcoma. Science. 1994;266(5192):1865–9.
16. Del Mistro A, Baboci L, Frayle-Salamanca H, Trevisan R, Bergamo E, Lignitto L, Sasset L, Cecchetto MG, Cattelan AM, Calabró ML. Oral human papillomavirus and human herpesvirus-8 infections among human immunodeficiency virus type 1-infected men and women in Italy. Sex Transm Dis. 2012;39(11):894–8.
17. www.cdc.gov/epstein-barr/about-ebv.html. Accessed 4 March 2014.
18. Pattle SB, Farrell PJ. The role of Epstein-Barr virus in cancer. Expert Opin Biol Ther. 2006;6(11):1193–205.
19. van Baarle D, Hovenkamp E, Dukers NH, et al. High prevalence of Epstein-Barr virus type 2 among homosexual men is caused by sexual transmission. J Infect Dis. 2000;181(6):2045–9.
20. www.cdc.gov/msmhealth/viral-hepatitis.htm. Accessed 8 March 2014.
21. www.cdc.gov/hepatitis/Populations/PDFs/HepGay-FactSheet.pdf. Accessed 8 March 2014.
22. Parkin DM. The global health burden of infection-associated cancers in the year 2002. IJC. 2006;118:3030–44.
23. Shiels MS, Pfeiffer RM, Gail MH, Hall HI, Li J, Chaturvedi AK, Bhatia K, Uldrick TS, Yarchoan R, Goedert JJ, Engels EA. Cancer burden in the HIV-infected population in the United States. J Natl Cancer Inst. 2011;103(9):753–62.
24. Shiels MS, Cole SR, Kirk GD, Poole C. A meta-analysis of the incidence of non-AIDS cancers in HIV-infected individuals. J Acquir Immune Defic Syndr. 2009;52(5):611–22.
25. Robbins HA, Shiels MS, Pfeiffer RM, Engels EA. Epidemiologic contributions to recent cancer trends among HIV-infected people in the United States. AIDS. 2014;28(6):881–90.
26. Simard EP, Pfeiffer RM, Engels EA. Cumulative incidence of cancer among individuals with acquired immunodeficiency syndrome in the United States. Cancer. 2011;117(5):1089–96.
27. Cutrell J, Bedimo R. Non-AIDS-defining cancers among HIV-infected patients. Curr HIV/AIDS Rep. 2013;10(3):207–16. doi:10.1007/s11904-013-0166-8.
28. Silverberg MJ, Chao C, Leyden WA, Xu L, Tang B, Horberg MA, Klein D, Quesenberry CP Jr, Towner WJ, Abrams DI. HIV infection and the risk of cancers with and without a known infectious cause. AIDS. 2009;23(17):2337–45.
29. Grulich AE, van Leeuwen MT, Falster MO, Vajdic CM. Incidence of cancers in people with HIV/AIDS compared with immunosuppressed transplant recipients: a meta-analysis. Lancet. 2007;370(9581):59–67.

30. Yanik EL, Tamburro K, Eron JJ, Damania B, Napravnik S, Dittmer DP. Recent cancer incidence trends in an observational clinical cohort of HIV-infected patients in the US, 2000 to 2011. Infect Agent Cancer. 2013;8(1):18.
31. Silverberg MJ, Leyden W, Warton EM, Quesenberry CP Jr, Engels EA, Asgari MM. HIV infection status, immunodeficiency, and the incidence of non-melanoma skin cancer. J Natl Cancer Inst. 2013;105(5):350–60.
32. Shebl FM, Engels EA, Goedert JJ, Chaturvedi AK. Pulmonary infections and risk of lung cancer among persons with AIDS. J Acquir Immune Defic Syndr. 2010;55(3):375–9.
33. Sigel K, Crothers K, Dubrow R, Krauskopf K, Jao J, Sigel C, Moskowitz A, Wisnivesky J. Prognosis in HIV-infected patients with non-small cell lung cancer. Br J Cancer. 2013;109(7):1974–80.
34. Persson EC, Shiels MS, Dawsey SM, Bhatia K, Anderson LA, Engels EA. Increased risk of stomach and esophageal malignancies in people with AIDS. Gastroenterology. 2012;143(4):943–50.
35. Beachler DC, D'Souza G, Sugar EA, Xiao W, Gillison ML. Natural history of anal vs oral HPV infection in HIV-infected men and women. J Infect Dis. 2013;208(2):330–9.
36. Berry JM, Jay N, Cranston RD, Darragh TM, Holly EA, Welton ML, Palefsky JM. Progression of anal high-grade squamous intraepithelial lesions to invasive anal cancer among HIV-infected men who have sex with men. Int J Cancer. 2014;134(5):1147–55.
37. Chiao EY, Krown SE, Stier EA, Schrag D. A population-based analysis of temporal trends in the incidence of squamous anal canal cancer in relation to the HIV epidemic. J Acquir Immune Defic Syndr. 2005;40:451–5.
38. Ryan DP, Compton CC, Mayer RJ. Review article: carcinoma of the anal canal. N Engl J Med. 2000;342:792–800.
39. Coromilas A, Brozovich A, Nelson J, Neu N. Epidemiology and prevalence of abnormal results for anal cytology screening in hiv-infected young men who have sex with men. LGBT Health. 2014:1(1):58–61.
40. Chaturvedi AK, Madeleine MM, Biggar RJ, Engels EA. Risk of human papillomavirus- associated cancers among persons with AIDS. J Natl Cancer Inst. 2009;101(16):1120–30.
41. Ioannou GN, Bryson CL, Weiss NS, Miller R, Scott JD, Boyko EJ. The prevalence of cirrhosis and hepatocellular carcinoma in patients with human immunodeficiency virus infection. Hepatology. 2013;57(1):249–57.
42. Shiels MS, Goedert JJ, Moore RD, Platz EA, Engels EA. Reduced risk of prostate cancer in U.S. Men with AIDS. Cancer Epidemiol Biomarkers Prev. 2010;19(11):2910–5.
43. D'Souza G, Carey TE, William WN Jr, Nguyen ML, Ko EC, Riddell J 4th, Pai SI, Gupta V, Walline HM, Lee JJ, Wolf GT, Shin DM, Grandis JR, Ferris RL. Epidemiology of head and neck squamous cell cancer among HIV-infected patients. (On behalf of the HNC SPORE HIV supplement consortium). J Acquir Immune Defic Syndr. 2014:65(5):603–10.
44. Gilbert PA, Brewer NT, Reiter PL. Association of human papillomavirus-related knowledge, attitudes, and beliefs with HIV status: a national study of gay men. J Low Genit Tract Dis. 2011;15(2):83–8.
45. Blackwell CW, Eden C. Human papillomavirus and anorectal carcinoma knowledge in men who have sex with men. J Assoc Nurses AIDS Care. 2011;22(6):444–53.
46. Rosa-Cunha I, Cardenas GA, Dickinson G, Metsch LR. Addressing anal health in the HIV primary care setting: a disappointing reality. AIDS Patient Care STDS. 2010;24(9):533–8.
47. Burkhalter JE, Hay JL, Coups E, Warren B, Li Y, Ostroff JS. Perceived risk for cancer in an urban sexual minority. J Behav Med. 2011;34(3):157–69.
48. Sanchez DM, Pathela P, Niccolai LM, Schillinger JA. Knowledge of human papillomavirus and anal cancer among men who have sex with men attending a New York City sexually transmitted diseases clinic. Int J STD AIDS. 2012;23(1):41–3.
49. FDA. Licensure of Quadrivalent Human Papillomavirus Vaccine (HPV4, Gardasil) for use in males and guidance from the Advisory Committee on Immunization Practices (ACIP). MMWR. 2010;59:630–2. http://www.cdc.gov/mmwr/preview/mmwrhtml/mm5920a5.htm.

50. Centers for Disease Control and Prevention (CDC). Recommendations on the use of quadrivalent human papillomavirus vaccine in males–Advisory Committee on Immunization Practices (ACIP), 2011. MMWR Morb Mortal Wkly Rep. 2011;60(50):1705–8.
51. Reiter PL, McRee AL, Pepper JK, Gilkey MB, Galbraith KV, Brewer NT. Longitudinal predictors of human papillomavirus vaccination among a national sample of adolescent males. Am J Public Health. 2013;103(8):1419–27.
52. Gilbert P1, Brewer NT, Reiter PL, Ng TW, Smith JS. HPV vaccine acceptability in heterosexual, gay, and bisexual men. Am J Mens Health. 2011;5(4):297–305.
53. Wheldon CW, Buhi ER, Daley EM. Gay and bisexual men's human papillomavirus vaccine intentions: a theory-based structural equation analysis. J Health Psychol. 2013;18(9):1177–86.
54. Wheldon CW, Daley EM, Buhi ER, Nyitray AG, Giuliano AR. Health beliefs and attitudes associated with HPV vaccine intention among young gay and bisexual men in the Southeastern United States. Vaccine. 2011;29(45):8060–5.
55. Kim JJ. Targeted human papillomavirus vaccination of men who have sex with men in the USA: a cost-effectiveness modelling analysis. Lancet Infect Dis. 2010;10(12):845–52.
56. MacKellar DA, Valleroy LA, Secura GM, McFarland W, Shehan D, Ford W, LaLota M, Celentano DD, Koblin BA, Torian LV, Thiede H, Janssen RS, Young Men's Survey Study Group. Two decades after vaccine license: hepatitis B immunization and infection among young men who have sex with men. Am J Public Health. 2001;91(6):965–71.
57. Gimenez F1, Costa-e-Silva IT, Daumas A, Araújo Jd, Medeiros SG, Ferreira L. The value of high-resolution anoscopy in the diagnosis of anal cancer precursor lesions in HIV-positive patients. Arq Gastroenterol. 2011;48(2):136–45.
58. Bean, SM, Chhieng, DC. Anal-Rectal Cytology. The Other Pap Test (2010) LabMedicine, 41, 168–71.
59. Cachay ER, Mathews WC. Human papillomavirus, anal cancer, and screening considerations among HIV-infected individuals. AIDS Rev. 2013;15(2):122–33.
60. Darragh TM, Tokugawa D, Castle PE, Follansbee S, Borgonovo S, LaMere BJ, Schwartz L, Gage JC, Fetterman B, Lorey T, Wentzensen N. Interrater agreement of anal cytology. Cancer Cytopathol. 2013;121(2):72–8.
61. Rosa-Cunha I, Degennaro VA, Hartmann R, Milikowski C, Irizarry A, Heitman B, Gomez-Marin O, Dickinson GM. Description of a pilot anal pap smear screening program among individuals attending a Veteran's Affairs HIV clinic. AIDS Patient Care STDS. 2011;25(4):213–9.
62. Tider DS, Caprio GR, Gaisa M, Klein RS, Goldstone SE. Successful initiation of an anal cancer screening and treatment program at a New York City HIV clinic AIDS. 2010;24(7):1085–6.
63. Czoski-Murray C, Karnon J, Jones R, Smith K, Kinghorn G. Cost-effectiveness of screening high-risk HIV-positive men who have sex with men (MSM) and HIV-positive women for anal cancer. Health Technol Assess. 2010;14(53):iii-iv, ix-x, 1–101.
64. Goldie SJ, Kuntz KM, Weinstein MC, et al. The clinical effectiveness and cost- effectiveness of screening for anal squamous intraepithelial lesions in homosexual and bisexual HIV-positive men. JAMA. 1999;281:1822–9.
65. Chiao EY, Dezube BJ, Krown SE, Wachsman W, Brock MV, Giordano TP, Mitsuyasu R, Pantanowitz L. Time for oncologists to opt in for routine opt-out HIV testing? JAMA. 2010;304(3):334–9.
66. Borges AH, Dubrow R, Silverberg MJ. Factors contributing to risk for cancer among HIV-infected individuals, and evidence that earlier combination antiretroviral therapy will alter this risk. Curr Opin HIV AIDS. 2014;9(1):34–40.
67. Chiao EY, Hartman CM, El-Serag HB, Giordano TP. The impact of HIV viral control on the incidence of HIV-associated anal cancer. J Acquir Immune Defic Syndr. 2013;63(5):631–8.
68. Assoumou SA, Mayer KH, Panther L, Linas BP, Kim J. Cost-effectiveness of surveillance strategies after treatment for high-grade anal dysplasia in high-risk patients. Sex Transm Dis. 2013;40(4):298–303.
69. Firnhaber C, Wilkin T. Human papillomavirus vaccines: where do they fit in HIV-infected individuals? Curr HIV/AIDS Rep. 2012;9(3):278–86.

70. Chao C, Xu L, Abrams DI, Towner WJ, Horberg MA, Leyden WA, Silverberg MJ. HMG-CoA reductase inhibitors (statins) use and risk of non-Hodgkin lymphoma in HIV-positive persons. AIDS. 2011;25(14):1771–7.
71. Engels EA, Biggar RJ, Hall HI, et al. Cancer risk in people infected with human immunodeficiency virus in the United States. Int J Cancer. 2008;123(1):187–94.
72. Engels EA, Pfeiffer RM, Goedert JJ, et al. Trends in cancer risk among people with AIDS in the United States 1980–2002. AIDS. 2006;20(12):1645–54.
73. Simard EP, Pfeiffer RM, Engels EA. Spectrum of cancer risk late after AIDS onset in the United States. Arch Intern Med. 2010;170(15):1337–45.
74. Simard EP, Engels EA. Cancer as a cause of death among people with AIDS in the United States. Clin Infect Dis. 2010;51(8):957–62.
75. Chao C, Leyden WA, Xu L, Horberg MA, Klein D, Towner WJ, Quesenberry CP Jr, Abrams DI, Silverberg MJ. Exposure to antiretroviral therapy and risk of cancer in HIV-infected persons.AIDS. 2012;26(17):2223–31.
76. Gopal S, Patel MR, Yanik EL, Cole SR, Achenbach CJ, Napravnik S, Burkholder GA, Reid EG, Rodriguez B, Deeks SG, Mayer KH, Moore RD, Kitahata MM, Eron JJ, Richards KL. Temporal trends in presentation and survival for HIV-associated lymphoma in the antiretroviral therapy era. J Natl Cancer Inst. 2013;105(16):1221–9.
77. Jiang Z, Jhunjhunwala S, Liu J, Haverty PM, Kennemer MI, Guan Y, et al. The effects of hepatitis B virus integration into the genomes of hepatocellular carcinoma patients. Genome Res. 2012;22:593–601.
78. Mollejo M, Menárguez J, Guisado-Vasco P, Bento L, Algara P, Montes-Moreno S, Rodriguez-Pinilla MS, Cruz MA, Casado F, Montalbán C, Piris MA. Hepatitis C virus-related lymphoproliferative disorders encompass a broader clinical and morphological spectrum than previously recognized: a clinicopathological study. Modern Pathol. 2014;27:281–93.
79. Hadjiandreou MM, Mitsis GD. Taking a break from chemotherapy to fight drug-resistance: The cases of Cancer and HIV/AIDS. Conf Proc IEEE Eng Med Biol Soc. 2013;2013:197–200.
80. Hooker CM, Meguid RA, Hulbert A, Taylor JT, Shin J, Wrangle J, Rodgers K, Lee B, Laskshmanan S, Brown T, Meneshian A, Sussman M, Keruly J, Moore RD, Yang SC, Brock MV. Human immunodeficiency virus infection as a prognostic factor in surgical patients with non-small cell lung cancer. Ann Thorac Surg. 2012;93(2):405–12.
81. Mourad WF, Hu KS, Shasha D, Concert C, Ishihara D, Lin W, Gamez ME, Lukens JJ, Shourbaji RA, Ryniak M, Li Z, Culliney BE, Khorsandi AS, Tran T, Jacobson A, Manolidis S, Schantz S, Urken M, Persky MS, Harrison LB. Long-term outcome of seropositive HIV patients with head and neck squamous cell carcinoma treated with radiation therapy and chemotherapy. Anticancer Res. 2013;33(12):5511–6.

Chapter 3
Understanding and Reducing Risks via Infection in LBT Women

J. Kathleen Tracy

Abstract Several infections are associated with increased risk of developing cancer. For example, persistent infection with high-risk strains of human papillomavirus causes cervical cancer. Our understanding of the association between infection and cancer in lesbian, bisexual and transgender (LBT) women is hampered by an absence of population-based data for LBT women. Formal epidemiologic studies of cancer, in general, and infection-associated cancer, in particular, among LBT individuals are lacking. This absence of robust epidemiologic data makes our understanding of infection-related cancer in the LBT women limited and speculative. This chapter attempts to summarize available epidemiologic data for infection-associated cancers in LBT women, highlight gaps in our knowledge, review interventions that have been used to reduce risk for infection-associated cancers in LBT women, and discuss challenges to research and policy that must be addressed in order prevent infection-associated cancers and reduce cancer disparities experienced by LBT women.

Our understanding of the role of infection in carcinogenesis has expanded greatly during the last half-century. In a recent review by De Martel et al. [1] it was noted that 16% of cancers that occurred globally in 2008 were attributable to infection, many of which are preventable. Infection-associated cancers typically follow a multi-step process during which most incident infections naturally resolve, while a relatively small fraction (e.g., approximately 10% of high-risk HPV infections) become persistent and result in pre-malignant stages that if untreated lead to disease. For most infection-associated cancers, there is a protracted latency period between acquisition of the infection and development of incident cancer, adding complexity to our understanding of etiology, carcinogenesis and prevention. Among sexual minority populations like LBT women, our understanding of the association between infection and cancer is further complicated by the fact that current population-based surveillance systems and registries do not include sexual orientation or gender identity as variables by which cancer incidence or risk can be characterized. In addition,

J. K. Tracy (✉)
Department of Epidemiology and Public Health, University of Maryland School of Medicine, Baltimore, MD, USA
e-mail: ktracy@epi.umaryland.edu

U. Boehmer, R. Elk (eds.), *Cancer and the LGBT Community*,
DOI 10.1007/978-3-319-15057-4_3

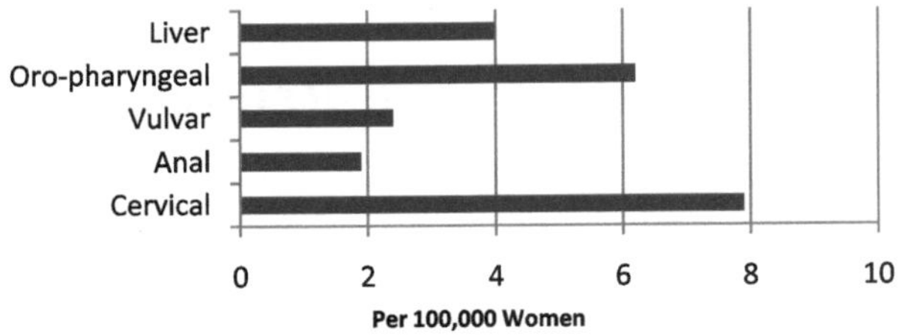

Fig. 3.1 Incidence rates for most common infection-associated cancers in US women

formal epidemiologic studies of cancer, in general, and infection-associated cancer, in particular, among LBT individuals are lacking. This absence of robust epidemiologic data makes our understanding of infection-related cancer in the LBT women limited and speculative.

Figure 3.1 presents cancer incidence data from the Surveillance Epidemiology and End Results (SEER) [2] program for US women. The most common infection-associated cancers among women in the US include cervical, oropharyngeal, liver, vulvar, and anal, respectively.

It is estimated that 4% of US women engage in sexual relationships with other women [3, 4]. Although population-level data are somewhat limited, it is estimated that 0.3% of individuals in the US identify as transgender, with a higher percentage of transgender women than men [4]. As previously mentioned, our knowledge of the most basic epidemiologic data for cancer in sexual minority women is hampered by the fact that the SEER program does not include reporting of sexual orientation or gender identity as essential demographic variables for use in characterizing cancer burden. While a number of studies have examined barriers to cancer prevention in lesbian and bisexual women (e.g., Tracy et al. [5, 6], Matthews et al. [7]), particularly breast and cervical cancer, no studies that we are aware of have characterized incidence, prevalence or mortality from these infection-associated cancers for sexual minority women as a population. Consequently, our discussion must focus on earlier disease endpoints such as incident and prevalent infections associated with cancer.

Causes and Prevalence of Sexually Transmitted Viruses

Bacterial infections have been linked to stomach cancer (*H. pylori)*, non-Hodgkin lymphoma (Epstein-Barr), and bladder cancer (*Schistosoma haematobium*); however, these cancers are relatively rare among women and are presumably even more rare when considered for sexual minority women who comprise such a small proportion of the general population. Of the viral pathogens associated with cancer, nearly all can be transmitted through sexual contact. Consequently, the focus in this chapter will be on cancers that are primarily associated with viral sexually transmitted infections (STIs) known to be associated with cancer (see Table 3.1).

Sexual minority women are at risk of many STIs through skin-to-skin contact, mucosal contact (e.g., mouth to vagina), exposure to vaginal fluids or menstrual

Table 3.1 Cancers associated with sexually transmitted viruses[a]

Cervical	Human papillomavirus (HPV), with or without HIV
Anogenital cancers	HPV, with or without HIV
Oropharyngeal	HPV, with or without tobacco and/or alcohol consumption
Liver	Hepatitis B (HBV), Hepatitis C (HCV)

[a] Classified as carcinogenic to humans in International Agency for Research on Cancer Monograph 100B.2

blood, and sharing of sex toys. While many STIs are less efficiently transmitted between same sex partners, less efficient transmission is not equivalent to zero risk. The remainder of this section reviews the basic epidemiology of viral STIs associated with cancer in women in general and when available LBT women.

HPV: HPV is a group of viruses that can be sexually transmitted via skin-to-skin contact, including oral-genital and/or digital-genital, and sharing of sex toys. There are more than 50 types of HPV that can infect the anogenital tract [8]; see Munoz et al. [9] for review. Infection with certain high-risk (i.e., oncogenic) strains of HPV can lead to cervical cancer; HPV has also been linked to increased risk of some anogenital (e.g., anal, vulvar, vaginal) and oropharyngeal cancers. Many, though not all, risk factors for HPV are related to sexual behavior. Sexual risk factors include unprotected sexual activity with an infected partner, number of lifetime sex partners and the partners' sexual history, early age of sexual debut, and inconsistent condom use [10]. Non-sexual risk factors include smoking, number of pregnancies, and genetic factors [10].

HPV infection is sufficiently ubiquitous, with lifetime prevalence of HPV infection estimated at 80% for women [11]. In a 2007 analysis of data from the National Health and Nutrition Survey (NHANES), Dunne et al. [11] reported an overall annual prevalence of genital HPV infection to be 26.8% among women between the ages of 14–59. There are relatively few studies that have directly assessed genital HPV infection among women who have sex with women (WSW). In a study of WSW, Marrazzo et al. detected HPV DNA in 30% of genital tract samples of participants and 19% of participants who reported no history of sexual intercourse with a male partner [12, 13]. Studies that have focused on the presence of serologic antibodies for HPV 6/11 or HPV 16/18 also confirm that HPV seropositivity did not differ among women with no history of sex with a male partner compared to women with no history of sex with a male partner. These findings suggest that while prevalence of HPV infection in WSW may be lower than what is observed in the general population, WSW are at risk of HPV infection, with and without history of sex with men. In fact, it is possible that WSW are at increased risk of developing HPV-associated cancers because of their behavioral risk profile.

HIV: HIV, the virus that causes Acquired Immune Deficiency Syndrome (AIDS), is a blood borne infection that can be transmitted via sexual contact and sharing of intravenous drug use (IVDU) paraphernalia. Risk factors for HIV infection include unprotected oral, vaginal or anal sexual activity with an HIV-infected partner, substance use, and number of lifetime sexual partners [14]. In 2011, the CDC estimated that 10,257 women 13 and older in the US were newly diagnosed with HIV [10], and approximately 0.5 % of US women are HIV positive [14]. Because female-to-female sexual contact is a much less efficient route for sexual transmission of HIV, the risk of HIV transmission among lesbians is believed to be low. Kwakwa and Ghobrial [15] reported a case of probable female-to-female transmission that was a hypothesized result of sharing of sex toys with an HIV-positive bisexual female partner. More recently, Chan et al. [16] reported a case of female-to-female HIV transmission in a serodiscordant couple from Texas; phylogenetic analysis of the HIV strains infecting each women revealed > 98 % sequence identity for three genes, providing persuasive evidence that HIV was transmitted from the HIV + women to her HIV- partner. As noted in the above section pertaining to risk for HPV infection, some lesbians do engage in high risk sexual behaviors that could increase risk of exposure to HIV. This includes high numbers of sexual partners, history of sexual activity with men, IVDU, and history of sexual activity with partners who are IVDU. Dworkin [17] reports that more than 20 % of IVDU are WSW. The reality is that WSW engage in a wide variety of sexual and other high risk behaviors that may lead to HIV infection with consequent increased risk of other infections associated with cancer.

HIV prevalence among transgender women is believed to be equal to or greater than that observed for other groups at high-risk for contracting HIV (e.g., men who have sex with men). Herbst et al. [18] reviewed studies published from 1990 through 2003 and found a laboratory-confirmed prevalence of 27.7 % among transgender women. More recently, Baral et al. [19] conducted a systematic review of studies published from 2000 to 2011 and noted an HIV prevalence of 21.6 % for transgender women in 5 high-income countries. These estimated rates are significantly higher than rates reported among lesbian, bisexual or heterosexual women.

HBV: Hepatitis B virus (HBV), like HIV, is a blood borne infection that is frequently sexually transmitted. Risk factors for HBV infection include unprotected sex with an infected person, history of multiple sex partners, co-occurring STI, men who have sex with men, IVDU share needles, syringes or other drug equipment, live with a person who has chronic HBV, occupationally exposed to blood, infants of infected mothers, hemodialysis, or travel to countries with moderate to high HBV rates [10]. Custer et al. [20] conducted a systematic review of published studies worldwide and noted that 5.4 % of the population has evidence of past or current HBV infection. More recently, NHANES analysis conducted by Wasley et al. [21] revealed that HBV infection among women is trending downward with a prevalence of 4.5 % for the period from 1988 to 1994 and 3.8 % for the period from 1999 to 2006. Studies of transmission of HBV between female partners are limited. Although not a study of sexual transmission per se, the previously mentioned study by Fethers et al. [22] found an HBV prevalence of approximately 5 % among WSW. This finding suggests that prevalence rates among WSW are similar to those observed for women in the general population; however, it is plausible that the Fethers study over-estimates the true prevalence of HBV in WSW because data for the study were derived from attendees at an Australian STI clinic who likely have a higher risk profile.

Prevalence data for HBV in transgender women is relatively sparse. A US-based study by Nuttbrock et al. reported HBV prevalences ranging from 6.5 to 36 % depending upon racial/ethnic group; HBV prevalence was highest among Hispanic and African American transgender women [23]. Similarly high prevalence of HBV was observed among transgender women from Argentina [19].

HCV: The CDC reports that hepatitis C virus (HCV) infection is the most common chronic blood borne infection in the United States [10]. HCV is most efficiently transmitted through large, repeated percutaneous exposures to infected blood (e.g., typically via IVDU). Although much less common, sexual exposures can also result in HCV transmission. Risk factors with sexual transmission of HVC infection include unprotected sex with an HCV-infected partner, history of multiple partners, presence of other STDs, or sex with trauma [10]. Non-sexual risk factors for HCV transmission include IVDU and sharing of IVDU equipment, needle stick injuries in health care settings, and sharing personal items (e.g., razor, toothbrush) that might be contaminated with traces of HCV-infected blood with an HCV-positive individual.

Analysis of NHANES data for the period from 1999 to 2002 indicates a prevalence of 1.1 % among US women [24]. There is relatively little research on the topic of HCV among lesbian and bisexual women. The largest available study that has examined HCV prevalence in lesbian and bisexual women is the Australian study by Fethers et al. [22]. This study noted a 5 % prevalence of HCV in lesbian and bisexual women seen at an STI clinic. These findings could be interpreted as reflecting greater risk of HBV and HCV in lesbian and bisexual women; however, it is more likely that the Fethers data overestimate the prevalence as women in that study were seeking care for STI and likely engaged in higher risk behaviors that in turn increased risk of these STIs.

As is the case for epidemiologic data for HBV among transgender women, prevalence data for HCV in transgender women is similarly scant. The previously mentioned study by Nuttrock et al. found HCV prevalence rates among transgender women in a US sample to range from 3.6 to 15.7 %, with higher rates observed among Hispanic and African American transgender women.

Genital Herpes: While genital herpes has not been linked directly to cancer, it has been noted that ulcerations that occur during outbreaks, increase the risk of acquiring other STIs, especially HIV [25, 26]. Infection with herpes simplex virus-2 (HSV-2) is the most common cause of genital herpes, although cases of genital herpes associated with herpes simplex-1 (HSV-1) have been reported. Genital herpes infection is typically transmitted via genital-genital contact or oral-genital contact. The biggest risk factor for contracting genital herpes infection is unprotected sexual activity with an infected partner. Other factors that increase risk of HSV-2 infection include early sexual debut, history of STI especially HIV, and number of lifetime sexual partners, and female sex [27–29].

The CDC reports an HSV-2 prevalence of 20.9 % in the general population of women [10]. Like epidemiologic data for HPV infection, the prevalence of HSV-2 among LBT is less well-known. In a study of nearly 400 lesbian and bisexual women, Marrazzo et al. [30] detected HSV-2 in 8 % of participants, most of whom were unaware of their HSV-2 status. In one of the few population-based studies of HSV among WSW Xu et al. used data from the National Health and Nutrition Survey (NHANES) to estimate HSV-2 infection in WSW. Xu et al. found an overall HSV-2 prevalence of 23.8 % and notably higher prevalences in WSW in the past year and WSW ever, 30.3 % and 36.2 %, respectively [31]. When prevalence was analyzed in conjunction with sexual orientation/identity, however, the authors found that among WSW ever, those who identified as lesbian had the lowest prevalence of HSV-2 (8.2 %), while HSV-2 prevalence among women who identified as heterosexual or bisexual was notably higher (45.6 % and 35.9 %, respectively). In a companion editorial, Marrazzo [32] noted that the complex associations between sexual behavior (i.e., WSW) and sexual identity (i.e., lesbian, bisexual, heterosexual) must be considered when evaluating population-level data for STIs as issues of wording, method of data collection, and focus on behavior vs. identity all potentially impact associations yielding over or under-estimates of the true prevalence of not only HSV-2 but presumably of other STIs as well.

Reasons for Differences in Rates from Heterosexual Population

In evaluating the epidemiologic data for the STIs of interest, it is noteworthy that although unique risk factors for each STI-associated cancer exist, there is a high degree of commonality for risk factors among STIs reviewed in this chapter. One of the most significant and consistent risk factors for all of the infectious agents reviewed in this chapter is unprotected sexual activity with an infected partner. Transmission dynamics for infectivity vary for same-sex and opposite-sex pairings, with infectivity appearing higher from male-female sexual encounters. However, two critical caveats must be considered. As noted earlier in this chapter a majority of women who self-define as lesbian have histories of sexual activity with male partners. Further, the work of Marrazzo et al. and the recent report by Chan et al. has provided compelling evidence that women with no history of sexual activity with a male partner can be infected with STIs through sole contact with an infected female partners. It is also noteworthy that WSW and transgender women report higher numbers of lifetime sexual partners than their heterosexual counterparts. Number of lifetime sex partners is another risk factor shared by all of the cancer-associated STIs.

Differences in STI rates among sexual minority women compared to heterosexual women appear to be largely explained by increased rates of STI risk behaviors such as greater number of lifetime partners [33, 35]; unprotected sexual activity with opposite sex partners [22] and same sex partners [35]; exchanging sex for money [36]; and history of intravenous drug use (IVDU) [34, 36, 37]. LBT women tend to report more lifetime sexual partners than heterosexual women. Beyond sexual risk behaviors, LBT women also have higher prevalence of alcohol and substances use [38–42] that may impair judgment in sexual situations leading to greater sexual risk taking. Among transgender women, there are particularly high rates of unprotected anal receptive intercourse and other high-risk sexual behaviors [43–45] (e.g., multiple causal partners, sex work, sex with MSM, alcohol and substance use) placing transgender women at elevated risk for STIs in general and particularly for blood borne STIs such as HIV, HBV, and HCV associated with cancer. Considered together, this suggests that LBT women, as a group, have a behavioral profile that may increase their risk for multiple STIs associated with cancer.

Interventions

Unlike many STIs, vaccines are currently available to prevent transmission of HBV and certain strains of HPV (e.g., strains 6, 11, 16, and 18). The HBV vaccine is recommended for all infants [46] with catch-up vaccination encouraged for children and adolescents born before infant vaccination became a recommendation. HPV vaccines are among those recommended for the general population of women between the ages of 9 to 26 years of age, but available data indicate uptake in the target age group has been modest [47], particularly in the United States. Review of public health efforts targeted to LBT women suggests that sexual minority populations are often not specifically encouraged to obtain such vaccines because their risk for STIs is poorly understood by medical and public health practitioners [48]. Although men who have sex with men (MSM) are viewed as a high-risk population that should obtain both of these vaccinations [49–51], the same perception is not widely held for LBT women. No studies or sexual programs were identified as part of the present review that expressly encouraged vaccination of LBT women with these two vaccines.

While health promotion materials exist that address safe sex practices for sexual minority women, these materials are not always easy to locate [52] and most have not been developed via evidence-based approaches. In a review of lesbian sexual health, Marrazzo [53] noted that no studies have directly assessed effectiveness or even acceptability of STI risk-reduction measures in lesbians. Barrier methods designed to reduce contact with cervicovaginal secretions (e.g., gloves, dental dams, female condoms) are likely effective in reducing risk of STI transmission. Harm reduction strategies for STI prevention include getting tested regularly for STIs and communicating STI status to partners, avoiding fluid exchange, avoiding unprotected contact, avoiding drug and alcohol use before sexual activity, and keeping nails short and groomed [54]. But again, evidence to suggest that LBT women are actively encouraged to engage in harm reduction strategies is currently lacking.

During the last decade, a limited number of small studies have evaluated interventions to reduce HIV and STI risk in transgender populations. Most of these interventions focused on awareness and education of prevention strategies that can reduce risk for STIs, especially HIV. One study found that a community-based sexual health curriculum was successful in improving attitudes about condom use and decreasing sexual risk behaviors [55]. A promising study by Taylor et al. [56]

evaluated the Girlfriends behavioral HIV intervention. Using a pre-post design to assess changes in sexual risk behaviors, Taylor et al. found that a group-style risk reduction intervention led to a decrease in number of sexual partners and less unprotected sexual encounters with both male and female partners [56]. In a recent Cochrane review of social marketing interventions to increase STI and HIV testing among MSM and transgender women, it was noted that multi-media social marketing efforts have been effective in increasing HIV testing among MSM, yet no studies have examined this in transgender women [57]. While there appears to be recognition of the unique risk of HIV and other STI transmission for transgender women, this awareness has not been translated into evidence-based interventions that have been broadly implemented.

In general, sexual minority women are not seen by mainstream health practitioners as a priority population for safe sex and STI prevention messages. For example, it has been noted that medical health professionals have poor knowledge of the sexual health needs of LBT women and often do not ask about sexual orientation, sexual behavior or gender identity when taking patient health histories [58].

Challenges and Implications

Several challenges must be addressed in order to advance our scientific study of STI-associated cancers in LBT women. To begin, we must acknowledge and address false assumptions about sexual identity, sexual behavior and gender identity at all levels of society. Among women who engage in sexual relationships with other women and who may or may not define themselves as lesbian, bisexual or transgender, a majority also report histories of sex with men [59] and may continue to have sexual contact with men. This fluidity of sexual behavior as it relates to sexual identity, sexual behavior and gender identity complicates our ability to draw firm conclusions about how the constructs of identity and behavior with members of the same sex or both sexes affects risk for infection-associated cancers. Studies have shown that sexual behavior (e.g., WSW, WSMW) does not always align with sexual orientation identity (e.g., lesbian) [60, 61] or gender identity. Few studies have examined STI among sexual minority women at the intersection of identity and behavior, but recent analysis by Everett demonstrated that approaches that examine both identity and behavior, offer new insights about STIs among LBT women [62]. This novel approach indicates, for example, that women who identify as lesbian and engage in sex with women, with or without a history of sex with men have lower odds of STI compared to women who identify as heterosexual or bisexual. Further, the study demonstrated that women who identify as bisexual and engage in sex with both men and women are at greater risk of STI, than women who identify as heterosexual (regardless of sexual behavior) or those who identify as lesbian (regardless of sexual behavior). A similar association was identified in Xu and colleagues' analysis of HSV-2 prevalence in NHANES participants. Future studies should strive to incorporate assessment of identity (sexual and gender) and sexual behavior in studies focused on infection-related cancers in LBT women. This approach will optimize our ability analyze risk at the intersection of identity and behavior.

We must also address misguided beliefs and stereotypes that hinder progress in research, policy and practice. There appears to be a somewhat tacit belief by some public policy makers, health providers and scientists that *women are women*, and that it is unnecessary to systematically explore subgroups of women that might be at disproportionate risk of cancer. A one-size-fits-all approach is often applied to recommendations for prevention without fully understanding how the risk profiles for LBT women differ from those of women in the general population or appreciating the unique cancer disparities that exist for LBT women. Brown and Tracy [63] noted that lesbians, in particular, have modifiable, behavioral risk factors for multiple cancers compared to women in the general population, suggesting that lesbians' risk of certain cancers may be disproportionately higher. The review of epidemiological data for STI-associated cancers presented in this chapter presents a similar picture for the constellation of behaviors that increase risk of STIs associated with cancer not only among lesbians but also among bisexual and transgender women. Taken together this suggests that sexual minority women may be at elevated risk of cancer, particularly STI-related cancers. This conclusion remains largely hypothetical for lack of available data and argues for empirical studies of this important question.

Many health care providers and public health practitioners incorrectly believe WSW and transgender women are at low risk for STIs, despite evidence that their STI rates are similar and sometimes higher than those of heterosexual women. McNair [64] presented practical suggestions for improving health care provider knowledge to facilitate sexual orientation and gender identity disclosure and culturally competent knowledge of STI risk and strategies for prevention for LBT women. For improvements to be made at the practice level, we must advocate for changes to occur in medical, nursing, allied health and public health education. Advocacy efforts should be targeted toward ensuring that LBT women's health is incorporated into the educational curricula of health care and public health professionals. In addition, there are many opportunities to increase efforts to implement and more broadly disseminate interventions that show promise for reducing risk for all STIs among LBT women and particularly STIs associated with cancer.

Finally, one of the greatest limitations to our understanding of cancer burden in LBT women is that of data collection about sexual orientation and gender identity. As was stated at the outset of this chapter, our knowledge of the most basic epidemiology of infection-associated cancers in LBT women is stymied by the fact that high quality, population-level data for cancer incidence, survival and mortality do not exist. Robust epidemiologic data to characterize disease burden, morbidity and mortality would provide the necessary scientific basis from which to address probable cancer disparities in general, and particularly for infection-associated cancers. Our approach to date in exploring the critical issue of understanding and reducing risks for infection-associated cancers in LBT women has, by necessity, been an approach in which scientists have had to cobble together cross-sectional evidence of varying quality across numerous studies to make the case that there are probable cancer disparities for LBT women. If we are to enhance our understanding of basic epidemiology of STI-associated cancers in LBT women, we must start by integrating data collection of sexual behavior, sexual identity and gender identity into our national surveillance systems as crucial demographic variables, and we must urge members of the scientific community to adopt standards for collecting demographic variables related to sexual identity, sexual behavior and gender identity so that results can be compared meaningfully across studies. Sell and Dunn [65] and Boehmer [66] have made compelling arguments for the inclusion of sexual orientation and gender identity as critical demographic variables that should be included in all surveillance and epidemiological research systems. This is a policy and research challenge we must overcome in order to more fully evaluate not only infection-associated cancer in LBT women but the burden of other cancers as well in LBT women.

References

1. de Martel C, Ferlay J, Franceschi S, Vignat J, Bray F, Forman D, et al. Global burden of cancers attributable to infections in 2008: A review and synthetic analysis. Lancet Oncol. 2012;13(6):607–15.
2. Seer*Stat–incidence [Internet]. www.seer.cancer.gov. Accessed 1 Feb 2014.
3. Mosher WD, Chandra A, Jones J. Sexual behavior and selected health measures: men and women 15–44 years of age, united states, 2002. Adv Data. 2005;15(362):1–55.
4. Gates GJ. How many people are lesbian, gay, bisexual and transgender? UCLA: The Williams Institute; 2011.
5. Tracy JK, Lydecker AD, Ireland L. Barriers to cervical cancer screening among lesbians. J Womens Health (Larchmt). 2010;19(2).
6. Tracy JK, Schluterman NH, Greenberg DR. Understanding cervical cancer screening among lesbians: a national survey. BMC Public Health. 2013;13(1):442.
7. Matthews AK, Brandenburg DL, Johnson TP, Hughes TL. Correlates of underutilization of gynecological cancer screening among lesbian and heterosexual women. Prev Med. 2004;38(1):105–13.
8. Schneider A, Koutsky LA. Natural history and epidemiological features of genital HPV infection. IARC Sci Publ. 1992;119:25–52.
9. Munoz N, Castellsague X, de Gonzalez AB, Gissmann L. Chapter 1: HPV in the etiology of human cancer. Vaccine. 2006;24 Suppl 3:S3/1–10.
10. Centers for disease control and prevention (CDC) [Internet]. (2014). www.cdc.gov. Accessed 1 Feb 2014.
11. Dunne EF, Unger ER, Sternberg M, McQuillan G, Swan DC, Patel SS, et al. Prevalence of HPV infection among females in the United States. JAMA. 2007;297(8):813–9.
12. Marrazzo JM, Koutsky LA, Stine KL, Kuypers JM, Grubert TA, Galloway DA, et al. Genital human papillomavirus infection in women who have sex with women. J Infect Dis. 1998;178(6):1604–9.
13. Marrazzo JM, Stine K, Koutsky LA. Genital human papillomavirus infection in women who have sex with women: a review. Am J Obstet Gynecol. 2000;183(3):770–4.
14. HIV-AIDS basics [Internet]. Washington, DC: US Department of Health and Human Services; (2012) [updated 6/6/2012]. http://www.aids.gov/hiv-aids-basics/. Accessed: 6 June 2012
15. Kwakwa HA, Ghobrial MW. Female-to-female transmission of human immunodeficiency virus. Clin Infect Dis. 2003;36(3):e40–1.
16. Chan SK, Thornton LR, Chronister KJ, Meyer J, Wolverton M, Johnson CK, et al. Likely female-to-female sexual transmission of HIV–Texas, 2012. MMWR Morb Mortal Wkly Rep. 2014;63(10):209–12.

17. Dworkin SL. Who is epidemiologically fathomable in the HIV/AIDS epidemic? Gender, sexuality, and intersectionality in public health. Cult Health Sex. 2005;7(6):615–23.
18. Herbst JH, Jacobs ED, Finlayson TJ, McKleroy VS, Neumann MS, Crepaz N, et al. Estimating HIV prevalence and risk behaviors of transgender persons in the United States: a systematic review. AIDS Behav. 2008;12(1):1–17.
19. Baral SD, Poteat T, Stromdahl S, Wirtz AL, Guadamuz TE, Beyrer C. Worldwide burden of HIV in transgender women: a systematic review and meta-analysis. Lancet Infect Dis. 2013;13(3):214–22.
20. Custer B, Sullivan SD, Hazlet TK, Iloeje U, Veenstra DL, Kowdley KV. Global epidemiology of hepatitis B virus. J Clin Gastroenterol. 2004;38(10 Suppl 3):S158–68.
21. Wasley A, Kruszon-Moran D, Kuhnert W, Simard EP, Finelli L, McQuillan G, et al. The prevalence of hepatitis B virus infection in the United States in the era of vaccination. J Infect Dis. 2010;202(2):192–201.
22. Fethers K, Marks C, Mindel A, Estcourt CS. Sexually transmitted infections and risk behaviours in women who have sex with women. Sex Transm Infect. 2000;76(5):345–9.
23. Nuttbrock L, Hwahng S, Bockting W, Rosenblum A, Mason M, Macri M, et al. Lifetime risk factors for HIV/sexually transmitted infections among male-to-female transgender persons. J Acquir Immune Defic Syndr. 2009;52(3):417–21.
24. Armstrong GL, Wasley A, Simard EP, McQuillan GM, Kuhnert WL, Alter MJ. The prevalence of hepatitis C virus infection in the United States, 1999 through 2002. Ann Intern Med. 2006;144(10):705–14.
25. Corey L, Wald A, Celum CL, Quinn TC. The effects of herpes simplex virus-2 on HIV-1 acquisition and transmission: A review of two overlapping epidemics. J Acquir Immune Defic Syndr. 2004;35(5):435–45.
26. Freeman EE, Weiss HA, Glynn JR, Cross PL, Whitworth JA, Hayes RJ. Herpes simplex virus 2 infection increases HIV acquisition in men and women: systematic review and meta-analysis of longitudinal studies. AIDS. 2006;20(1):73–83.
27. Corey L. The current trend in genital herpes. Progress in prevention. Sex Transm Dis. 1994;21(2 Suppl):S38–44.
28. Ashley RL, Wald A. Genital herpes: review of the epidemic and potential use of type-specific serology. Clin Microbiol Rev. 1999;12(1):1–8.
29. Roberts C. Genital herpes in young adults: changing sexual behaviours, epidemiology and management. Herpes. 2005;12(1):10–4.
30. Marrazzo JM, Stine K, Wald A. Prevalence and risk factors for infection with herpes simplex virus type-1 and -2 among lesbians. Sex Transm Dis. 2003;30(12):890–5.
31. Xu F, Sternberg MR, Markowitz LE. Women who have sex with women in the united states: Prevalence, sexual behavior and prevalence of herpes simplex virus type 2 infection-results from national health and nutrition examination survey 2001–2006. Sex Transm Dis. 2010;37(7):407–13.
32. Marrazzo JM. Even NHANES evolves: some surprising findings about women who have sex with women. Sex Transm Dis. 2010;37(7):414–5.
33. Rosario M, Meyer-Bahlburg HF, Hunter J, Gwadz M. Sexual risk behaviors of gay, lesbian, and bisexual youths in New York city: prevalence and correlates. AIDS Educ Prev. 1999;11(6):476–96.
34. Bauer GR, Welles SL. Beyond assumptions of negligible risk: sexually transmitted diseases and women who have sex with women. Am J Public Health. 2001;91(8):1282–6.
35. Rowen TS, Breyer BN, Lin TC, Li CS, Robertson PA, Shindel AW. Use of barrier protection for sexual activity among women who have sex with women. Int J Gynaecol Obstet. 2013;120(1):42–5.
36. Scheer S, Peterson I, Page-Shafer K, Delgado V, Gleghorn A, Ruiz J, et al. Sexual and drug use behavior among women who have sex with both women and men: results of a population-based survey. Am J Public Health. 2002;92(7):1110–2.
37. Bauer GR, Jairam JA, Baidoobonso SM. Sexual health, risk behaviors, and substance use in heterosexual-identified women with female sex partners: 2002 US national survey of family growth. Sex Transm Dis. 2010;37(9):531–7.

38. Roberts SJ, Grindel CG, Patsdaughter CA, DeMarco R, Tarmina MS. Lesbian use and abuse of alcohol: results of the Boston lesbian health project II. Subst Abus. 2004;25(4):1–9.
39. Drabble L, Trocki K. Alcohol consumption, alcohol-related problems, and other substance use among lesbian and bisexual women. J Lesbian Stud. 2005;9(3):19–30.
40. Hyde Z, Comfort J, McManus A, Brown G, Howat P. Alcohol, tobacco and illicit drug use amongst same-sex attracted women: results from the western australian lesbian and bisexual women's health and well-being survey. BMC Public Health. 2009;9:317,2458-9-317.
41. Chappin SR, Tross S, Sanchez JP, Dermatis H, Galanter M. Alcohol consumption patterns: gay and lesbian urban ethnic minority members. Subst Abus. 2010;31(1):71–3.
42. Newcomb ME, Heinz AJ, Mustanski B. Examining risk and protective factors for alcohol use in lesbian, gay, bisexual, and transgender youth: a longitudinal multilevel analysis. J Stud Alcohol Drugs. 2012;73(5):783–93.
43. Feldman J, Bockting W. Transgender health. Minn Med. 2003;86(7):25–32.
44. Nemoto T, Operario D, Keatley J, Nguyen H, Sugano E. Promoting health for transgender women: transgender resources and neighborhood space (TRANS) program in san francisco. Am J Public Health. 2005;95(3):382–4.
45. Nemoto T, Bodeker B, Iwamoto M, Sakata M. Practices of receptive and insertive anal sex among transgender women in relation to partner types, sociocultural factors, and background variables. AIDS Care. 2014;26(4):434–40.
46. Advisory committee on immunization practices (ACIP) [Internet]. Atlanta, GA: Centers for Disease Control; 2014 [updated February 27, 2014]. http://www.cdc.gov/vaccines/acip/. Accessed 1 March 2014.
47. Jemal A, Simard EP, Dorell C, Noone AM, Markowitz LE, Kohler B, et al. Annual report to the nation on the status of cancer, 1975–2009, featuring the burden and trends in human papillomavirus(HPV)-associated cancers and HPV vaccination coverage levels. J Natl Cancer Inst. 2013;105(3):175–201.
48. Deol AK, Heath-Toby A. HIV risk for lesbians, bisexuals and other women who have sex with women. Whitepaper. Gay Men's Health Crisis; 2009.
49. Kim JJ. Targeted human papillomavirus vaccination of men who have sex with men in the USA: a cost-effectiveness modelling analysis. Lancet Infect Dis. 2010;10(12):845–52.
50. Kim JJ. Focus on research: weighing the benefits and costs of HPV vaccination of young men. N Engl J Med. 2011;364(5):393–5.
51. Kim JJ. Weighing the benefits and costs of HPV vaccination of young men. N Engl J Med. 2011;364(5):393–5.
52. Cox P, McNair R. Risk reduction as an accepted framework for safer-sex promotion among women who have sex with women. Sex Health. 2009;6(1):15–8.
53. Marrazzo JM. "Can I get herpes from my girlfriend?" Lesbians' sexual health. In: Dibble SL, Robertson PA, editors. Lesbian health 101: a clinician's guide. San Francisco: UCSF Nursing Press; 2010. p. 55–66.
54. Marrazzo JM, Coffey P, Bingham A. Sexual practices, risk perception and knowledge of sexually transmitted disease risk among lesbian and bisexual women. Perspect Sex Reprod Health. 2005;37(1):6–12.
55. Bockting WO, Robinson BE, Forberg J, Scheltema K. Evaluation of a sexual health approach to reducing HIV/STD risk in the transgender community. AIDS Care. 2005;17(3):289–303.
56. Taylor RD, Bimbi DS, Joseph HA, Margolis AD, Parsons JT. Girlfriends: evaluation of an HIV-risk reduction intervention for adult transgender women. AIDS Educ Prev. 2011;23(5):469–78.
57. Wei C, Herrick A, Raymond HF, Anglemyer A, Gerbase A, Noar SM. Social marketing interventions to increase HIV/STI testing uptake among men who have sex with men and male-to-female transgender women. Cochrane Database Syst Rev. 2011;9:CD009337. doi(9):CD009337.
58. McNair R. Risks and prevention of sexually transmissible infections among women who have sex with women. Sex Health. 2005;2(4):209–17.

59. Mercer CH, Bailey JV, Johnson AM, Erens B, Wellings K, Fenton KA, et al. Women who report having sex with women: British national probability data on prevalence, sexual behaviors, and health outcomes. Am J Public Health. 2007;97(6):1126–33.
60. Laumann EO, Gagnon J, Michael R, Michaels S. The social organization of sexuality: sexual practices in the United States. Chicago: University of Chicago Press; 1994.
61. Bauer GR, Jairam JA. Are lesbians really women who have sex with women (WSW)? Methodological concerns in measuring sexual orientation in health research. Women Health. 2008;48(4):383–408.
62. Everett BG. Sexual orientation disparities in sexually transmitted infections: examining the intersection between sexual identity and sexual behavior. Arch Sex Behav. 2013;42(2):225–36.
63. Brown JP, Tracy JK. Lesbians and cancer: an overlooked health disparity. Cancer Causes Control. 2008;19(10).
64. McNair R. Lesbian and bisexual women's sexual health. Aust Fam Physician. 2009;38(6):388–93.
65. Sell RL, Dunn PM. Inclusion of lesbian, gay, bisexual and transgender people in tobacco use-related surveillance and epidemiological research. J LGBT Health Res. 2008;4(1):27–42.
66. Boehmer U, Miao X, Ozonoff A. Cancer survivorship and sexual orientation. Cancer. 2011;117(16):3796–804.

Chapter 4
Addressing Behavioral Cancer Risks from a LGBT Health Equity Perspective

Karen I. Fredriksen-Goldsen, Charles P. Hoy-Ellis and Maria Brown

Abstract Accounting for individual, community, and societal factors, as well as historical context and life-course events, we utilize a Health Equity model to consider behavioral risks and identify social determinants that may influence cancer risks in LGBT populations. Based on data from available research, we provide estimates of the prevalence of behavioral risks in LGBT communities, including excessive drinking and substance abuse, obesity, poor nutrition and diet, and physical inactivity. Both upstream and downstream factors that may elevate such behavioral risks for cancer among LGBT populations, including those unique to particular subgroups, are discussed. Examples of innovative programs and interventions designed for LGBT communities to target cancer-related behavioral risks are briefly described. We conclude with research, practice, and policy recommendations that are needed to promote health equity and reduce the disparate cancer burden in LGBT communities.

Introduction

In *Healthy People 2020* lesbian, gay, bisexual, and transgender (LGBT) people are for the first time identified as U.S. national health priorities [1]. The Centers for Disease Control and Prevention [2] conclude that sexual orientation is a primary gap in health disparities research, which result from social, economic, and environmental disadvantage. Current research indicates that LGBT people experience higher rates of disability [3], physical limitations [3–6], poor general health [3–5], and psychological distress [3–5].

The American Cancer Society [7] recognizes cancer as a significant health issue in the LGBT community. It is estimated that there are more than a million LGBT people living with cancer in the United States [8]. Cancer risks occur at many lev-

K. I. Fredriksen-Goldsen (✉) · C. P. Hoy-Ellis
School of Social Work, University of Washington, Seattle, Washington, USA
e-mail: fredrikk@u.washington.edu

M. Brown
Syracuse University, NY, USA

U. Boehmer, R. Elk (eds.), *Cancer and the LGBT Community*,
DOI 10.1007/978-3-319-15057-4_4

els, from cells to society—from biological and genetic, to behavioral to environmental risks. As a result of a distinct cluster of risk factors (such as higher rates of smoking, excessive alcohol use, and obesity), emerging evidence suggests there is an elevated cancer burden in the LGBT community [8–15].

Although research suggests elevated levels of cancer risks in this population, to date there is a lack of concrete data regarding the incidence and prevalence of cancer in LGBT communities [14]. Because sexual orientation and gender identity data are not included in national cancer registries, our understanding of cancer in these communities remains limited. In recent years only a few state-level population-based health surveys have included sexual orientation questions, providing preliminary data to estimate the cancer risk in lesbian, gay, and bisexual populations, although not in transgender populations. Yet, cancer prevalence and risks vary considerably between states and regions [16], requiring broader, more comprehensive data collection to better understand the cancer risks faced by LGBT populations across the country.

Social contextual factors, such as social networks, cultural norms, discrimination, and victimization are shaped by socio-demographic characteristics, such as race/ethnicity and sexual orientation [17] and strongly influence behavior [18]. *Behavioral risk factors* are personal behaviors that impact health outcomes, such as diet, physical activity, and tobacco and alcohol use, to name just a few [19]. Such behavioral risk factors, including over-eating, excessive drinking, substance use, poor diet and nutrition, and physical inactivity, are critical to identify and fully consider, since they are potentially modifiable and may be amenable to change. Furthermore, behavioral risk factors can increase the risk of multiple types of cancer [20], and can operate synergistically with other risk factors, dramatically increasing the overall risk of cancer [7, 8].

This chapter will examine available evidence on the prevalence and potential causes of cancer-related behavioral risk factors in LGBT populations, including excessive drinking and substance use, physical inactivity and obesity, and diet and poor nutrition. When available, we will also examine prevalence rates for subgroups in these populations and the influence of demographic characteristics. Based on a Health Equity model, we will discuss potential factors associated with these behavioral risks, and highlight innovative programs and interventions that have been developed to reduce these risks. Lastly, we will identify the unique challenges that exist in addressing behavioral cancer risks in LGBT communities and implications for future practice, policy and research.

Social, Contextual, and Behavioral Risks

It is important to recognize that there are numerous types and subtypes of cancer, and that some risk factors are common to multiple types of cancers while others are more specific to a particular type. Equally important is that some risk factors are synergistic. For example, obesity or being overweight, inadequate nutrition, and lack of physical activity are related and together account for approximately a third of U.S. cancer mortality [21]. Such behavioral risks for cancer, along with excessive drinking and substance use, have been found to be elevated among various subgroups in LGBT populations [14]. Smoking as a primary behavioral risk for cancer will be discussed in-depth in a subsequent chapter so is not addressed here. The health-wealth gradient (i.e., lower income, education, and social status being associated with worse health) is also found in cancer risk [17], and the larger social context has both direct and indirect effects. For example, experiences of discrimination have been implicated in poor general health among older LGBT adults [22, 23], while the stress associated with concealment of minority identity may affect psychoneuroimmunological functioning [24]. For example, the functionality of immune-system cells may foster metastasis of breast cancer to other organs and body-systems [25]. At the same time, individuals may use alcohol as a way to cope with stress [26].

It is also important to recognize that some health risks may have their origins much earlier in life. For example, sexual minority women and men report significantly higher rates of physical [27, 28], sexual [27, 28], and psychological abuse [27] in childhood. Sexual minorities also report higher rates of victimization in adulthood than heterosexuals [27, 28], and these higher rates of victimization are associated with excessive alcohol use [28] and other drug abuse [29]. In the general population, childhood victimization is also associated with adult obesity, physical inactivity, victimization, and multiple serious illnesses, among several other poor health outcomes [30–32]. Transgender adults also report significant rates of childhood victimization [33]. Recent research suggests that adverse childhood events such as these may also have a link to cancer in adulthood through alterations of biological systems [34]. Two such examples are the dysregulation of the hypothalamic-pituitary-adrenal (HPA) axis and subsequent allostatic load, and epigenetics, the process whereby environmental factors, including stress, induce methylation to literally switch genes on or off to result in disease [34–36]. Such an epigenetic "switch" has recently been identified in relation to breast cancer and the ATF3 gene [25].

Health Equity Model

Most LGBT health research has focused on health disparities [37–39], with limited attention to the full continuum of health outcomes in these communities. In this chapter we utilize the *Health Equity model*, which addresses the full health potential of LGBT people [40]. Health disparities are differences in population-level disease incidence and prevalence resulting from marginalization and economic, environmental, or social disadvantage [38]. A health equity approach aims to not only reduce disparities, but to fully maximize efforts embedded within social contexts so that all people can attain their health potential [40, 41]. The behavioral risks and resources that influence LGBT health must be examined in order to develop services and interventions that promote health equity and improve health and well-being in these communities.

From this perspective, LGBT health can best be understood in the context of a multidimensional framework, highlighting how (a) social positions and (b) structural and environmental context intersect with (c) adverse and health-promoting pathways to influence the full range of health outcomes in LGBT communities [40]. The pathways influencing health as identified in this perspective include behavioral, social, psychological, and biological mechanisms [40]. This model expands upon earlier conceptualizations by taking into account the historical and cultural contexts over the life course, including generational and cohort effects, as well as the intersectionality of broader social positions and health-promoting and adverse mechanisms, including health behaviors. Utilizing the Health Equity model is important in order to understand the complexity and range of the risks and resources and health indicators that influence LGBT health across the life course.

Excessive Drinking

Excessive use of alcohol increases the risk for several types of cancer, including oral, esophageal, breast, liver, and colorectal [42]. Alcohol is broken down through metabolic processes into other compounds which are toxic (e.g., acetaldehyde), and oxygen reactive, both of which can damage DNA; it can also increase the risk for cancer through interfering with the body's ability to absorb many important vitamins and nutrients, as well as increasing serum estrogen, which has been linked to breast cancer [42].

Several studies provide evidence that LGBT populations drink alcohol excessively and/or have higher rates of drug use than do heterosexuals [5, 6, 29, 43]. Data from the 2000 National Alcohol Survey (NAS) indicates that 12% of lesbians and 17% of bisexual women met *DSM-IV* criteria for alcohol dependence (past-year), compared to 2% of heterosexual women and 4% of women who identified as heterosexual but also reported same-sex behavior in the previous 5 years [44]. This same study found that 10% of gay men and 6% of bisexual men met the criteria, compared to 6% of heterosexual men and 11% of men who identified as heterosexual but also reported same-sex behavior in the previous five years; the differences among women were significant, while those among men were not [44].

Data from the Washington State Behavioral Risk Factor Surveillance System (BRFSS) indicates that older lesbian and bisexual women (8%) are significantly more likely to drink excessively than heterosexual women (5%), as are older gay and bisexual men (17%), compared to 11% of older heterosexual men [4]. Conversely, California Health Interview Survey (CHIS) data indicates that on average among adults of all ages, heterosexual men drink more than gay and bisexual men [45]. It may be that these conflicting findings reflect differences in the ages of the respective samples, or other regional sociodemographic differences (e.g., race/ethnicity). Population-based data from New Mexico indicates that bisexual and heterosexual men binge-drink at similar rates (20%), although the rate among bisexual women (24%) is significantly higher than heterosexual women (8%) [46]. Nearly half (46%) of lesbian, gay, and bisexual high school youth in Massachusetts report binge-drinking in the past month, compared to 33% of their heterosexual peers

[47]. Significantly higher rates of excessive drinking and other substance use by lesbian, gay, and bisexual youth has been found across several population-based studies [47].

In addition to important differences by sexual orientation and gender, it also appears there may be important differences by sexual orientation and age. For example, evidence suggests that bisexual women may be at greater risk than either lesbian or heterosexual women [48]. Similarly, in contrast to comparably aged heterosexual women, lesbian and bisexual women younger than aged 50 may be more likely to drink excessively [9, 49], while lesbians aged 50 and older appear more likely to drink excessively than bisexual women of the same age [4]. Because research on older sexual minorities as a distinct population is still rare, these findings are preliminary. There are several studies that include young, middle-aged, and older adults, but very few make comparisons between cohorts. On the other hand, there has been significantly more research on younger sexual minorities, which suggests that results for this age group may be more robust. The evidence indicates that alcohol and drug use are more prevalent among lesbian, gay, and bisexual youth than among their heterosexual peers. Lesbian, gay, and bisexual youth are more likely than their heterosexual peers to use alcohol and cocaine before the age of 13 [47]. Substance use before age 18 is strongly associated with increased risk of abuse and dependency in adulthood [50].

Discrimination, internalized stigma, and expectations of rejection have been associated with increased alcohol use among sexual minority and transgender individuals [51, 52]. There is some evidence that internalized heterosexism may also be associated with alcohol use and alcohol-related problems among lesbians [53], and more experiences of rejection subsequent to disclosure of sexual orientation among sexual minority youth [54]. One in four transgender participants in a large community-based survey report abusing alcohol, after experiencing discrimination in the workplace [55]. Childhood maltreatment is among the stressors associated with earlier onset and greater prevalence of alcohol use among adults [51], which is one of the significant risk factors for multiple types of cancer. Risk of excessive drinking may also result from the significance of bars as both an important historical and contemporary social venue in LGBT communities [56]. This is further exacerbated by targeted marketing practices; "...alcohol and tobacco advertising works on LGBT audiences because gay-targeted ads make them feel desired, understood, safer, and more comfortable doing business with brands that recognized them for who they were" (Double Platinum, n.d., as cited in [57]).

Other Drugs

Unlike excessive drinking, substance abuse includes a wide variety of other drugs that are composed of numerous chemical compounds. Studying the relationships between drug use and cancer risk is further confounded by the fact that many drugs (e.g., cocaine, methamphetamine, heroin) are often "cut" or diluted with a variety of other substances, from mannitol, which is a diuretic, to strychnine, a commonly used rodent poison; such toxic substances may be used in the manufacturing and processing of some drugs [58]. Thus, the relationship between drug use and cancer risk is complex and difficult to study. A review of epidemiological studies found conflicting results in the relationship between marijuana use and the risk of different types of cancer [59]. Some carcinogens found in tobacco smoke are also present in marijuana smoke [59], although compounds in marijuana have also shown to have anti-inflammatory and anti-carcinogenic properties [59, 60].

The lack of attention to sexual orientation and gender identity in most national surveys creates significant challenge in understanding the prevalence of drug abuse among LGBT people. It has been suggested that the rate of drug abuse among LGBT people ranges from 20 to 30 %, which is substantially higher than the 9 % estimated in the overall population [61]. A Washington State study of heterosexual and LGBT individuals seeking publicly-funded drug abuse treatment found that the four most common drugs for which treatment was sought were the same, although differences in prevalence of other abused drugs were noted [62]. The most commonly reported drugs used among LGBT versus heterosexual clients respectively were alcohol (50 vs. 37 %), methamphetamine (21 % vs. 14 %), marijuana (13 % each), and heroin (14 % vs. 11 %). This same study found that heterosexual women and men were more likely to seek treatment for alcohol; lesbian, bisexual, and transgender women were more likely to seek treatment for heroin; and gay, bisexual, and transgender men were more likely to do so for methamphetamine [62].

Data from the National Epidemiologic Survey on Alcohol and Related Conditions (NESARC) indicates that lesbian (26 %) and bisexual women (24 %) have significantly higher rates of past-year drug abuse disorders than heterosexual women (6 %), as do gay (31 %) and bisexual men (28 %) compared to heterosexual men (16 %) [43]. Data from the Massachusetts BRFSS indicates that among adults aged 40 and older, 24 % of gay men, 10 % of lesbians, 20 % of bisexual men, and 39 % of bisexual women used illicit drugs in the past 30 days, compared to 10 % of heterosexual men and 5 % of heterosexual women [6]. High rates of substance use, as well as hormone therapy among transgender individuals have been noted in large-scale surveys, thus they may be at elevated risk for some cancers than non-transgender people [63].

Discrimination, internalized stigma, and expectations of rejection have been associated with increased use of drugs among bereaved gay men [64]. The experience of LGBT-based victimization (verbal and physical assaults) has been associated with greater risk of lifetime drug abuse problems [65]. Lesbian, gay, and bisexual young adults who are rejected by their families are more than three times as likely to abuse illicit drugs as those who are not [66]. More than half (57 %) of transgender participants have been rejected by their families [55]. As a result of employment discrimination, transgender individuals may end up working in the "street economy," which places them at increased risk for drug abuse and interpersonal victimization [55].

Obesity

Obesity and being overweight are connected to as many as 20% of cancer mortalities in the U.S. [21], and have been positively linked with breast cancer (among post-menopausal women), colorectal, endometrial (uterine lining), esophageal, and kidney cancers, and may increase the risk for cancers of the gallbladder, liver, ovaries, cervix, aggressive prostate, as well as non-Hodgkin lymphoma and multiple myeloma. Having a large waistline, whether or not one is overweight or obese, is associated with greater risk of colorectal cancers and likely with pancreatic, endometrial, and breast (among postmenopausal women) cancers [21]. The underlying mechanisms of risk seem to vary by cancer type, but may include inflammation, immune system functioning, hormone levels, and how the body regulates hormones, as well as substances involved in cellular division, such as insulin-like growth factor-1 (IGF-1). Sedentary lifestyles (i.e., physical inactivity) and poor nutrition are significant predictors of adult obesity [67].

Lesbian and bisexual women have higher rates of being overweight or obese than their heterosexual peers [4, 5, 68]; and, lesbians may have higher rates of obesity than bisexual women [69]. Washington State data indicates that 36% of lesbians and bisexual women 50 years of age and older are obese, compared to 26% of older heterosexual women; 23% of older gay and bisexual men are obese, compared to 27% of older heterosexual men [4]. The lower rates of obesity among gay and bisexual men mirror findings from the CHIS [45]. Interestingly, New Mexico data indicates non-significant differences in the rates of obesity among gay men (35%) as compared to heterosexual men (24%) [46].

In a study comparing lesbian and heterosexual sisters, lesbians had greater waist circumferences, waist-to-hip ratios, higher body-mass indices, and more extensive weight-cycling [70]. Demographic factors associated with being overweight or obese among lesbian and bisexual women include older age, less education, living with a partner, and poor general health [71]; African American lesbians, and lesbians that reside in urban or rural areas (as opposed to suburban) are also at higher risk for obesity [48]. In attempting to obscure anatomical differences in the chest and hips, transgender men may elect to intentionally gain extra weight [72].

Obesity is generally considered to result from individual characteristics (e.g., genetics) and behaviors (e.g., overeating, poor nutrition, and lack of exercise). While these factors are important, recent research strongly suggests that obesity also spreads through social network ties, particularly friendships that are of the same-sex [73]. Being in a cohabiting relationship is a risk factor for obesity and overweight among lesbian and bisexual women [71]. Modifiable risk factors in controlling excess weight and obesity include more physical activity, consumption of more fresh fruits and vegetables and less sugary foods and drinks, and eating smaller portions [67]. Increasing physical activity in structured environments, such as fitness centers or exercise classes, may be more difficult for sexual minority women, as many fitness facilities do not offer family memberships to same-sex headed families, and physical activity groups tend not to be lesbian-specific [48].

Many lesbians who do wish to lose weight frame weight loss in the context of becoming healthier, rather than in the context of improving their appearance [74], and they may therefore be amenable to modifying nutrition and exercise to improve overall health and decrease cancer risk. There is some evidence of a weight loss benefit to participating in a mostly lesbian group, which was found in an internationally-franchised weight loss program, even when the program itself is not focused on sexual minority issues [74].

Diet and Nutrition

Diet and poor nutrition are related to being overweight and obese, and are also independent risk factors for cancer [75]. The actual role that diet and nutrition plays in cancer has been investigated but remains somewhat unclear [76], in part, because foods contain many compounds and the ways in which foods are prepared may also be important. Diets high in vegetables and fruits likely decrease the risk of oral, esophageal, stomach, pancreatic, prostate, and lung cancers, possibly through the antioxidant properties of phytochemicals that occur naturally in plants; whole grain fiber has been associated with decreased risk of colorectal cancers [76]. Large intake of red meats, especially fatty cuts, and processed meats (e.g., bologna, hotdogs) have been linked with increased risk of colorectal cancer; dairy products, such as milk, may decrease the risk of colorectal and bladder cancers but may increase the risk of prostate cancer [76]. Fatty foods in general, and foods prepared in fat and through frying have also been linked to increased risk of cancer [76]. Skipping meals and eating fast food are also associated with poor nutrition [77]. Again, although clear associations between nutrition and numerous cancers have been established, the underlying mechanisms of risk continue to be studied [76].

"Food insecurity is generally defined as having limited or uncertain availability of nutritionally adequate and safe foods or limited or uncertain ability to acquire acceptable foods in socially acceptable ways" [78]. Compilation of data from the Gallup Daily Tracking Survey (GDTS), the National Survey of Family Growth (NSFG), and the American Community Survey (ACS) indicates that regardless of gender, race/ethnicity, age, and educational achievement, LGBT adults (29 %) are significantly more likely than their heterosexual peers (18 %) to have experienced food insecurity in the past year [78]. New Mexico data indicates that only 16 % of lesbians and gay men meet nutritional guidelines for fruits and vegetables, compared to 21 % of heterosexuals, and 29 % of bisexuals, although these differences are not significant [46]. Although percentages were not provided, CHIS data indicates that gay and bisexual men's nutritional habits are similar to heterosexual men's [45].

While sexual minority women may be aware that diet is important, they may not know what constitutes a healthy diet [79]. Lesbian and bisexual women are more likely to skip breakfast than heterosexual women [80], and are less likely to include fresh fruits and vegetables in their diets [68]. Lesbians, but not bisexual women aged 50 and older are less likely than heterosexual women of the same age to consume five or more servings of fresh fruits and vegetables daily; no differences have been noted between gay, bisexual, and heterosexual men [9]. There is no difference in reported fruit and vegetable consumption between sexual minority and heterosexual women according to CHIS data [81]. Compared to non-LGBT heterosexual adults aged 18 and older, across LGBT demographic groups, women, Native, Hispanic, African, and Hawaiian Americans, those who identify as multiracial, those with less than a 4-year degree, and those who are younger are at particular risk for food insecurity [78].

Transgender individuals may have unique dietary issues, as some foods are involved in the production of hormones; thus, some may adjust their diets in feminizing and masculinizing efforts [72]. Transgender men on testosterone therapy may experience deficiencies in protein, micronutrients, certain vitamins, and insufficient calories in their diets; some transgender women may diet excessively to appear more feminine [72]. Modifiable factors related to better diet and nutrition are similar to those related to obesity, such as eating more fresh fruits and vegetables, avoiding foods high in fat and sugar [67], reducing red meat and eliminating processed meats, utilizing cooking methods other than frying in food preparation [76], avoiding fast food, and not missing meals, whenever possible.

Physical Activity

Lack of physical activity is an important factor in being overweight or obese, as well as an independent risk factor for cancer [21, 75]. Regular physical activity improves immune system functioning, levels and regulation of certain hormones (e.g., estrogen, insulin), and reduces inflammation [82]. Regular physical activity has been linked to decreased risk of breast, colon, uterine, and lung cancers [82]. People with disabilities and physical limitations have a significantly increased risk for being physically inactive [83]. A diet poor in fruits and vegetables, low/intermediate levels of routine physical activity, and being a current or recent smoker each independently increase the risk of disability [84].

Lifetime experiences of discrimination and internalized heterosexism have been associated with increased risk of disability among older lesbian, gay, bisexual [22], and transgender adults [23]. Data on adults aged 50 and older indicates that 44% of lesbian and bisexual women have a disability, compared to 37% of heterosexual women, and 38% of gay and bisexual men, compared to 34% of heterosexual men; not only are these differences significant after accounting for age, income, and education, but it appears that lesbian, gay, and bisexual adults experience the onset of disability at younger ages than do their heterosexual peers [4].

A study comparing lesbians to heterosexual women noted that about a third of each group had been physically inactive during the past month, but among those who were physically active, 37% of lesbians had engaged in regular vigorous physical activity, compared to only 14% of heterosexual women [85]. Data from another study indicates that bisexual women and men are more likely to meet standards for physical activity (71 %) than are their heterosexual counterparts (54 %), as are lesbians and gay men (60 %), although the latter is non-significant [48]. Percentages were not provided, but CHIS data indicates that gay and bisexual men's exercise habits are similar to heterosexual men's [45]. A convenience sample of transgender men found that more than half (55 %) were physically inactive [86], although a large-scale survey found that 74 % of transgender and 82 % of lesbian, gay, and bisexual older adults engage in moderate physical activity on a weekly basis [87].

Several studies have shown that at least some subgroups of sexual minorities may be more likely to engage in physical activity, which may reduce risk for cancer. For example, Boehmer and colleagues [9] report that lesbians younger than 50 are more likely to engage in moderate physical activities and bisexual women are more likely to engage in muscle-strengthening activities than heterosexual women of similar age. Brown and Grossman's [88] analysis of data from the National Social Life, Health, and Aging Project (NSHAP) suggests that respondents who report a history of same-sex sexual relationships are more likely to be physically active than their sexual majority peers.

Boehmer and Bowen's [81] examination of California Women's Health Survey (CWHS) data indicates that women who only have sex with women are the most physically active, while women who have sex with both men and women are the least physically active, although the difference is not statistically significant. Compared to heterosexuals of similar age, gay men less than 50-years old seem to have a higher probability of engaging in exercise that builds muscle, and bisexual men 50-years old and older seem to have a higher probability of engaging in vigorous activities [9]. Fredriksen-Goldsen, Kim and colleagues [4] find that lesbian, gay, and bisexual adults aged 50 and older do not differ from older heterosexual adults in their levels of moderate physical activity. Sexual minority youth, especially boys, may be at increased risk for physical inactivity [89]. Emerging evidence suggests that transgender women and men may be hesitant to exercise for a variety of reasons related to bodily appearance, comfort, and perceived gender norms [72].

Cross Cutting Risks and Strengths

Although risks for cancer and many other serious diseases are often attributed in part to individual genetic and behavioral factors, a health equity perspective identifies how larger structural factors are also important [90, 91]. Alcohol is a good example, since LGBT people are specifically targeted for marketing; in a featured article in the *New York Times*, Absolut® vodka "celebrated 30 years of marketing" to the LGBT community [92]. LGBT individuals may abuse alcohol and other drugs in part as a response to such exposure, as well as in response to their experiences with discrimination [93]; even today it is still legal to discriminate against lesbians, gay men, and bisexual women and men in 29 states, and against transgender women and men in 32 [94]. An alarming finding is that sexual minorities living in communities with high levels of anti-gay prejudice have an estimated 12-year shorter life expectancy, as well as higher rates of cardiovascular disease (CVD) [95], which is significantly associated with stress. Lesbian, gay, and bisexual populations living in states that have passed anti-LGBT legislation experience significant increases in psychological distress as a result of stress [96].

Another structural risk factor is that LGBT people experience discrimination in healthcare settings, which can lead them to delay treatment and/or conceal their sexual and gender identities [97], which in turn can directly and negatively impact the timeliness, type and quality of care provided [98]. Healthcare providers' prejudicial attitudes are also a barrier to health promotion through healthcare access, such as preventive screenings that are critical to early detection, intervention and treatment [14]. In addition to missed opportunities for education about risky health behaviors, irregular access to healthcare may actually increase the odds of health risk behaviors [99, 100].

A recent study that pooled data from the 2005–2007 Youth Risk Behavior Surveys (YRBS) found that lesbian, gay, and bisexual youth in 9th to 12th grades in high school scored significantly higher than their heterosexual peers on 11 of 12 behavioral risks for cancer [89]. LGBT individuals who experienced physical, psychological, or sexual abuse or other adverse events in childhood may be at heightened risk for cancer [34]. This risk may be even greater in that childhood victimization has been associated with increased numbers of sexual partners and other high risk sexual behaviors as an adult [32], which increases the risk of cancers associated with human papilloma viruses (HPV), including oral, cervical, and anal [101].

Based on the Health Equity model it is imperative that we recognize the strengths and resources of LGBT people and the protective behaviors that promote good health. LGBT individuals and communities are resilient, despite the challenges and adversity that they may face. The human agency of LGBT people and the LGBT community are important resources, as was seen during the height of the AIDS pandemic. LGBT health activism can be traced back to the 1970s, "…when the American Psychiatric Association (APA)—under siege from activists disrupting the association's meetings—voted to change the classification [of homosexuality as a sociopathic personality disorder]" [102]. When HIV and the modes of transmission were identified, LGBT people and communities rallied from within to promote health and reduce risk behaviors [103]. Such health activism has continued, from lesbian and bisexual women's active engagement in raising awareness about breast cancer, to transgender women and men's work to recognize "the need for serious research on biological processes related to [their] … life circumstances" [102], and most recently the advocacy efforts that have led to LGBT health being prioritized in the national health objectives in *Healthy People 2020* [1].

Consider the role of similar advocacy efforts in the marriage equality movement. While the federal Defense of Marriage Act (DOMA) was passed by majorities of both Houses of Congress and was signed into law by President Clinton in 1996, Massachusetts became the first state to recognize same-sex marriage only seven years later in 2003; in 2013 the Supreme Court struck down a major provision of DOMA, requiring the federal government to recognize same-sex marriages [104].

Currently, 19 states and the District of Columbia recognize same-sex marriages, with litigation pending in the remaining states and in Puerto Rico [105].

Marriage has been shown to be a protective factor in terms of both mental and physical health, a protective mechanism that extends to same-sex marriage [106]. Marriage equality is still relatively recent and while some studies have examined its positive relationship to health outcomes [107], research is needed to assess its influence on health behaviors. A recent research synthesis on the "effect of [traditional] marriage and health behaviors" commissioned by the U.S. Department of Health and Human Services [108] found that, among other things: the frequency of excessive drinking in the year prior to and the year after first marriage declined by around 50% for men and 25% for women; both women and men experience modest gains in weight, as well as somewhat smaller gains in physical activity; and increased health care access and utilization.

Community-level factors are also important in the Health Equity model. Lesbian, gay, and bisexual youth who live in communities with supportive environments have fewer problems with alcohol abuse than their peers who reside in non-supportive communities [109]. Similarly, being active in HIV/AIDS organizations, as well as LGBT-specific community organizations, appears to moderate the relationship between stigma, engaging in sex under the influence, and consequent risky sex among gay, bisexual, and transgender Latino men [110].

LGBT individuals and their social relations and networks are important strengths; supportive social relationships can facilitate positive changes in health risk behaviors [18]. The LIVESTRONG Foundation™ (http://www.livestrong.org/) seeks to support and advocate for those affected by cancer. In a recent survey of cancer survivors, the foundation notes those who identify as LGBT are significantly less likely than heterosexuals to list biological family members as sources of support, instead listing members of their families of choice [111]. LGBT young adults who are accepted by their families of origin are at decreased risk for substance abuse [112].

Some studies suggest that lesbians and bisexual women are more likely to seek help for an alcohol problem than are heterosexual women [44], and they may also be more likely than their heterosexual sisters to exercise on a weekly basis [70]. Although gay men's concerns with body image is often seen as a negative and may increase their risk for eating disorders, it may also lead them to pay closer attention to their diet [113]. Lesbian and bisexual women and gay and bisexual men are significantly more likely than their heterosexual peers to engage in both professional mental health treatment and self-help groups [114]. Results of a large community-based survey indicate that 75% of transgender participants have received counseling, and another 14% intend to do so [55]. Such positive help-seeking behaviors across LGBT subgroups suggest that they may be amenable to engagement in programs or services designed to promote the behavioral change necessary to promote good health.

Innovative Programs and Interventions Designed to Reduce Risks

While there is a significant body of literature discussing the need for culturally sensitive, tailored interventions to reduce behavioral risks among LGBT people [115–117], there is limited evaluation of tailored interventions in modifying cancer-related risk behaviors. Although LGBT populations are increasingly being recognized as having disproportionate risks for some cancers, there appears to be a dearth of programs designed to address their specific behavioral risks, and very limited research on the programs that do exist. For example, only 6% of the nearly 14,000 substance abuse treatment centers in the U.S. provide programs specifically targeting lesbian and gay clients, and because many treatment groups are gender-specific, transgender adults likely encounter significant challenges accessing appropriate treatment [48]. Below we describe some innovative programs that have been designed to reduce behavioral risks and promote good health in LGBT communities. Each of these programs described below is free of charge in order to increase accessibility.

Obesity, Nutrition, Physical Activity The *SHE* (Strong. Healthy. Energized.) program offered by SAGE (Services & Advocacy for Gay, Lesbian, Bisexual & Transgender Elders) and other agencies that serve the LGBT community consists of 12 weekly in-person sessions designed to help older lesbian and bisexual women who are overweight or obese to work toward fitness goals (http://sageusa.org/newsevents/events.cfm?ID=627). Each session combines information about nutrition and cooking with exercise and topical discussions. In a "comfortable, fun atmosphere" participants learn about the relationships between weight, nutrition, and physical activity to lead happier, healthier lives.

Reduction of Excessive Use of Alcohol Canadian high schools that have long-standing (i.e., 3 or more years) Gay-Straight Alliances (GSAs) and LGB-specific anti-bullying policies have been shown to have a positive impact on lesbian and bisexual female adolescent problem alcohol use and its consequences, as well as that of heterosexual female and male adolescents [118].

The *Over the Influence Book Club* utilizes a harm reduction model [119], incorporating the principle "that people do engage in high-risk behaviors and to commit to helping those people reduce the harm associated with their behavior" [120]. In the *Over the Influence Book Club* in San Francisco (http://new.sfaf.org/stonewall/assets/doc/secular-alternatives-or.pdf), instead of reading a different book each month, the participants "read and chat" about the book *Over the Influence: The Harm Reduction Guide for Managing Drugs and Alcohol* [121]. The group's "come as you are" philosophy provides a safe supportive space where facilitated discussions help participants learn about various harm reduction tools and strategies, as well as themselves.

Drug Abuse Seattle's *Project NEON* (Needle Exchange and Sex Education Outreach Network) is also a harm reduction program that targets gay, bisexual, and transgender men who are engaged in methamphetamine use (http://www.projectneon.org/home.html). In addition to raising awareness about the relationships between methamphetamine use and an array of health concerns, this program seeks to change community norms. An effective aspect of this program is the use of Peer Educators who go out into the community to provide needle exchange and bleach kits, and educate active users about both the importance of safer drug use (e.g., clean needles) as well as safer sex practices. Peer Educators undergo training and are supervised by professional staff, and because they are current and/or former users themselves, they are trusted in the community.

Research

The National Cancer Institute's Surveillance Epidemiology and End Results (SEER) database does not collect information on either sexual or gender identity, which presents a significant barrier to understanding cancer in LGBT communities [14]. The recent inclusion of a sexual identity question in the National Health Interview Survey (NHIS) will be instrumental in assessing cancer risk factors for lesbian, gay, and bisexual people at the national level, but no national health survey asks gender identity questions, so the prevalence of risk factors for cancer for the transgender population will remain unknown. In fact, even most existing state-level health surveys (e.g., the Washington BRFSS and the CHIS) that assess sexual orientation do not include gender identity questions, with the exception of Massachusetts's BRFSS [122]. Including these questions in both state and national health surveys will be instrumental in identifying the incidence, prevalence, and geographic variations in cancer and behavioral cancer risks among LGBT populations.

Research is needed that further delineates pathways by which health outcomes can be influenced by risk factors resulting from sexual and gender minority status. Based on the Minority Stress Model [24] both discriminatory acts and internal minority stressors (i.e., expectations of rejection, concealment of minority identity, internalized stigma) can create stress resulting from one's sexual and/or gender identity minority status [23, 24, 123–125]. Based on the Health Equity model, the interplay of structural factors such as social exclusion and discrimination, in combination with the presence or absence of personal and social resources may also result in adverse health behaviors [37, 40], some of which have been linked to the etiology of cancer. Continued research is needed to test the efficacy of such models in identifying multi-level pathways of risk.

Research must also be responsive to the identification of new risk factors as they emerge, such as the recent recognition that lack of sleep may create cancer risk [126]. A study using a convenience sample has examined the relationship between sexual orientation and sleep; results suggest that lesbians and gay men have shorter sleep durations than their heterosexual peers [127]. One of the main diagnostic criteria for depressive and anxiety disorders is sleep disturbances [128], and population studies have documented higher rates of these disorders among lesbians, gay men, and bisexual women and men [129].

More research is clearly needed to investigate linkages between stress and cancer. Through epigenetics and the gene-environment interaction, researchers have recently identified that the ATF3 gene is activated by stress, which affects the functionality of immune-system cells and may foster metastasis of breast cancer to other organs and body-systems, and independently predicts consequent morbidity [25]. Another line of research has identified a possible link between adverse childhood experiences, such as abuse, and cancer, which is not accounted for by other factors, such as smoking [34]. To date most of the extant research on LGBT cancer is cross-sectional in nature. While these studies provide helpful insights, findings are limited in terms of understanding health trajectories and addressing risk reduction. Longitudinal studies and those which include biological markers may significantly contribute to our understanding of underlying pathways of cancer risk.

Practice

Programs and interventions must address the heterogeneity of LGBT populations. In fact, programs have rarely been developed to attend to the unique needs of bisexual and transgender people, yet research demonstrates that they are vulnerable and may have distinct unmet needs [23, 55, 87, 130]. It is also imperative that intersecting social positions and identities of LGBT people be considered in order to develop culturally responsive interventions. In developing behavioral interventions, trust and credibility of providers are important considerations [131]. It is also important to consider the inclusion of members of the targeted population in the early development of tailored interventions for LGBT communities. It has also been suggested that social and recreational activities may be important to supplement the specific focus on behavior change [132].

Because of a long history of discrimination and marginalization, many LGBT people are fearful of accessing healthcare, both in the larger community and *within* LGBT communities [87]. Many who have accessed care have either been denied care or received inferior care because of their perceived sexual orientation or gender identity [87]. As a result, significant numbers of LGBT people have not disclosed their sexual orientation or gender identity to their medical providers [87], which can have serious negative consequences for health [98]. When LGBT people do disclose, they are at heightened risk for discrimination; medical providers themselves acknowledge discrimination exists within medical settings [133, 134]. Delay in accessing healthcare can have serious consequences for cancer-related mortality, as early detection can make a significant difference in cancer treatment and outcomes [20].

Experiences of heterosexism and homophobia in health care settings, and barriers to health insurance and access, may contribute to the under-utilization of cancer screenings by lesbian and bisexual women [135–141]. The experience of discrimination in medical settings based on sexual orientation may be further complicated by racial discrimination. Gay and bisexual men are more likely to be tested for colorectal cancer than are heterosexual men, but with the exception of gay and bisexual men living alone, there is no difference in prostate-specific antigen (PSA) testing based on sexual orientation [142]. However, gay and bisexual African American men are less likely to be screened than either heterosexual African American men or gay and bisexual Non-Hispanic White men [142]. Furthermore, lack of recognition of the unique needs of transgender people in healthcare settings can result in compromised quality of care and under-utilization [143].

The experiences of LGBT patients in health care settings can be improved by training medical students and providers. This may result in more LGBT-friendly healthcare settings and opportunities for LGBT patients to safely disclose their sexual orientation and gender identity and confide in providers about health-related issues they would not discuss if they perceived a hostile or insensitive setting. Exposure to LGBT patients during clinical training has been shown to positively affect medical students' attitudes about LGBT patients, knowledge about LGBT healthcare concerns, and clinical interactions with LGBT patients [144].

Surveyed LGBT cancer patients suggest that healthcare workers providing cancer care be educated about the following issues pertaining to being LGBT and being diagnosed with cancer: the role that stigma plays in LGBT healthcare; the influence that the local healthcare environment has on the LGBT patient experience, and how highly variable environments can be; the degree to which disclosure about sexual orientation or gender identity is influenced by a patient's sense of perceived safety; the fact that respecting LGBT patients must also include respecting their support teams; the way that LGBT cancer patients are alienated by pervasive expectations of gender conformity; and the need of LGBT cancer survivors for culturally appropriate information and support [145].

There are unique challenges in addressing risk within LGBT communities, and risk reduction and prevention more generally. For example, some risk behaviors (e.g., alcohol and drug use) have been a normative aspect of LGBT culture and community in the past, which should be considered in treatment. LGBT individuals as "a group" may not be comfortable in drug abuse treatment programs in the general community, due to anti-LGBT attitudes and behaviors of providers, other group members, and agencies themselves. The "one size fits all" assumption implicit in grouping LGBT people under the same umbrella may also create significant challenges. Furthermore, lesbian and bisexual women and gay and bisexual men may be uncomfortable in drug abuse treatment groups that are not segregated by sex. Another challenge is heterosexism in mainstream behavioral risk reduction programs. For example, many physical fitness programs designed for adults are held in organizations which may be overtly or covertly hostile to LGBT people. Similarly, sports and other organized physical fitness activities may be anti-LGBT, even at younger ages [146].

Patients and providers need to be aware of cancer related resources available within the LGBT community. For example, the National LGBT Cancer Network (http://www.cancer-network.org/) provides access to online LGBT cancer support groups, cultural competence training modules, and a database for "LGBT-friendly cancer treatment facilities." The Lesbian Cancer Initiative (http://www.gaycenter.org/health/lci) of the Lesbian, Gay, Bisexual, and Transgender Community Center in New York provides in-person services (e.g., mammography, support groups).

Policy

Because sexual orientation and gender identity information is not included in the National Cancer Institute's SEER registry [14], policymakers do not have vital information necessary to make informed decisions regarding the allocation of resources to address cancer and behavioral cancer risks in LGBT communities. Similarly, the Institute of Medicine [14] strongly recommends including sexual orientation and gender identity in electronic health records as an important avenue for collecting patient-level data and information on LGBT populations.

Multi-level interventions are needed to confront structural and environmental factors that may be linked to cancer risk in LGBT communities. Although most interventions target individual behavior change, it is equally important to develop an upstream approach and target larger systems and environmental and structural change to promote better health outcomes. To this end, policy studies are needed to assess health changes resulting from shifting structural and environmental contexts. Changing community norms and behaviors, as potential intervention points, may be used to enhance social capital to promote behavior change. For example, identifying additional sponsors and funding sources that promote healthy products at community events can influence community norms by creating healthy options as well as reducing reliance on alcohol and tobacco-related companies as they market to LGBT people.

Unlike the general population, wherein biological and legal family members provide the majority of informal caregiving, including caring for loved ones with cancer, LGBT people tend to provide such care to and for each other [87]. Yet, because these relationships are generally not recognized as such, important instrumental support may be denied [147]. Less than 40% of LGBT adults have executed legal documents such as durable power of attorney for healthcare or living wills that allow someone else to make healthcare decisions on their behalf [148]. This will have profound implications for end of life care, in terms of both palliative and hospice care. Older lesbians and gay men living in states that do not recognize same-sex relationships are significantly more likely to be afraid of both dying alone and dying in pain than their counterparts residing in states that do recognize such relationships [149]. Policy change at local, state, and national levels are needed to recognize same-sex relationships and the role of friends and others in providing both instrumental and respite support for members of the LGBT community living with, or caring for someone with cancer.

Policies also impact LGBT cancer risks in other important ways. For example, alcohol and drug abuse programs and media tend to target younger LGBT people, despite evidence that LGBT older adults also drink excessively and use illicit drugs at disproportionately high rates. For example, while the Healthy People 2010 chapter on alcohol and drug abuse among LGBT populations opens with the statement, "substance abuse is pervasive and affects all populations, youth to elderly, in the United States" [150], the chapter is overwhelmingly targeting LGBT youth, including the recommendations. Programs that do promote risk reduction among older adults, such as physical activity, tend to target heterosexuals.

Even within LGBT communities, policies by and large fail to recognize cancer risk as a serious health issue. Agencies and programs that serve LGBT people are ideally situated to communicate cancer risks that LGBT people face. In addition to communicating this information, it is necessary to provide free or low-cost cancer screenings specific to uninsured or underinsured subpopulations at risk (e.g., breast and cervical cancer for lesbians and bisexual women and transgender men, prostate cancer for gay and bisexual men and transgender women). Policies supporting prevention and early detection are also needed, as both policymakers and individuals in high-risk groups may be unaware of their risk. The returns of such a public health approach are evident in the impact that free screenings for HIV have had in the United States. Overcoming barriers increases the likelihood of early detection and treatment of cancer. By making free or low-cost screenings more readily available, cultural and social norms to access such services may be positively influenced with long-term public health benefits. Mainstream agencies and programs should also engage in targeted outreach efforts, using communications (e.g., language and imagery) that are culturally sensitive to LGBT people and their families.

Conclusion

This chapter illustrates cancer-related behavioral risks in LGBT populations. Based on the Health Equity model, the risks identified result from behavioral factors as well as larger sociocultural forces. Excessive use of alcohol and other drugs, weight management, diet, and physical activity are all related to cancer risks and are critical determinants of morbidity and mortality in the general population. It is imperative to better understand the complex ways in which individual behaviors, community norms, and larger social contexts interact to create and maintain cancer risks in LGBT communities. It is imperative that tailored community-based prevention efforts and interventions be designed and tested to improve health and promote health equity in these communities.

References

1. U. S. Department of Health and Human Services. Healthy people 2020 objectives: lesbian, gay, bisexual, and transgender health. 2011. http://www.healthypeople.gov/2020/topicsobjectives2020/overview.aspx?topicid=25. Accessed 26. Oct. 2011.
2. Centers for Disease Control and Prevention. CDC health disparities and inequalities report United States, 2011. MMWR *2011*. 2011;60(Suppl):1–116.

3. Wallace SP, Cochran SD, Durazo EM, Ford CL. The health of aging lesbian, gay and bisexual adults in California. Los Angeles: UCLA Center for Health Policy Research; 2011 Contract No.: PB2011-2.
4. Fredriksen-Goldsen KI, Kim H-J, Barkan SE, Muraco A, Hoy-Ellis CP. Health disparities among lesbian, gay male and bisexual older adults: results from a population-based study. Am J Pub Health. 2013;103(10):1802–9.
5. Dilley JA, Simmons KW, Boysun MJ, Pizacani BA, Stark MJ. Demonstrating the importance and feasibility of including sexual orientation in public health surveys: health disparities in the Pacific Northwest. Am. J Pub Health. 2010;100(3):460–7.
6. Conron KJ, Mimiaga MJ, Landers SJ. A population-based study of sexual orientation identity and gender differences in adult health. Am J Pub Health. 2010;100(10):1953–60.
7. American Cancer Society. Cancer facts for gay and bisexual men. Atlanta: American Cancer Society; 2013. http://www.cancer.org/healthy/findcancerearly/menshealth/cancer-facts-for-gay-and-bisexual-men. Accessed 17. Dec. 2013.
8. National LGBT Cancer Network. The LGBT Community's Disproportionate Cancer Burden. New York: National LGBT Cancer Network; 2013. http://www.cancer-network.org/cancer_information/cancer_and_the_lgbt_community/the_lgbt_communitys_disproportionate_cancer_burden.php. Accessed 17. Dec. 2013.
9. Boehmer U, Miao X, Linkletter C, Clark MA. Adult health behaviors over the life course by sexual orientation. Am J Pub Health. 2012;102(2):292–300.
10. Brandenburg DL, Matthews AK, Johnson TP, Hughes TL. Breast cancer risk and screening: a comparison of lesbian and heterosexual women. Women Health. 2007;45(4):109–30.
11. Case P, Austin SB, Hunter DJ, Manson JE, Malspeis S, Willett WC, et al. Sexual orientation, health risk factors, and physical functioning in the Nurses' Health Study II. J Women's Health (Larchmt). 2004;13(9):1033–147.
12. Cochran SD, Mays VM. Risk of breast cancer mortality among women cohabiting with same sex partners: findings from the National Health Interview Survey, 1997–2003. J Women's Health. 2012;21(5):528–33.
13. Dibble SL, Roberts SA, Nussey B. Comparing breast cancer risk between lesbians and their heterosexual sisters. Women's Health Issues. 2004;14(2):60–8.
14. Institute of Medicine. The health of lesbian, gay, bisexual, and transgender people: building a foundation for better understanding. Washington, DC: The National Academies Press; 2011. p. 347.
15. Zaritsky E, Dibble SL. Risk factors for reproductive and breast cancers among older lesbians. J Women's Health (Larchmt). 2010;19(1):125–31.
16. U.S. Cancer Statistics Working Group. United States Cancer Statistics: 1999–2010 Incidence and Mortality Web-Based Report. Atlanta: U.S. Department of Health and Human Services, Centers for Disease Control and Prevention, National Cancer Institute; 2013. http://www.cdc.gov/uscs. Accessed 17. March 2014.
17. Sorensen G, Emmons K, Hunt MK, Barbeau E, Goldman R, Peterson K, et al. Model for incorporating social context in health behavior interventions: applications for cancer prevention for working-class, multiethnic populations. Preventive Med. 2003;37(3):188–97.
18. Wilkinson RG, Marmot MG. Social determinants of health: the solid facts. Copenhagen: World Health Organization, 2003.
19. Centers for Disease Control and Prevention. Behavioral risk factor surveillance system. 2012. http://www.cdc.gov/brfss/. Accessed 24. Feb. 2012.
20. Centers for Disease Control and Prevention. Other ways to reduce cancer risk. Atlanta: Centers for Disease Control and Prevention; 2013. http://www.cdc.gov/cancer/dcpc/prevention/other.htm. Accessed 17. Dec. 2013.
21. American Cancer Society. Body weight and cancer risk. Washington, DC: American Cancer Society; 2013. http://www.cancer.org/cancer/cancercauses/dietandphysicalactivity/bodyweightandcancerrisk/body-weight-and-cancer-risk-effects. Accessed 18. March 2014.
22. Fredriksen-Goldsen KI, Emlet CA, Kim H-J, Muraco A, Erosheva EA, Goldsen J, et al. The physical and mental health of lesbian, gay male, and bisexual (LGB) older adults: the role of key health indicators and risk and protective factors. Gerontologist. 2013;53(4):664–75.

23. Fredriksen-Goldsen KI, Cook-Daniels L, Kim H-J, Erosheva EA, Emlet CA, Hoy-Ellis CP, et al. Physical and mental health of transgender older adults: an at-risk and underserved population. Gerontologist. 2013;53(4):664–75.
24. Meyer IH. Prejudice, social stress, and mental health in lesbian, gay, and bisexual populations: conceptual issues and research evidence. Psychol Bull. 2003;129(5):674–97.
25. Wolford CC, McConoughey SJ, Jalgaonkar SP, Leon M, Merchant AS, Dominick JL, et al. Transcription factor ATF3 links host adaptive response to breast cancer metastasis. J Clin Invest. 2013;123(7):2893–906.
26. Dawson DA, Grant BF, Stinson FS, Chou PS, Huang B, Ruan WJ. Recovery from DSM-IV alcohol dependence: United States, 2001–2002. Addiction. 2005;100(3):281–92.
27. Balsam KF, Rothblum ED, Beauchaine TP. Victimization over the life span: a comparison of lesbian, gay, bisexual, and heterosexual siblings. J Consulting Clin Psychol. 2005;73(3):477–87.
28. Drabble L, Trocki KF, Hughes TL, Korcha RA, Lown AE. Sexual orientation differences in the relationship between victimization and hazardous drinking among women in the National Alcohol Survey. Psychol Addict Behav. 2013;27(3):639–48.
29. Hughes T, McCabe SE, Wilsnack SC, West BT, Boyd CJ. Victimization and substance use disorders in a national sample of heterosexual and sexual minority women and men. Addiction. 2010;105(12):2130–40.
30. Alvy LM, Hughes TL, Kristjanson AF, Wilsnack SC. Sexual identity group differences in child abuse and neglect. J Interpers Violence. 2013;28(10):2088–111.
31. Springer KW, Sheridan J, Kuo D, Carnes M. Long-term physical and mental health consequences of childhood physical abuse: results from a large population-based sample of men and women. Child Abuse Negl. 2007;31(5):517–30.
32. Springer KW, Sheridan J, Kuo D, Carnes M. The long-term health outcomes of childhood abuse: an overview and a call to action. J Gen Internal Med. 2003;18(10):864–70.
33. Bandini E, Fisher AD, Ricca V, Ristori J, Meriggiola MC, Jannini EA, et al. Childhood maltreatment in subjects with male-to-female gender identity disorder. Intern J Impot Res. 2011;23(6):276–85.
34. Kelly-Irving M, Mabile L, Grosclaude P, Lang T, Delpierre C. The embodiment of adverse childhood experiences and cancer development: potential biological mechanisms and pathways across the life course. Intern J Pub Health. 2013;58(1):3–11.
35. Murgatroyd C, Spengler D. Epigenetics of early child development. Front Psychiatry. 2011;2:16.
36. Juster R-P, McEwen BS, Lupien SJ. Allostatic load biomarkers of chronic stress and impact on health and cognition. Neurosci Biobehav Rev. 2010;35(1):2–16.
37. Fredriksen-Goldsen KI. Health, aging, and sexuality in marginalized communities: LGBT older adults emerging from the margins. Invitational keynote address presented at the 7th Annual Chicago Workshop on Biomarkers in Population-Based Health and Aging Research (CCBAR); Chicago, IL; 2013, October.
38. Centers for Disease Control and Prevention. Social determinants of health. Atlanta: Centers for Disease Control and Prevention; 2011. http://www.cdc.gov/socialdeterminants/Definitions.html. Accessed 17. Oct. 2012.
39. U. S. Department of Health and Human Services. Foundation health measures: disparities, healthy people 2020. Washington, DC: U.S. Department of Health and Human Services; 2010. http://www.healthypeople.gov/2020/about/disparitiesAbout.aspx. Accessed 26. Oct. 2011.
40. Fredriksen-Goldsen KI, Simoni JM, Walters KL, Kim H-J, Lehavot K, Yang J, et al. Reconceptualization of health disparities by sexual orientation and gender identity: *LGBTQ Health Equity Model*. Am J Orthopsychiatr. 2014;84(6):653–63.
41. Braveman P. What is health equity: and how does a life-course approach take us further toward it? Matern Child Health J. 2014;18(2):366–72.

42. National Cancer Institute. Alcohol and Cancer Risk. Washington, DC: National Cancer Institute; 2013. http://www.cancer.gov/cancertopics/factsheet/Risk/alcohol. Accessed 17. March 2014.
43. McCabe SE, Hughes TL, Bostwick WB, West BT, Boyd CJ. Sexual orientation, substance use behaviors and substance dependence in the United States. Addiction. 2009;104(8):1333–45.
44. Drabble L, Midanik LT, Trocki K. Reports of alcohol consumption and alcohol-related problems among homosexual, bisexual and heterosexual respondents: results from the 2000 National Alcohol Survey. J Stud Alcohol. 2005;66(1):111–20.
45. Deputy NP, Boehmer U. Determinants of body weight among men of different sexual orientation. Prev Med. 2010;51(2):129–31.
46. VanKim NA, Padilla JL. New Mexico's progress in collecting lesbian, gay, bisexual, and transgender health data and its implications for addressing health disparities. Albuquerque: New Mexico Department of Health; 2010.
47. Garofalo R, Wolf RC, Kessel S, Palfrey SJ, DuRant RH. The association between health risk behaviors and sexual orientation among a school-based sample of adolescents. Pediatrics. 1998;101(5):895–902.
48. Substance Abuse and Mental Health Services Administration. Top health issues for LGBT populations information and resource kit. Rockville: Substance Abuse and Mental Health Services Administration, 2012. Contract No.: HHS Publication No. (SMA) 12-4684.
49. Gruskin EP, Hart S, Gordon N, Ackerson L. Patterns of cigarette smoking and alcohol use among lesbians and bisexual women enrolled in a large health maintenance organization. Am J Pub Health. 2001;91(6):976–9.
50. Hawkins JD, Catalano RF, Miller JY. Risk and protective factors for alcohol and other drug problems in adolescence and early adulthood: implications for substance abuse prevention. Psychol Bull. 1992;112(1):64–105.
51. Keyes KM, Hatzenbuehler ML, Hasin DS. Stressful life experiences, alcohol consumption, and alcohol use disorders: the epidemiologic evidence for four main types of stressors. Psychopharmacology. 2011;218(1):1–17.
52. Bradford J, Reisner SL, Honnold JA, Xavier J. Experiences of transgender-related discrimination and implications for health: results from the Virginia Transgender Health Initiative Study. Am J Pub Health. 2012;103(10):1820–29.
53. Amadio DM. Internalized heterosexism, alcohol use, and alcohol-related problems among lesbians and gay men. Addict Behav. 2006;31(7):1153–62.
54. Rosario M, Schrimshaw EW, Hunter J. Disclosure of sexual orientation and subsequent substance use and abuse among lesbian, gay, and bisexual youths: critical role of disclosure reactions. Psychol Addict Behav. 2009;23(1):175–84.
55. Grant JM, Mottet LA, Tanis J, Harrison J, Herman JL, Keisling M. Injustice at every turn: a report of the National Transgender Discrimination Survey. Washington, DC: National Center for Transgender Equality and National Gay and Lesbian Task Force; 2011.
56. Cochran SD, Keenan C, Schober C, Mays VM. Estimates of alcohol use and clinical treatment needs among homosexually active men and women in the US population. J Consulting Clin Psychol. 2000;68(6):1062–71.
57. Eliason MJ. Environmental strategies to address LGBT alcohol, tobacco, and drug use. San Francisco: LGBT-TRISTAR; 2010.
58. Cole C, Jones L, McVeigh J, Kicman A, Syed Q, Bellis MA. Cut: a guide to adulterants, bulking agents and other contaminants found in illicit drugs. Liverpool: Centre for Public Health; 2010.
59. Hashibe M, Straif K, Tashkin DP, Morgenstern H, Greenland S, Zhang ZF. Epidemiologic review of marijuana use and cancer risk. Alcohol. 2005;35(3):265–75.
60. National Cancer Institute. Laboratory/animal/preclinical studies. Bethesda: National Cancer Institute; 2013. http://www.cancer.gov/cancertopics/pdq/cam/cannabis/healthprofessional/page4. Accessed 26. March 2014.

61. Hunt J. Why the gay and transgender population experiences higher rates of substance use: many use to cope with discrimination and prejudice. Washington, DC: Center for American Progress; 2012.
62. Cochran BN, Cauce AM. Characteristics of lesbian, gay, bisexual, and transgender individuals entering substance abuse treatment. J Subst Abuse Treat. 2006;30(2):135–46.
63. Ashbee O, Goldberg JM. Trans people and cancer. Vancouver: Transgender Health Program; 2006.
64. Hatzenbuehler ML, Nolen-Hoeksema S, Erickson SJ. Minority stress predictors of HIV risk behavior, substance use, and depressive symptoms: results from a prospective study of bereaved gay men. Health Psychol. 2008;27(4):455–62.
65. Mereish EH, O'Cleirigh C, Bradford JB. Interrelationships between LGBT-based victimization, suicide, and substance use problems in a diverse sample of sexual and gender minorities. Psychol Health Med. 2014;19(1):1–13.
66. Ryan C, Huebner D, Diaz RM, Sanchez J. Family rejection as a predictor of negative health outcomes in white and Latino lesbian, gay, and bisexual young adults. Pediatrics. 2009;123(1):346–52.
67. Centers for Disease Control and Prevention. Obesity: halting the epidemic by making health easier, at a glance 2011. Atlanta: Centers for Disease Control and Prevention; 2011. http://www.cdc.gov/chronicdisease/resources/publications/aag/obesity.htm. Accessed 7. Dec. 2011.
68. Valanis BG, Bowen DJ, Bassford T, Whitlock E, Charney P, Carter RA. Sexual orientation and health: comparisons in the women's health initiative sample. Arch Fam Med. 2000;9(9):843–53.
69. Boehmer U, Bowen DJ, Bauer GR. Overweight and obesity in sexual-minority women: evidence from population-based data. Am J Pub Health. 2007;97(6):1134–40.
70. Roberts SA, Dibble SL, Nussey B, Casey K. Cardiovascular disease risk in lesbian women. Womens Health Issues. 2003;13(4):167–74.
71. Yancey AK, Cochran SD, Corliss HL, Mays VM. Correlates of overweight and obesity among lesbian and bisexual women. Prev Med. 2003;36(6):676–83.
72. Center of Excellence for Transgender Health. General Prevention and Screening San Francisco, CA: University of California Center of Excellence for Transgender Health; 2014. http://transhealth.ucsf.edu/trans?page=protocol-screening#S4X. Accessed 3. April 2014.
73. Christakis NA, Fowler JH. The spread of obesity in a large social network over 32 years. N Engl J Med. 2007;357(4):370–9.
74. Fogel S, Young L, Dietrich M, Blakemore D. Weight loss and related behavior changes among lesbians. J Homosex. 2012;59(5):689–702.
75. National Cancer Institute. Risk factors. Washington, DC: National Institutes of Health; 2006. http://www.cancer.gov/cancertopics/wyntk/cancer/page3. Accessed 17. Dec. 2013.
76. American Society of Clinical Oncology. The role of major nutrients in cancer prevention. Alexandria: American Society of Clinical Oncology; 2012. http://www.cancer.net/navigating-cancer-care/prevention-and-healthy-living/diet-and-nutrition/role-major-nutrients-cancer-prevention. Accessed 25. March 2014.
77. Veugelers PJ, Fitzgerald AL, Johnston E. Dietary intake and risk factors for poor diet quality among children in Nova Scotia. Can J Pub Health. 2005;96(3):212–6.
78. Gates GJ. Food insecurity and SNAP participation (Food Stamps) in LGBT communities. Los Angeles: Williams Institute, UCLA School of Law; 2014.
79. Bowen DJ, Balsam KF, Diergaarde B, Russo M, Escamilla GM. Healthy eating, exercise, and weight: impressions of sexual minority women. Women Health. 2006;44(1):79–93.
80. Brown SG, Morrison LA, Calibuso MJ, Christiansen TM. The menstrual cycle and sexual behavior: relationship to eating, exercise, sleep, and health patterns. Women Health. 2008;48(4):429–44.
81. Boehmer U, Bowen DJ. Examining factors linked to overweight and obesity in women of different sexual orientations. Prev Med. 2009;48(4):357–61.

82. American Society of Clinical Oncology. Physical activity and cancer risk. Alexandria: American Society of Clinical Oncology; 2013. http://www.cancer.net/navigating-cancer-care/prevention-and-healthy-living/physical-activity/physical-activity-and-cancer-risk. Accessed 18. March 2014.
83. Centers for Disease Control and Prevention. Physical inactivity and people with disabilities: a tip sheet for public health professionals. Atlanta: Centers for Disease Control and Prevention; 2010. http://www.cdc.gov/ncbddd/documents/physical-inactivity-tip-sheet-_phpa_1.pdf. Accessed 26. March 2014.
84. Artaud F, Dugravot A, Sabia S, Singh-Manoux A, Tzourio C, Elbaz A. Unhealthy behaviours and disability in older adults: three-City Dijon cohort study. Br Med J. 2013;347:f4240.
85. Aaron DJ, Markovic N, Danielson ME, Honnold JA, Janosky JE, Schmidt NJ. Behavioral risk factors for disease and preventive health practices among lesbians. Am J Pub Health. 2001;91(6):972–5.
86. Reisner SL, Gamarel KE, Dunham E, Hopwood R, Hwahng S. Female-to-male transmasculine adult health: a mixed-methods community-based needs assessment. J Am Psychiatr Nurses Assoc. 2013;19(5):293–303.
87. Fredriksen-Goldsen KI, Kim H-J, Emlet CA, Muraco A, Erosheva EA, Hoy-Ellis CP, et al. The aging and health report: disparities and resilience among lesbian, gay, bisexual, and transgender older adults. Seattle: Institute for Multigenerational Health; 2011.
88. Brown MT, Grossman BR. Same-sex sexual relationships in the national social life, health and aging project: making a case for data collection. J Gerontol Soc Work. 2014; 57(2–4):108–29.
89. Rosario M, Corliss HL, Everett BG, Reisner SL, Austin SB, Buchting FO, et al. Sexual orientation disparities in cancer-related risk behaviors of tobacco, alcohol, sexual behaviors, and diet and physical activity: pooled youth risk behavior surveys. Am J Public Health. 2014;104(2):245–54.
90. Hatzenbuehler ML, Phelan JC, Link BG. Stigma as a fundamental cause of population health inequalities. Am J Public Health. 2013;103(5):813–21.
91. Williams DR, Costa MV, Odunlami AO, Mohammed SA. Moving upstream: how interventions that address the social determinants of health can improve health and reduce disparities. J Public Health Manage. 2008;14(Suppl):S8–17.
92. Elliott S. Absolut celebrates its 30 years of marketing to gay consumers. New York Times [Internet]; (Business Day Media & Advertising). 2011. http://www.nytimes.com/2011/10/27/business/media/absolut-heralds-its-marketing-to-gay-consumers.html?_r=0.
93. McCabe SE, Bostwick WB, Hughes TL, West BT, Boyd CJ. The relationship between discrimination and substance use disorders among lesbian, gay, and bisexual adults in the United States. Am J Public Health. 2010;100(10):1946–52.
94. Human Rights Campaign. Employment Non-Discrimination Act. Human Rights Campaign, Washington DC. 2014. http://www.hrc.org/laws-and-legislation/federal-legislation/employment-non-discrimination-act. Accessed 19. May 2014.
95. Hatzenbuehler ML, Bellatorre A, Lee Y, Finch BK, Muennig P, Fiscella K. Structural stigma and all-cause mortality in sexual minority populations. Soc Sci Med. 2014;103:33–41.
96. Rostosky SS, Riggle EDB, Horne SG, Miller AD. Marriage amendments and psychological distress in lesbian, gay, and bisexual (LGB) adults. J Couns Psychol. 2009;56(1):56–66.
97. Eliason MJ, Dibble S, Dejoseph J. Nursing's silence on lesbian, gay, bisexual, and transgender issues: the need for emancipatory efforts. ANS Adv Nurs Sci. 2010;33(3):206–18.
98. American Medical Association. AMA policies on GLBT issues: H-65.973 health care disparities in same-sex partner households. American Medical Association, Washington, DC. 2013. http://www.ama-assn.org//ama/pub/about-ama/our-people/member-groups-sections/glbt-advisory-committee/ama-policy-regarding-sexual-orientation.page. Accessed 1. Nov. 2013.
99. Fisher JD, Cornman DH, Osborn CY, Amico KR, Fisher WA, Friedland GA. Clinician-initiated HIV risk reduction intervention for HIV-positive persons: formative research, acceptability, and fidelity of the options project. J Acquir Immune Defic Syndr. 2004;37(Suppl 2):S78–87.

100. Fisher JD, Fisher WA, Cornman DH, Amico RK, Bryan A, Friedland GH. Clinician-delivered intervention during routine clinical care reduces unprotected sexual behavior among HIV-infected patients. J Acquir Immune Defic Syndr. 2006;41(1):44–52.
101. National Cancer Institute. HPV and cancer. National Institutes of Health, Rockville. 2012. http://www.cancer.gov/cancertopics/factsheet/Risk/HPV. Accessed 11. July 2014.
102. Epstein S. Sexualizing governance and medicalizing identities: the emergence of 'state-centered' LGBT health politics in the United States. Sexualities. 2003;6(2):131–71.
103. Rofes E. Dry bones breathe: gay men creating post-AIDS identities and cultures. Harrington Park Press: New York; 1998.
104. Knauer NJ. Navigating a post-Windsor world: the promise and limits of marriage equality. Georget J Gend Law. 2014.
105. Freedom to Marry. Marriage Litigation. Freedom to Marry, New York. 2014. http://www.freedomtomarry.org/litigation. Accessed 14. July 2014.
106. Herek GM. Legal recognition of same-sex relationships in the United States: a social science perspective. Am Psychol. 2006;61(6):607–21.
107. Wight RG, LeBlanc AJ, de Vries B, Detels R. Stress and mental health among midlife and older gay-identified men. Am J Public Health. 2012;102(3):503–10.
108. Wood RG, Goesling B, Avellar S, Mathematica Research. The effects of marriage on health: a synthesis of recent research evidence. U.S. Department of Health and Human Services & Office of the Assistant Secretary for Planning and Evaluation, Washington, DC; 2007.
109. Hatzenbuehler ML, Pachankis JE, Wolff J. Religious climate and health risk behaviors in sexual minority youths: a population-based study. Am J Public Health. 2012;102(4):657–63.
110. Ramirez-Valles J, Kuhns LM, Campbell RT, Diaz RM. Social integration and health: community involvement, stigmatized identities, and sexual risk in Latino sexual minorities. J Health Soc Behav. 2010;51(1):30–47.
111. LIVESTRONG Foundation. Families of choice: sources of support for LGBT cancer survivors. LIVESTRONG Foundation, Austin. 2013. http://blog.livestrong.org/2013/03/25/families-of-choice-sources-of-support-for-lgbt-cancer-survivors/. Accessed 2. April 2014.
112. Ryan C, Russell ST, Huebner D, Diaz R, Sanchez J. Family acceptance in adolescence and the health of LGBT young adults. J Child Adolesc Psychiatr Nurs. 2010;23(4):205–13.
113. Kaminski PL, Chapman BP, Haynes SD, Own L. Body image, eating behaviors, and attitudes toward exercise among gay and straight men. Eat Behav. 2005;6(3):179–87.
114. Cochran SD, Sullivan JG, Mays VM. Prevalence of mental disorders, psychological distress, and mental health services use among lesbian, gay, and bisexual adults in the United States. J Clin Consult Psychol. 2003;71(1):53–61.
115. Cochran BN, Peavy KM, Robohm JS. Do specialized services exist for LGBT individuals seeking treatment for substance misuse? A study of available treatment programs. Subst Use Misuse. 2007;42(1):161–76.
116. Nemoto T, Operario D, Keatley J, Nguyen H, Sugano E. Promoting health for transgender women: Transgender Resources and Neighborhood Space (TRANS) program in San Francisco. Am J Public Health. 2005;95(3):382–4.
117. Nuttbrock L, Bockting W, Rosenblum A, Hwahng S, Mason M, Macri M, et al. Gender abuse, depressive symptoms, and HIV and other sexually transmitted infections among male-to-female transgender persons: a three-year prospective study. Am J Public Health. 2013;103(2):300–7.
118. Konishi C, Saewyc E, Homma Y, Poon C. Population-level evaluation of school-based interventions to prevent problem substance use among gay, lesbian and bisexual adolescents in Canada. Prev Med. 2013;57(6):929–33.
119. van Wormer K, McKinney R. What schools can do to help gay/lesbian/bisexual youth: a harm reduction approach. Adolescence. 2003;38(151):409–20.
120. Denning P. Practicing harm reduction psychotherapy: an alternative approach to addictions. vol xxv. Guilford Press: New York; 2000. p 262.

121. Denning P, Little J, Glickman A. Over the influence: the harm reduction guide for managing drugs and alcohol. vol xix. Guilford Press: New York; 2004. p 328.
122. Massachusetts Department of Public Health. The health of lesbian, gay, bisexual, and transgender (LGBT) persons with their heterosexual and non-transgender counterparts. Massachusetts: Massachusetts Department of Public Health; 2009.
123. Hendricks ML, Testa RJ. A conceptual framework for clinical work with transgender and gender noncomforming clients: an adaptation of the minority stress model. Prof Psychol: Res Pract. 2012;43(5):460–7.
124. Bockting WO, Miner MH, Swinburne Romine RE, Hamilton A, Coleman E. Stigma, mental health, and resilience in an online sample of the U.S. transgender population. Am J Public Health. 2013;103(5):943–51.
125. Szymanski DM, Sung MR. Minority stress and psychological distress among Asian American sexual minority persons. Couns Psychol. 2010;38(6):848–72.
126. Davis S, Mirick DK. Circadian disruption, shift work and the risk of cancer: a summary of the evidence and studies in Seattle. Cancer Causes Control. 2006;17(4):539–45.
127. Rahman Q, Silber K. Sexual orientation and the sleep-wake cycle: a preliminary investigation. Arch Sex Behav. 2000;29(2):127–34.
128. American Psychiatric Association, DSM-5 Task Force. Diagnostic and statistical manual of mental disorders: DSM-5. 5th ed. Arlington: American Psychiatric Association; 2013.
129. King M, Semlyen J, Tai SS, Killaspy H, Osborn D, Popelyuk D, et al. A systematic review of mental disorder, suicide, and deliberate self harm in lesbian, gay and bisexual people. BMC Psychiatry. 2008;8:70.
130. Sephton S, Spiegel D. Circadian disruption in cancer: a neuroendocrine-immune pathway from stress to disease? Brain Behav Immun. 2003;17(5):321–8.
131. Schwappach DL. Smoking behavior, to quit, and preferences toward cessation programs among gay men in Zurich, Switzerland. Nicotine Tob Res. 2008;10(12):1783–7.
132. Remafedi G, Carol H. Preventing tobacco use among lesbian, gay, bisexual, and transgender youths. Nicotine Tob Res. 2005;7(2):249–56.
133. Eliason MJ, Dibble SL, Robertson PA. Lesbian, gay, bisexual, and transgender (LGBT) physicians' experiences in the workplace. J Homosex. 2011;58(10):1355–71.
134. Eliason MJ, Dejoseph J, Dibble S, Deevey S, Chinn P. Lesbian, gay, bisexual, transgender, and queer/questioning nurses' experiences in the workplace. J Prof Nurs. 2011;27(4):237–44.
135. Buchmueller T, Carpenter CS. Disparities in health insurance coverage, access, and outcomes for individuals in same-sex versus different-sex relationships, 2000–2007. Am J Public Health. 2010;100(3):489–95.
136. Cochran SD, Mays VM, Bowen D, Gage S, Bybee D, Roberts SJ, et al. Cancer-related risk indicators and preventive screening behaviors among lesbians and bisexual women. Am J Public Health. 2001;91(4):591–7.
137. Harcourt J. Current issues in lesbian, gay, bisexual, and transgender (LGBT) health. J Homosex. 2006;51(1):1–11.
138. Kerker BD, Mostashari F, Thorpe L. Health care access and utilization among women who have sex with women: sexual behavior and identity. J Urban Health. 2006;83(5):970–9.
139. Roberts SJ, Patsdaughter CA, Grindel CG, Tarmina MS. Health related behaviors and cancer screening of lesbians: results of the Boston Lesbian Health Project II. Women Health. 2004;39(4):41–55.
140. Tracy JK, Lydecker AD, Ireland L. Barriers to cervical cancer screening among lesbians. J Women's Health (Larchmt). 2010;19(2):229–37.
141. Charlton BM, Corliss HL, Missmer SA, Frazier AL, Rosario M, Kahn JA, et al. Reproductive health screening disparities and sexual orientation in a cohort study of U.S. adolescent and young adult females. J Adolesc Health. 2011;49(5):505–10.
142. Heslin KC, Gore JL, King WD, Fox SA. Sexual orientation and testing for prostate and colorectal cancers among men in California. Med Care. 2008;46(12):1240–8.

143. Bauer GR, Hammond R, Travers R, Kaay M, Hohenadel KM, Boyce M. "I don't think this is theoretical; this is our lives": how erasure impacts health care for transgender people. J Assoc Nurs AIDS Care. 2009;20(5):348–61.
144. Sanchez NF, Rabatin J, Sanchez JP, Hubbard S, Kalet A. Medical students' ability to care for lesbian, gay, bisexual, and transgendered patients. Fam Med. 2006;38(1):21–7.
145. Margolies L, Scout N. LGBT patient-centered outcomes: cancer survivors teach us how to care for all. Washington, DC: National LGBT Cancer Network, Network for LGBT Health Equity; 2013.
146. Gill DL, Morrow RG, Collins KE, Lucey AB, Schultz AM. Perceived climate in physical activity settings. J Homosex. 2010;57(7):895–913.
147. Cahill S, South K, Spade J. Outing age: public policy issues affecting gay, lesbian, bisexual and transgender elders. Washington, DC: National Gay and Lesbian Task Force; 2000.
148. Metlife Mature Market Institute, American Society on Aging. Still out, still aging: the metlife study of lesbian, gay, bisexual, and transgender baby boomers. New York: Metlife Mature Market Institute and American Society on Aging; 2010.
149. de Vries B, Mason AM, Quam J, Aquaviva K. State recognition of same-sex relationships and preparations for end of life among lesbian and gay boomers. Sex Res Soc Policy. 2009;6(1):90–101.
150. U.S. Department of Health and Human Services. Healthy People 2010: lesbian, gay, bisexual, and transgender health: substance abuse. Washington, DC: U.S. Department of Health and Human Services; 2000.

Chapter 5
Smoking in the LGBT Community

Jack E. Burkhalter

Abstract Tobacco use is the single most preventable cause of cancer. Smoking prevalence among lesbian, gay, bisexual, and transgender (LGBT) persons is significantly higher than in the general U.S. population. This health disparity likely originates during sexual minority adolescence, when smoking initiation occurs earlier and maintains at higher rates than for their heterosexual peers. Among youth, identifying as bisexual and being female, and experiencing more victimization increase risk for smoking. For LGBT adults, alcohol, substance use, and depression are often associated with smoking. One hypothesis proposes that disparate LGBT tobacco use is driven by sexual minority stress resulting from externally imposed and internally incorporated stigma and victimization. If true, does engagement in a validating LGBT community protect against the risk of smoking? Research findings suggest a more complex question, depending upon age of the person, number and type of LGBT organizations, and perhaps whether they have active tobacco control programs. Definitive answers await further research. LGBT tobacco control advocates have developed community-based smoking cessation programs, such as The Last Drag, tailored to LGBT persons, held in LGBT-serving venues, and assuring a supportive context for smoking cessation. Evaluations of community-based programs are encouraging. A marked paucity of LGBT-tailored or targeted randomized controlled cessation trials exist, and some studies not tailored or limited to LGBT smokers show cessation rates equivalent for LGBT and heterosexual persons. Multi-site studies encompassing different regions of the country beyond the two coasts could address the likely complex efficacy issues of tailored vs. non-tailored smoking cessation interventions for LGBT smokers.

Tobacco use is the single most preventable cause of disease, disability, and death in the United States [14] and the single most preventable cause of cancer [73]. The 2014 U.S. Surgeon General's Report increased the number of cancers caused by smoking to include liver and colorectal cancers, bringing the total to nearly 20 different cancers linked to tobacco use[65]. In 2012, 18.1% of the general U.S. population smoked cigarettes, the prevalent form of tobacco use [16]. Given the

J. E. Burkhalter (✉)
Memorial Sloan Kettering Cancer Center, New York, NY, USA
e-mail: burkhalj@mskcc.org

U. Boehmer, R. Elk (eds.), *Cancer and the LGBT Community*,
DOI 10.1007/978-3-319-15057-4_5

toll of smoking on the nation's health, disparities in the burden of smoking in subpopulations are of particular concern. Evidence began to emerge in the 1990's that smoking was significantly more prevalent in the LGBT community than in the general U.S. population. Over the last two decades LGBT individuals and tobacco prevention and control advocates and experts have organized and responded from the grassroots, research, treatment and policy spheres to address the community's tobacco use problem. This chapter provides an overview of the history of the tobacco control movement in the LGBT community, empirical support for smoking disparities, factors related to LGBT tobacco use, theoretical frameworks for understanding disparities, cessation interventions targeting the community, and a discussion of opportunities and challenges that lie ahead.

History

In the U.S. during the late 1980's, smoking bans on domestic airlines, accumulating evidence of the harms of involuntary smoke exposure [72] and a growing list of cities and states enacting indoor and outdoor smoking restrictions provided momentum for critical public health events in the next decade. The decade of the 1990's saw increasing convergence of legal actions and policy advances at the federal, state, and community levels to propel forward tobacco prevention and control activities within and outside the LGBT community. Among these were the 1992 U.S. Environmental Protection Agency's report on the adverse effects of secondhand smoke [75], the FDA's 1995 attempt to regulate tobacco products, California becoming the first state to pass a comprehensive, statewide smoke-free air law (1998), and the landmark Master Settlement Agreement in 1998 between the attorneys general of 46 states and the tobacco industry to reimburse state governments for tobacco-related health costs and to fund tobacco prevention and control programs [49]. In 1991, the Coalition of Lavender-Americans on Smoking and Health (CLASH) was formed in San Francisco and provided "The Last Drag," the first known community-based cessation program targeted to LGBT smokers and using evidence-based strategies [25, 69]. This multi-session group program has been disseminated through training to other states and cities and remains active to this day.

During the same period, published research was emerging that showed elevated prevalence of smoking among lesbian and bisexual women [6, 23]and gay and bisexual men [67], when compared to the general population or their heterosexual counterparts, further raising awareness of the tobacco problem in community and academic settings. In parallel with the larger public discourse about the impact of cigarette marketing on smoking among U.S. youth and other subpopulations, policy experts, researchers and the LGBT community became more conscious and critical of LGBT-targeted cigarette marketing [28, 77], further bolstering tobacco control efforts. The release of tobacco industry internal documents as part of the Master Settlement revealed that over a period from 1995 to 1997, R.J. Reynolds intended to increase its Camel brand's share of the market in San Francisco via subculture urban marketing that included gay people in the Castro district, called "Project SCUM," [71]. The disrespect embedded in the project name and the targeting of the LGBT community fueled critical response, counter-advertising [77], and provided a potent weapon for anti-tobacco organizations, e.g., Legacy's "truth" campaign [1] and advocates in the LGBT community.

Tobacco control became entangled in the activities of the AIDS Coalition to Unleash Power (ACTUP) [22], which sought ways to counter the work of then senator Jesse Helms of North Carolina, an ardent foe of AIDS and LGBT activists [54]. Philip Morris, the cigarette manufacturer and owner of Miller Brewing, provided financial support to Helms. ACT-UP led a national boycott of the company's tobacco products and then expanded this to Miller beer. The two parties settled the boycott in 1991, with Philip Morris agreeing to provide financial support for AIDS organizations but continuing support for Helms. Soon after, Philip Morris placed its first advertisement in a gay magazine [55]. Ironically, this agreement provided a doorway to sometimes closer relations between the tobacco industry and cash-starved LGBT organizations, which gained a benefactor [54]. As Offen et al. [53] documented in interviews with leaders of 76 LGBT organizations across the U.S. from 2002 to 2004, that arrangement fostered normalization of tobacco use. They found that 22 % of these leaders had accepted tobacco industry money, and only 24 % of those interviewed said smoking was a priority concern. This period also saw the advent of "gay vague" advertisements in LGBT publications, in which a 3rd person was introduced into a smoking scene, creating ambiguity about whether the attraction was between two of the same sex, different sex, or both, enabling LGBT viewers to perceive the former while providing cover for the advertiser to deny such an interpretation [50]. Providing visibility, no matter how ambiguous, could be seen as progress for the LGBT community fighting for acknowledgement of its existence and rights at that time, while opening up an untapped market for tobacco products.

Early voices in the tobacco control and LGBT community, such as CLASH, [28, 54, 77] warned of the impact of the tobacco industry targeting the community. In 2002, the American Legacy Foundation (now called Legacy) awarded grants to diverse LGBT organizations to prevent and reduce tobacco use [2]. Under the leadership of Scout at the Fenway Institute, the National LGBT Tobacco Control Network was founded with support from the Centers for Disease Control (CDC) and became a locus for organizing and promoting LGBT tobacco control efforts in communities across the nation, including sponsorship of the national LGBT tobacco summits [70]. In 2004, the Network issued The National LGBT Communities Tobacco Action Plan: *Research, Prevention, and Cessation,* which has served as a blueprint for initiating and maintaining tobacco prevention and control programs and activities in the LGBT community. Many LGBT community-based organizations offer tobacco cessation programs that provide a welcoming environment and tailored support for smokers to pursue abstinence, as well as fostering new generations of tobacco control activists, researchers, and policy experts. Next, the scope of the smoking and tobacco use problem for the LGBT community is presented.

Prevalence of Smoking in LGBT Community

The gold standard for collecting prevalence data on a disease risk factor such as smoking is to use *population-based sampling methods* that assure that the sample of individuals drawn from the general population represent important characteristics of the general population, meaning here the U.S. population. Population-based samples can be contrasted with "convenience samples" whereby data are collected from a group of individuals who can be more easily accessed but who may not represent the characteristics of the larger population to which they belong [47]. Presented below are definitions of statistical terminology [51], as diverse statistical terms are used by different researchers in presenting smoking data. *Median* is the middle value of a sequence of ordered data, the value where 50 % of data are below and 50 % of data are above that value. A *prevalence rate* is the total number of cases, for example, of current cigarette smoking, existing in a population divided by the total population number, including both smokers and nonsmokers. Prevalence is influenced by initiation of smoking and rates of cessation. An *odds ratio* (OR) is a measure of association between a risk factor (e.g., being LGBT) and an outcome (e.g., smoking). The OR represents the odds that an outcome (e.g., smoking) will occur given a particular risk factor (e.g., being LGBT), compared to the odds of the outcome occurring in the absence of that risk factor (being heterosexual) [68]. An odds ratio is reported along with its *95 % confidence interval (95 % CI)*, which is used to estimate the precision of the OR. It is common practice to interpret the OR association as being statistically significant if the 95 % CI range of values does not include the "null value" of 1, which would indicate, for example, that being LGBT was associated with a 50/50 odds of being a smoker, or OR = 1. A larger CI denotes a lower level of precision of the OR, while a smaller CI indicates a higher precision of the OR.

The methods by which sexual orientation and gender identity are assessed often vary across studies, and the definitions of "current smoking" may also vary, making cross-study comparisons difficult. When only subgroups of the LGBT community are studied, this will be indicated by using subgroup acronyms. Fortunately, in recent years the more widespread incorporation of standard assessment items for sexual and gender identities and tobacco use have aided interpretation of new findings in relation to prior data. To aid in interpretation, this chapter places more weight on studies using population-based sampling methods, standard measures of tobacco use, and commonly used measures of sexual orientation and gender identity than it does other studies. Next, prevalence data for youth and then adults are presented.

Youth For the purposes of this chapter, studies that included those younger than age 18 years (but could include young adults) or students at high school level or lower are cited. The disparities in smoking prevalence observed in the adult LGBT population likely originate during adolescence and emerging adulthood. Early on, Garofalo et al. [27] observed higher rates of smoking among Massachusetts youth in grades 9–12, who identified as gay, lesbian, or bisexual in the state's Youth Risk Behavior Surveillance Survey (YRBSS) [13], a CDC-designed, state-based survey of health risk behaviors of youth in the U.S. They found that 59.3 % of LGB youth were current smokers compared to 35.2 % of the non-LGB youth. This tobacco use disparity in Massachusetts was confirmed subsequently by YRBSS findings in Colorado [10].

In 2011, researchers at the CDC reported prevalence of LGB risk behaviors assessed through YRBSS surveys conducted in seven states and six large urban school districts [15], a marked expansion of efforts to understand LGBT youth health disparities. Population-based sampling was used and data were collected on both sexual identity and sexual contacts, i.e., same sex only, opposite sex only, or both sexes. Among the many health behaviors assessed, 12 measures of tobacco use or attempts to quit were reported, as adolescent and young adults often experiment with tobacco and may not have stable patterns of smoking typical for most adult smokers [11]. Median current cigarette use (smoked on at least 1 day in the 30 days before the survey) was as follows: lesbian and gay, 30.5 %; bisexuals, 30.8 %; heterosexuals, 13.6 %, and; unsure, 18.2 %. Current frequent cigarette use, in which cigarettes are smoked 20 or more days during the prior 30 days before the survey, was, for lesbian and gay, 15.5 %; bisexuals, 16.7 %; heterosexuals, 5.1 %, and; unsure, 7.3 %. Similar patterns of elevated prevalence for LGB youth were observed for having ever smoked a cigarette, having smoked a cigarette before age 13 years, having smoked > 10 cigarettes per day (CPD) on days when they smoked in the prior 30 days, and smokeless tobacco and cigar use. Any current tobacco use (current cigarette use, smokeless tobacco use, or cigar use) figures were for lesbian and gay, 35.4 %; bisexuals, 39.6 %; heterosexuals, 18.9 %, and; unsure, 20.5 %. Prevalence data for bisexuals were not markedly different than for gay and lesbian youth. Analyses using sexual contacts (behavior rather than sexual identity) yielded somewhat different results, but they confirmed the overall pattern of tobacco use disparities. Finally, youth were asked if they had tried to quit smoking during the 12 months before the survey, and for lesbian and gay, 52.3 % had tried; bisexuals, 55.5 %; heterosexuals, 54.4 %, and; for those unsure, 66.2 % reported trying to quit. Thus, there is some promising news in that LGB youth appear to be trying to quit at rates similar to those seen with heterosexual youth, despite the more prevalent tobacco use.

More recently, Corliss et al. [20] also used YRBS survey data from 13 jurisdictions and found similar overall results as Kann et al. [15] above regarding tobacco use disparities by sexual orientation identity and the sex of sexual contacts, but they also examined interactions of race, ethnicity, gender, and age with sexual orientation identity. Across five different smoking variables, they observed that Black and Asian/Pacific Island LG youth, when compared to their respective race or ethnic heterosexual counterparts, were at elevated risk for cigarette use. Bisexual females, compared to bisexual males, and adolescent girls reporting sexual contacts with both sexes, compared to those reporting only opposite-sex contacts, were also at higher risk for cigarette use. These data support the value of larger datasets that capture not only sexual orientation data but enable the exploration of the intersection of race, ethnicity, age, and gender variables with tobacco use and the identification of disparities within these subgroups.

The strengths of the YRBS survey data include population-based sampling, large samples of youth, and standard questions that enable comparisons across states and years, but they are cross-sectional data, do not include homeless youth and those not in public schools, and the data are generalizable only to the states participating. Although some state YRBS surveys assess more than one facet of sexual identity, e.g., items about sexual orientation identity and the sex of those with whom they have had sexual contact, most studies examining smoking prevalence and correlates measure sexual orientation by assessing self-identity. Recently, researchers [7] found lack of concordance among methods used to assess sexual orientation—self-identity, sexual attraction, and sexual experience—in their study of $n=3{,}963$ youth ages 15–24 years in the National Survey of Family Growth. Sexual experience rather than identity or attraction was the most consistent predictor of substance use, including tobacco. Thus, particularly among youth, sexual identity is a work in progress and relying on only one measure of sexual orientation may not accurately describe their patterns and the correlates of tobacco use. Future research of sexual minority youth's tobacco use can contribute to a more nuanced understanding by incorporating a multidimensional assessment of sexual identity and the perspectives of developmental-stage theories of identity development [24].

In summary, the cumulative population-based survey data indicate disparate tobacco use among LGB youth compared to their heterosexual counterparts, although data are often limited to certain regions of the country. LGB racial, ethnic, and gender subgroups are at higher risk for smoking than their heterosexual peers. Smoking data are lacking for transgender and gender nonconforming youth.

Adults A solid and growing body of published research using national, population-based sampling indicates that the prevalence of smoking among lesbians, gay men, and bisexual men and women is significantly elevated when compared to smoking prevalence for their heterosexual counterparts. Smoking prevalence data for transgender persons have not been collected [42] in most population-based surveys, and the existing studies that do use varying methods to sample the transgender subpopulation. A systematic review of the tobacco research literature conducted by Lee et al. [42], and spanning nearly two decades up to mid-2007, found that sexual minority men and women have 1.5 to 2.5 times the odds of being current smokers when compared to their heterosexual counterparts. More recent tobacco use data from 10 states participating in the CDC Behavioral Risk Factor Surveillance Survey (BRFSS) [4] and assessing sexual orientation and gender identity in 2010, are consistent with that review. Specifically, lesbians had nearly twice the odds of being a current smoker compared to heterosexual women (OR = 1.91, 95 % CI = 1.26, 2.91). Bisexual women had over twice the odds of being a smoker (OR = 2.13, 95 % CI = 1.33, 3.42). In terms of smoking prevalence, 19.1 % of lesbians were current smokers, whereas 29.7 % of bisexual women and 11.7 % of heterosexual women smoked. Both gay men and bisexual men had nearly twice the odds of being a current smoker compared to heterosexual men (respectively, OR = 1.93, 95 % CI = 1.27, 2.93; OR = 1.92, 95 % CI = 1.04, 3.53) [4]. The prevalence of current smoking was 22.9 % for gay men, 33.3 % for bisexual men, and 15.8 % for heterosexual men. As the authors noted, the limitation of these data include the absence of any southern state among the 10 states reporting BRFSS data; therefore, they are not representative of the U.S. population, and assessment of sexual orientation varied across states.

The strongest evidence for smoking disparities for transgender persons comes from the 2004 California Tobacco Use Survey, which used a strong sampling methodology to adequately sample the LGBT population in that state [9]. Smoking prevalence for transgender respondents was 30.7%, compared to 30.4% for the LGBT sample overall, indicating prevalence nearly double that of the general California population at 15.4%. Showing data consistent with the California findings but using a very different sampling approach was the 2010 National Transgender Discrimination Survey [31]. The survey was conducted by contacting over 800 transgender-led or -serving community-based organizations in the U.S., and the outreach yielded 6,450 valid survey responses from all 50 states. Some 88% of the sample identified as either female-to-male or male-to-female. Thirty percent of the transgender sample reported daily or occasional smoking, compared to the U.S. general population adult smoking prevalence of 20.6% at the time of the survey. Notably, 70% reported wanting to quit smoking, similar to national population data [74]. A third study reported in a conference abstract secondary analyses from an internet-based HIV risk reduction intervention targeting transgender persons [38]. The sample size was $n=1{,}106$, 80.3% Caucasian, with a mean age of 33 years, and over 80% had some post-high school education. Smoking prevalence was 41% overall, with higher prevalence among the female-to-male (FTM) subgroup (47.5%) compared to the male-to-female (MTF) subgroup (36.1%). These three studies begin to fill the data gap on smoking prevalence for transgender persons. Using different sampling methods, they have arrived at prevalence figures indicating smoking rates substantially higher than seen in the general population and equivalent to or higher than rates for LGB persons.

Rath et al. [59] reported fine-grained data on characteristics associated with LGB tobacco use and diverse types of tobacco products in the Legacy Young Adults Cohort, a nationally representative longitudinal sample of young adults ages 18–34. Prevalence of current cigarette use within the past 30 days was significantly higher for LGB respondents: 35% for lesbians and gay men; 27% for bisexuals, and; 18% for heterosexuals. LGB young adults, compared to heterosexual counterparts, were more likely to have ever visited a hookah bar or restaurant, and used cigars, little cigars, cigarillos, or bidis, and dissolvable tobacco products.

In conclusion, consistent findings using population-based sampling or intensive community sampling indicates significantly higher smoking prevalence in all LGBT subpopulations compared to heterosexuals. Within the LGBT population, bisexuals and transgender persons may be at higher risk for tobacco use.

Factors Associated with Smoking in the LGBT Community

Identifying the correlates of tobacco use and potential causes of elevated prevalence of smoking in the LGBT community is important because doing so provides actionable information for increasing awareness of the tobacco problem within the

LGBT community by advocates, arming tobacco control experts, and motivating funding sources to address the problem. As Blosnich et al. [3] observed in their review of risk factors and correlates of tobacco use in the LGB population, these can be divided into two broad categories: Factors unique in type or intensity for sexual minorities, and factors common to both sexual minorities and the general population. This approach is helpful in thinking about future tobacco use prevention programs targeted or tailored to LGBT youth, as well as cessation interventions for current smokers. Comparisons of LGBT smokers and nonsmokers across sociodemographic and psychosocial characteristics may also shed light on protective and risk factors for smoking.

Youth LGB adolescents compared to heterosexual youth are more likely to start smoking at an earlier age and report current smoking [19, 20]. In general, adolescents who smoke compared to those who don't are at greater risk to become regular smokers in adulthood [17]. There is variability in risks for smoking within sexual minority subgroups. A meta-analysis of 18 studies examining sexual orientation and adolescent substance use found that being female (vs. male) or bisexual (vs. gay or lesbian) were associated with higher risk for smoking [49]. Bisexual identity, compared to lesbian/gay or heterosexual identity, as a risk factor for higher risk for tobacco use and other risk behaviors [49] was confirmed in later YRBSS data [11]. Victimization, such as verbal or physical harassment due to being LGB, is longitudinally associated with LGB smoking status [52], and LGBQ (queer-identified youths were included) youths experiencing high victimization levels also had higher smoking levels and other health risk behavior compared with heterosexual youths reporting low levels of victimization [5]. In the latter study, LGBQ youth who reported low levels of victimization had health risk behavior profiles similar to heterosexual youth, and LGBQ youth reporting the highest victimization were at higher risk than heterosexual youth also reporting high victimization [5]. Approaching the influence of social environment on smoking risk from an alternative perspective, Hatzenbuehler et al. [35] found that among 11th graders in Oregon, a greater supportive social environment for LGB youth (e.g., presence of gay-straight alliances, school nondiscrimination and anti-bullying policies that specifically protected LGB students) was associated with *reduced* tobacco use. The potential mitigating effect of supportive school environments on LGBT youths' risk for tobacco use, along with the link between victimization and risk for smoking, strongly suggest that social stigma, harassment, and absence of clear support for LGBT identity are potent risk factors for smoking in these youth. Parallel to these data are consistent findings across studies that use of other substances and levels of other high risk health behaviors are elevated among LGB youth [11, 44]. Interviews with LGBT youths about smoking have highlighted the perceived utility of smoking in managing stressors and stress reactions [60], although other data suggest that smoking can amplify the association between stress burden and subsequent psychological distress [62].

In summary LGB youth, compared to heterosexual youth, start smoking at a younger age. Identifying as bisexual and being female, and experiencing more victimization are associated with greater risk for smoking. Factors associated with adult LGBT smoking are now presented.

Adults A 2011 systematic review of publications reporting sociodemographic, behavioral, and mental health associations with smoking among sexual minorities noted a fragmented research literature lacking coherence in sampling methods, measures, and definitions of sexual orientation and smoking. The reviewers stated "the current evidence base constructs an incomplete and challenging glimpse into the etiology of smoking disparities among sexual minorities," ([3], p. 4). Although some progress has been made since, their statement largely holds. That review identified alcohol use, depression or depressive symptoms, younger age, and lower education level as associated with LGB tobacco use, all of which are also associated with current smoking in the general population [3, 12, 30, 56]. Similarly, the Legacy Young Adults Cohort study [59] conducted multivariate logistic regressions to determine covariates of tobacco use by sexual identity. Current cigarette use by LGB young adults was significantly associated with having a high school education (vs. some college or greater), OR=4.27 (95% CI: 1.51–12.12); current alcohol use, OR=12.65 (95% CI: 2.99–53.54); and current other drug use, OR=9.67 (95% CI: 2.22–42.09). The same three covariates were significant in the statistical model using any current tobacco use as the outcome variable. Notably, when the same statistical models were developed for heterosexuals, two of the three variables significant for LGB youth, i.e., high school education and current alcohol use, were significant for them as well. As the authors noted, current alcohol use was most strongly associated with current cigarette and any tobacco use by LGB young adults.

Being HIV-infected is strongly associated with current smoking, as smoking prevalence is some two to three times the rates in the general population [48]. Men who have sex with men, largely gay-identified men but including bisexual- and heterosexual-identified men, are the largest risk group among those living with HIV/AIDS [12]. As the HIV-infected population ages, both aging- and tobacco-related cancer risks have increased [66].

Quitting smoking is considered the optimal outcome in tobacco control, but smokers may not be ready to quit and therefore not receptive to cessation messages and programs. Several studies have examined readiness, motivation, or intentions to quit smoking, as interventions may be required to bolster motivation to seek treatment. For example, more positive attitudes about cessation and specific beliefs that cessation would make LGBT smokers feel more like their ideal selves and improve health and longevity were related to greater intention to quit [8]. Studies examining LGBT smokers' treatment preferences have found support for the concept of tailoring cessation interventions to the population, enhancing receptivity to treatment [25, 43, 64, 76].

Theoretical Frameworks for Understanding Tobacco Use Disparities Stress, psychological distress, and discrimination are associated with higher risk for smoking in both general population and racial minority samples ([41, 57]; Landrine and Klonoff 2000). Given the overlap of correlates for tobacco use for LGBT and heterosexual smokers, what is unique about being LGBT that may account for disparate smoking prevalence? A prominent hypothesis, the minority stress model, posits that higher smoking prevalence and smoking rate in the LGBT population, as well as other adverse health behaviors and mental health, are driven by sexual minority stress resulting from externally imposed and internally incorporated stigma, and victimization [36, 46]. In this hypothesis, smoking is seen as a means by which to cope with this added layer of sexual minority stressors and the increased psychological distress ensuing from the higher stress burden. Extending the minority stress model, Hatzenbuehler [34] has proposed a psychological mediation model that holds that the impact of social stressors specific to LGBT persons is mediated via general psychological processes. This mediation model integrates findings from research on stress and stigma and posits that increased exposure to stressors engenders emotion dysregulation, social and interpersonal problems, and dysfunctional cognitions that confer increased risk for psychopathology, creating observed mental health and substance use disparities for LGBT persons. LGBT persons who identify as women, transgender, or bisexual may experience additional stressors related to their gender identity, or in the case of bisexuals, a lack of social support within and outside the LGBT community [40], leading to greater vulnerability to adverse mental health and substance use outcomes, as data presented on smoking above support.

Evidence for a smoking-stigma association has been mixed, despite findings clearly indicating higher levels of distress in the LGBT community (e.g., [18]). For example, Newcomb et al. [52] found that LGBT-based victimization was associated with higher odds of smoking when assessed at the same time period and also predicted subsequent smoking rate in their longitudinal cohort study of 248 youth ages 16–20 years. Blosnich and Horn [3] observed in their college student sample that although the LGB students reported much higher prevalence of discrimination, this was not associated with current smoking status. However, LGB students who were in physical fights or were physically assaulted had greater odds of being a smoker compared to LGB smokers who did not experience these stressors. It may be that violent victimization, in contrast to perceived discrimination per se, is more closely associated with smoking in LGB adults. Transgender persons may be an exception to this speculation, as Humfleet et al. [38] found that tobacco use was associated with self-reported employment and housing discrimination in the FTM subgroup of their internet-based study, but among MTF participants tobacco use was related to sexual abuse and assault. In both subgroups verbal abuse and harassment were associated with tobacco use.

If the dominant heterosexual culture inflicts sexual minority stress, does engagement with the LGBT community buffer the risk of smoking? Arguably, since the prevalence of smoking is elevated in the LGBT community, more engagement with the community may encourage or normalize the uptake or maintenance of smoking, such as a qualitative study of LGBTQ young adults observed [70]. On the other hand, there is evidence that greater involvement in the LGBT community can be protective in a number of ways, such as buffering from loneliness and depression [58], which may reduce the risk of using smoking as a strategy for coping with psychological distress. A study of young sexual minority women ages 18–24 explicitly examined the role of community connectedness (one item asking how much personally they see themselves as being part of the local LGBTQ community) as it relates to smoking and found that study participants who were more connected were significantly less likely to smoke [39]. Interestingly, organizational membership (one item asking how many LGBTQ organizations they have belonged to in the past year) had the opposite relationship—the higher the organizational membership the greater the odds of being a smoker. Actual participation in LGBTQ community activities was not associated with smoking status. Thus, assessing different components of LGBT community involvement can yield different relationships with smoking status, and given the changing concept of community to include internet-based communities [63], warrants further exploration. It is also worth considering in future research the potential impact on motivation to quit smoking and smoking status of those LGBT youth or adults who are engaged in community organizations that actively promote smoking prevention and cessation and provide cessation services on-site.

Fortunately, progress in documenting the tobacco disparities and correlates of smoking among LGBT persons and developing theoretical frameworks to explain them has been accompanied by efforts to develop and test cessation programs to reduce those disparities. The next section reviews community-based smoking cessation programs tailored to LGBT smokers and research-focused cessation interventions targeting or including LGBT smokers.

LGBT-Focused Smoking Cessation Interventions

Community-based Cessation Programs The first known smoking cessation program designed for LGBT smokers, The Last Drag, was conducted in 1991 by CLASH at the Lyon-Martin Women's Health Center in San Francisco [25]. The Last Drag program typically comprises seven sequential, group format classes 2 h each, delivered over 6 weeks, and facilitated by an LGBT community member who has been certified by the American Lung Association's *Freedom from Smoking* Program. Smoking cessation medications, such as nicotine replacement therapies (NRT; e.g., nicotine gum, patch) are not provided but participants may use them during the program. Three publications on characteristics of participants and cessation outcomes for The Last Drag support the approach of holding cessation classes in an LGBT venue and having LGBT community members as facilitators trained in tobacco cessation [25, 32, 76]. One report analyzed data on 233 participants over multiple classes [25], and self-reported quit rates at the end of treatment for those who attended more than one session ranged from 28 to 89 %, with the median value at 52 %. Those who attended more classes, were Hispanic, or were non-Hispanic white participants, were more likely to be quit than other ethnicities. The larger study followed up program participants six months later and found cessation rates declining to 36 % [25], a rate that compares favorably to the estimated rate of 26.9 % for cessation treatment that combines medication and 4–8 sessions of behavioral counseling [26]. Greenwood and colleagues standardized The Last Drag program in a treatment manual and conducted a pilot study yielding a post-treatment quit rate of 40 % [32]. Although tailored to the LGBT community, for example, by educating participants about marketing targeted to the community and the specific impact of tobacco on the LGBT community, what effects this tailoring has on cessation outcomes is unknown and would require an explicit test of tailored vs. non-tailored interventions, and perhaps different settings. For example, is the setting the most critical factor, i.e., holding the program in an LGBT-serving venue, thereby reducing barriers to access and assuring an LGBT-validating environment? Or could an LGBT-tailored program be just as effective in a non-LGBT but neutral setting, all other factors being equal?

Matthews et al. [45] reported on a community-based, culturally-tailored smoking cessation group treatment program for LGBT smokers. Of the $n = 198$ participants, 42 % completed treatment and of those, 32.3 % reported smoking abstinence at the post-treatment assessment. Cultural tailoring was defined in terms of holding the programs at LGBT venues, having LGBT-identified program facilitators, branding program materials with LGBT-specific images, and including relevant content such as discussion of HIV/AIDS and the interaction of hormone use with smoking on health risks for transgender smokers. Greater treatment program attendance, the use of NRT, and lower nicotine dependency were positively associated with smoking abstinence.

Besides the lack of biochemical verification of smoking status to adjust for possible misreporting of smoking status, limitations in the published reports are that the bulk of data come from the San Francisco-based program, limiting generalizability, and drop-out rates can be substantial. Nonetheless, notable strengths of The Last Drag are its longevity, indicating a high level of acceptance by the LGBT community and the commitment of its creators to disseminate the program nationally, and its reliance on evidence-based treatment components. The U.S. Public Health Service Clinical Practice Guideline for Treating Tobacco Use and Dependence [26] calls for research on tailored treatments for LGBT smokers. Future work comparing an LGBT community-tailored cessation intervention like The Last Drag program with a non-tailored approach and in different settings could illuminate how these factors impact treatment uptake, retention, and abstinence outcomes, contributing to the broader discourse about the benefits of culturally-tailored interventions [61].

Academic-based Cessation Studies These studies typically are based in academic settings with more experimental control, and often with random assignment to treatment conditions. Within this category of studies are two subcategories:Those studies with aims specifically targeting LGBT smokers, and those that report secondary findings based on sexual orientation but do not tailor the interventions or have research aims specific to LGBT smokers.

Although not a randomized clinical trial, one of the earliest LGBT-focused studies was a pilot project from British researchers who aimed to bridge the dissemination gap between evidence-based smoking cessation treatments and communities in need, here gay men [33]. The 98 men participating were recruited through the gay press, largely white and well-educated, and 25 % qualified for no-cost government-supported cessation medication. The intervention was for 7 weeks and included large and small group support by forming "quit cells" of 3–4 participants, education about nicotine withdrawal and cessation medications, and creating a welcoming space for the men to discuss sexuality, HIV concerns, drug use and other relevant topics, and group discussion was focused on contexts specific to gay men. At the end of treatment, 58 % of those who attended the first session had quit, verified by a carbon monoxide breath test, a rate higher than the 53 % cessation rate reported nation-wide. In multivariate analyses the only baseline predictor of quitting success was higher number of prior quit attempts.

The only other study focused exclusively on LGBT smokers was conducted by Humfleet et al. [37], in which preliminary data were reported at a conference, so few details are available. They conducted a large, randomized trial ($n=356$ LGBT smokers) in which all participants received via mail a smoking cessation self-help treatment manual (MST), and were randomized to one of four intervention conditions: MST only, MST+ internet-based treatment, MST+ proactive telephone counseling, and MST+ combined internet-based and telephone counseling. They hypothesized that the combined treatment would produce the highest quit rates. The abstinence rates at 6 months for the four treatment conditions were 15, 21, 34, and 29 %, respectively. Contrary to their hypothesis, there was no difference between the combined and the MST+ telephone counseling conditions, but there was a main effect for MST+ telephone counseling vs. those not receiving telephone counseling. Use of the internet-based intervention was low, and 48 % of those assigned to proactive telephone counseling declined participation. This study holds promise for developing further treatment modalities to reach diverse LGBT smokers with different treatment preferences.

Two published studies not using LGBT-tailored interventions collected sexual orientation data, enabling comparisons of abstinence outcomes with those of heterosexuals. Covey [21] conducted an 8-week open treatment intervention with nicotine patch, bupropion, and counseling with 297 men, 54 (18 %) of whom were gay or bisexual (GB). There were no smoking history, psychiatric or psychological differences between heterosexual and GB men at baseline, except the latter were younger, reported lower body mass index, and included more professional white collar workers. There were no differences between the two groups of men in terms of adverse drug effects or adherence to treatment. GB men had significantly higher quit rates than heterosexual men 2 weeks after quitting (77 vs. 68 %, respectively), but at the end of treatment the quit rates were equivalent (59 vs. 57 %). A second report was on secondary analyses presented in a conference abstract [29]. In this report data from two different studies were combined, with each examining extended treatment combinations of medication (NRT or bupropion) or counseling, for a combined sample of 810 participants, 17 % of whom ($n=138$) identified as LGBT. Abstinence rates assessed at 12, 24, 52, 64, and 104 weeks did not differ significantly by sexual orientation, e.g., at week 12, heterosexual men's abstinence rate was 62 %, and GB men's was 55 %, and; at 104 weeks, 40 and 38 % were abstinent, respectively. Thus, in both studies presenting abstinence data on non-tailored interventions, LGBT smokers quit at rates similar to heterosexuals. As the authors noted, however, these findings may not generalize to other locations (beyond San Francisco and New York) where access to treatment is limited or stigma is higher.

In summary, the LGBT community has longstanding tailored smoking cessation programs that have been evaluated, but relatively few randomized smoking cessation intervention trials have been conducted with LGBT smokers. Capitalizing on community-grounded experience in developing and delivering well-received cessation programs, investigators need to design scientifically rigorous studies comparing LGBT tailored vs. non-tailored cessation interventions to answer the question of whether, or to what extent, such tailoring impacts study uptake, retention, and cessation outcomes. The work of Covey [21] and Grady above [29] suggests that when treatment access is high in large urban areas with large LGBT populations, non-tailored interventions may be as efficacious for LGBT persons as for heterosexuals. Although not investigated, in regions where LGBT persons are more stigmatized, LGBT-tailored interventions could be more efficacious because they assure a safe, validating environment that enhances receptivity to treatment and cessation. Multi-site studies encompassing different regions of the country beyond the two coasts could address this hypothesis.

Summary and Future Directions

Because of the default absence of sexual orientation and gender identity questions in most state and federal tobacco use surveys and all cancer registries, we are still catching up to other minorities in understanding the full impact of tobacco use on the health of the LGBT community. Provisions of the Affordable Care Act begin to address this critical lack of data in its broader role of addressing health disparities. Once LGBT cancer disparities are identified and this information is made widely available, the community and its allies will be further empowered to act on the root causes: social inequity, stigma, and discrimination. That smoking is more prevalent among LGB adolescents and at a younger age strongly supports targeted efforts to mitigate early risk through assuring school and community environments that support and validate LGBT identity, counter stigma, and prevent victimization. Evidence-based tobacco prevention programs targeting vulnerable populations such as LGBT youth are also effective cancer prevention interventions. As discussed, how tailored to the LGBT community tobacco prevention and cessation interventions need to be to reach the community and impact tobacco use is largely unknown. In the meantime, tobacco control activists, researchers, policy experts, and clinicians in the LGBT community are likely to continue leading the effort to eliminate this health disparity.

References

1. American Legacy Foundation: American Legacy Foundation Pulls Back the "Orange Curtain" on Project SCUM. Produces truthsm ad for teens on tobacco company targeting of gay and homeless communities (Press Release). http://tobaccodocuments.org/landman/518021121.html. Accessed 16 March 2014.
2. American Legacy Foundation: American Legacy Foundation Awards Small Innovative Grants to Five Community Organizations Across the United States In: Press Releases. 2014. http://www.legacyforhealth.org/newsroom/press-releases/american-legacy-foundation-awards-small-innovative-grants-to-five-community-organizations-across-the-united-states/(language)/eng-US. Accessed 16 March 2014.

3. Blosnich JR, Horn K. Associations of discrimination and violence with smoking among emerging adults: differences by gender and sexual orientation. Nicotine Tob Res. 2011;13(12):1284–95. doi:10.1093/ntr/ntr183.
4. Blosnich JR, Farmer GW, Lee JGL, Silenzio VMB, Bowen DJ. Health inequalities among sexual minority adults evidence from ten U.S. states, 2010. Am J Prev Med. 2014;46(4).
5. Bontempo D, D'Augelli A. Effects of at-school victimization and sexual orientation on lesbian, gay, or bisexual youths' health risk behavior. J Adolesc Health. 2002;30(5):364–74.
6. Bradford J, Ryan C, Rothblum ED. National Lesbian Health Care Survey: implications for mental health care. J Consult Clin Psychol. 1994;62(2):228–42.
7. Brewster KL. Sexual orientation and substance use among adolescents and young adults. Am J Public Health (1971). 2012;102(6):1168–76. doi:10.2105/AJPH.2011.300261.
8. Burkhalter JE, Warren B, Shuk E, Primavera L, Ostroff JS. Intention to quit smoking among lesbian, gay, bisexual, and transgender smokers. Nicotine Tob Res. 2009;11(11):1312–20. doi:ntp140 [pii]10.1093/ntr/ntp140.
9. Bye L, Gruskin E, Greenwood G, Albright V, Krotki K. California Lesbians, Gays, Bisexuals, and Transgender (LGBT) tobacco use survey—2004. Sacramento: California Department of Health Services; 2005.
10. Centers for Disease Control and Prevention: 2003 Youth risk behavior surveillance system by sexual orientation: Boulder County, Colorado. In: Local Risk Behavior Data. 2003. http://www.bouldercounty.org/family/youth/pages/yrbsresultslinks.aspx. Accessed 16 March 2014.
11. Center for Disease Control and Prevention: Current cigarette smoking among adults—United States, 2011. Morb Mortal Wkly Rep. 2012;61(44):889–94.
12. Centers for Disease Control and Prevention: Estimated HIV incidence in the United States, 2007–2010. HIV Surveillance Supplemental Report 2012. 2012.
13. Centers for Disease Control and Prevention: Youth Risk Behavior Surveillance System (YRBSS). Division of Adolescent and School Health 2014.
14. Centers for Disease Control and Prevention, Adhikari B, Kahende J, Malarcher A, Pechacek T, Tong V. Smoking-attributable mortality, years of potential life lost, and productivity losses—United States, 2000–2004. MMWR; 2008.
15. Centers for Disease Control and Prevention, Kann L, O'Malley Olsen E, McManus T, Kinchen S, Chyen D, et al. Sexual identity, sex of sexual contacts, and health-risk behaviors among students in grades 9–12—youth risk behavior surveillance, selected sites, United States, 2001–2009. MMWR; 2011.
16. Centers for Disease Control and Prevention, Agaku IT, King BA, Dube SR. Current cigarette smoking among adults—United States, 2005–2012. MMWR; 2014.
17. Chassin L, Presson CC, Rose JS, Sherman SJ. The natural history of cigarette smoking from adolescence to adulthood: demographic predictors of continuity and change. Health Psychol. 1996;15(6):478–84.
18. Cochran SD, Sullivan JG, Mays VM. Prevalence of mental disorders, psychological distress, and mental health services use among lesbian, gay, and bisexual adults in the United States. J Consult Clin Psychol. 2003;71(1):53–61. doi:10.1037/0022-006x.71.1.53.
19. Corliss HL, Wadler BM, Jun HJ, Rosario M, Wypij D, Frazier AL, et al. Sexual-orientation disparities in cigarette smoking in a longitudinal cohort study of adolescents. Nicotine Tob Res. 2013;15(1):213–22. doi:10.1093/ntr/nts114.
20. Corliss HL, Rosario M, Birkett MA, Newcomb ME, Buchting FO, Matthews AK. Sexual orientation disparities in adolescent cigarette smoking: intersections with race/ethnicity, gender, and age. Am J Public Health. 2014;104(6):1137–47. doi:10.2105/AJPH.2013.301819.
21. Covey LS, Weissman J, LoDuca C, Duan N. A comparison of abstinence outcomes among gay/bisexual and heterosexual male smokers in an intensive, non-tailored smoking cessation study. Nicotine Tob Res. 2009;11(11):1374–7. doi:10.1093/ntr/ntp137.
22. Crimp D, Rolston A. AIDS demo graphics. Seattle: Bay Press; 1990.
23. Diamant AL, Wold C, Spritzer K, Gelberg L. Health behaviors, health status, and access to and use of health care: a population-based study of lesbian, bisexual, and heterosexual women. Arch Fam Med. 2000;9(10):1043–51.

24. Eliason M, Schope R. Shifting sands or solid foundation? Lesbian, gay, bisexual, and transgender identity formation. In: Meyer I, Northridge M, editors. The health of sexual minorities. New York: Springer US; 2007. pp. 3–26.
25. Eliason MJ, Dibble SL, Gordon R, Soliz GB. The last drag: an evaluation of an LGBT-specific smoking intervention. J Homosex. 2012;59(6):864–78. doi:10.1080/00918369.2012.694770.
26. Fiore MC, Jaén CR, Baker TB, Bailey WC, Benowitz N, Curry SJ, et al. Treating tobacco use and dependence: 2008 update. Clinical Practice Guideline In: US Department of Health and Human Services. Public Health Service, editor. Rockville MDMay; 2008.
27. Garofalo R, Wolf RC, Kessel S, Palfrey SJ, DuRant RH. The association between health risk behaviors and sexual orientation among a school-based sample of adolescents. Pediatrics. 1998;101(5):895–902.
28. Goebel K. Lesbian and gays face tobacco targeting. Tob Control. 1994;3(1):65–7. doi:10.1136/tc.3.1.65.
29. Grady ES, Humfleet GL, Hall SM, Reus VI, Munoz RF. Smoking cessation outcomes among LGBT and heterosexual smokers in extended smoking treatments. Society for Research on Nicotine and Tobacco 19th Annual International Meeting; Westin Boston Waterfront Hotel in Boston, Massachusetts: Poster Session POS1-169; March 13–16, 2013. p. 109.
30. Grant BF, Hasin DS, Chou SP, Stinson FS, Dawson DA. Nicotine dependence and psychiatric disorders in the United States: results from the national epidemiologic survey on alcohol and related conditions. Arch Gen Psychiatry. 2004;61(11):1107–15. doi:10.1001/archpsyc.61.11.1107.
31. Grant JM, Mottet LA, Tanis J. National Transgender Discrimination Survey Report on health and health care. In: Herman JL, Harrison J, Keisling M, editors. Findings of a Study by the National Center for Transgender Equality and the National Gay and Lesbian Task Force. October; 2010.
32. Greenwood G. Queertip: smoking cessation interventions in San Francisco's Queer communities. Prevention: University of California San Francisco (UCSF); 2002.
33. Harding R, Bensley J, Corrigan N. Targeting smoking cessation to high prevalence communities: outcomes from a pilot intervention for gay men. BMC Public Health. 2004;4:43.
34. Hatzenbuehler ML. How does sexual minority stigma "get under the skin"? A psychological mediation framework. Psychol Bull. 2009;135(5):707–30. doi:10.1037/a0016441.
35. Hatzenbuehler M, Wieringa N, Keyes K. Community-level determinants of tobacco use disparities in lesbian, gay, and bisexual youth: results from a population-based study. Arch Pediatr Adolesc Med. 2011;165(6):527–32.
36. Herek GM, Gillis JR, Cogan JC. Internalized stigma among sexual minority adults: insights from a social psychological perspective. J Couns Psychol. 2009;56(1):32–43.
37. Humfleet G, Hall SM. Using telephone-based and internet-based smoking treatments with LGBT smokers: preliminary findings. Society for Research on Nicotine and Tobacco 18th Annual Meeting; Hilton Americas Houston Hotel, Houston, Texas: Paper Session PA7-3; March 13–16, 2012. p. 26.
38. Humfleet GL, Swinburne Romine RE, Ott M, Bockting WO. Tobacco use and correlates in a large sample of transgender americans. Society for Research on Nicotine and Tobacco 19th Annual International Meeting; Boston, Massachusetts: Poster Session POS2-99; March 13–16, 2013. p. 140.
39. Johns MM, Pingel ES, Youatt EJ, Soler JH, McClelland SI, Bauermeister JA. LGBT community, social network characteristics, and smoking behaviors in young sexual minority women. Am J Community Psychol. 2013;52(1–2):141–54. doi:10.1007/s10464-013-9584-4.
40. Kertzner RM, Meyer IH, Frost DM, Stirratt MJ. Social and psychological well-being in lesbians, gay men, and bisexuals: the effects of race, gender, age, and sexual identity. Am J Orthopsychiatr. 2009;79(4):500–10. doi:10.1037/a0016848.
41. Landrine, H. and E.A. Klonoff, Racial discrimination and cigarette smoking among Blacks: findings from two studies. Ethnicity & Disease. 2000;10(2):195–202.

42. Lee JGL, Griffin GK, Melvin CL. Tobacco use among sexual minorities in the USA, 1987 to May 2007: a systematic review. Tob Control. 2009;18(4):275–82. doi:10.1136/tc.2008.028241.
43. Levinson AH. Smoking cessation treatment preferences, intentions, and behaviors among a large sample of colorado gay, lesbian, bisexual, and transgendered smokers. Nicotine Tob Res. 2012;14(8):910–8. doi:10.1093/ntr/ntr303.
44. Marshal MP, Friedman MS, Stall R, King KM, Miles J, Gold MA, et al. Sexual orientation and adolescent substance use: a meta-analysis and methodological review. Addiction. 2008;103(4):546–56. doi:10.1111/j.1360-0443.2008.02149.x.
45. Matthews AK, Li CC, Kuhns LM, Tasker TB, Cesario JA. Results from a community-based smoking cessation treatment program for LGBT smokers. J Environ Public Health. 2013;2013:Article ID 984508. doi:10.1155/2013/984508.
46. Meyer IH. Prejudice, social stress, and mental health in lesbian, gay, and bisexual populations: conceptual issues and research evidence. Psychol Bull. 2003;129(5):674–97.
47. Meyer IH, Wilson PA. Sampling lesbian, gay, and bisexual populations. J Couns Psychol. 2009;56(1):23–31. doi:10.1037/A0014587.
48. Nahvi S, Cooperman NA. Review: the need for smoking cessation among HIV-positive smokers. AIDS Educ Prev. 2009;21(3):14–27.
49. National Association of Attorneys General: The Tobacco Master Settlement Agreement (MSA). November. 1998. http://www.naag.org/backpages/naag/tobacco/msa/msa-pdf/. Accessed 16 Feb 2014.
50. National LGBT Tobacco Control Network: Tobacco marketing to LGBTs. In: The Fenway Institute at Fenway Health: Resources/Resource Library. 2014. http://www.lgbttobacco.org/resources.php?ID=24#33. Accessed Feb 22.
51. New York State Department of Health: Chronic diseases; basic statistics: about incidence, prevalence, morbidity, and mortality—statistics teaching tools. 2014. http://www.health.ny.gov/diseases/chronic/basicstat.htm. Accessed 8 March.
52. Newcomb ME, Heinz AJ, Birkett M, Mustanski B. A longitudinal examination of risk and protective factors for cigarette smoking among lesbian, gay, bisexual, and transgender youth. J Adolesc Health. 2014. doi:10.1016/j.jadohealth.2013.10.208.
53. Offen N. Is tobacco a gay issue? Interviews with leaders of the lesbian, gay, bisexual and transgender community. Cult Health Sex. 2008;10(2):143–57. doi:10.1080/13691050701656284.
54. Offen N, Smith EA, Malone RE. From adversary to target market: the ACT-UP boycott of Philip Morris. Tob Control. 2003;12(2):203–7.
55. Offen N, Smith EA, Malone RE. Tobacco industry targeting of the lesbian, gay, bisexual, and transgender community: a white paper. 2008.
56. Pratt LA, Brody DJ. Depression and smoking in the U.S. household population aged 20 and over, 2005–2008. NCHS data brief, no 34. Hyattsville, MD: National Center for Health Statistics. 2010.
57. Purnell JQ, Peppone LJ, Alcaraz K, McQueen A, Guido JJ, Carroll JK, et al. Perceived discrimination, psychological distress, and current smoking status: results from the Behavioral Risk Factor Surveillance System Reactions to Race module, 2004–2008. Am J Public Health. 2012;102(5):844–51. doi:10.2105/AJPH.2012.300694.
58. Ramirez-Valles J, Fergus S, Reisen CA, Poppen PJ, Zea MC. Confronting stigma: community involvement and psychological well-being among HIV-positive Latino gay men. Hisp J Behav Sci. 2005;27(1):101–19. doi:10.1177/0739986304270232.
59. Rath JM, Villanti AC, Rubenstein RA, Vallone DM. Tobacco use by sexual identity among young adults in the United States. Nicotine Tob Res. 2013;15(11):1822–31. doi:10.1093/ntr/ntt062.
60. Remafedi G. Lesbian, gay, bisexual, and transgender youths: who smokes, and why? Nicotine Tob Res. 2007;9(Suppl 1):S65–71. doi:769874221 [pii] 10.1080/14622200601083491.
61. Resnicow K, Baranowski T, Ahluwalia JS, Braithwaite RL. Cultural sensitivity in public health: defined and demystified. Ethn Dis. 1999;9(1):10–21.

62. Rosario M, Schrimshaw EW, Hunter J. Cigarette smoking as a coping strategy: negative implications for subsequent psychological distress among lesbian, gay, and bisexual youths. J Pediatr Psychol. 2011;36(7):731–42. doi:10.1093/jpepsy/jsp141.
63. Ross MW, Tikkanen R, Berg RC. Gay community involvement: its interrelationships and associations with Internet use and HIV risk behaviors in Swedish men who have sex with men. J Homosex. 2014;61(2):323–33. doi:10.1080/00918369.2013.839916.
64. Schwappach DL. Smoking behavior, intention to quit, and preferences toward cessation programs among gay men in Zurich, Switzerland. Nicotine Tob Res. 2008;10(12):1783–7. doi:10.1080/14622200802443502.
65. Secretan B, Straif K, Baan R, Grosse Y, El Ghissassi F, Bouvard V, et al. A review of human carcinogens–Part E: tobacco, areca nut, alcohol, coal smoke, and salted fish. Lancet Oncol. 2009;10(11):1033–4.
66. Shiels MS, Pfeiffer RM, Gail MH, Hall HI, Li J, Chaturvedi AK, et al. Cancer burden in the HIV-infected population in the United States. J Natl Cancer Inst. 2011;103(9):753–62. doi:10.1093/jnci/djr076.
67. Stall RD, Greenwood GL, Acree M, Paul J, Coates TJ. Cigarette smoking among gay and bisexual men. Am J Public Health. 1999;89(12):1875–8.
68. Szumilas M. Explaining odds ratios. J Can Acad Child Adolesc Psychiatry. 2010;19(3):227–9.
69. The Last Drag: A free 7-session quit smoking class for lesbian, gay, bisexual, transgender and HIV+ smokers held in San Francisco. 2014. http://www.lastdrag.org/. Accessed 22 March 2014.
70. The National Youth Advocacy Coalition: Coming out about smoking: A report from the National LGBTQ Young Adult Tobacco Project. Washington, DC. 2010. http://lgbttobacco.org/files/Coming_Out_About_Smoking_NYAC.pdf. Accessed 22 March 2014.
71. Tobaccodocuments.org: "Project Scum". 2014. http://tobaccodocuments.org/landman/518021121.html. Accessed 22 March.
72. U.S. Department of Health and Human Services: A Report of the Surgeon General. Department of Health and Human Services, Centers for Disease Control, Center for Health Promotion and Education, Office on Smoking and Health. Department of Health and Human Services: Public Health Service, Centers for Disease Control, Center for Health Promotion and Education, Office on Smoking and Health, The Health Consequences of Involuntary Smoking. DHHS Publication No. (CDC) 87-8398. Rockville (MD): U.S. 1986.
73. U.S. Department of Health and Human Services: How Tobacco Smoke Causes Disease: The Biology and Behavioral Basis for Smoking-Attributable Disease: A Report of the Surgeon General. Atlanta, GA: U.S. Department of Health and Human Services, Centers for Disease Control and Prevention, National Center for Chronic Disease Prevention and Health Promotion, Office on Smoking and Health; 2010.
74. U.S. Department of Health and Human Services: The Health Consequences of Smoking—50 Years of Progress: A Report of the Surgeon General.—Atlanta, GA. http://www.surgeongeneral.gov/library/reports/50-years-of-progress/index.html#fact. Rockville, MD: U.S. Department of Health and Human Services, Public Health Service, Office of the Surgeon General; Centers for Disease Control and Prevention, National Center for Chronic Disease Prevention and Health Promotion, Office on Smoking and Health; 2014.
75. U.S. Environmental Protection Agency: Framework for Ecological Risk Assessment. In: U.S. Environmental Protection Agency—Risk Assessment Forum, editor. Washington, DC, EPA/630/R-92/0011992.
76. Walls NE, Wisneski H. Evaluation of smoking cessation classes for the lesbian, gay, bisexual, and transgender community. J Soc Serv Res. 2011;37(1):99–111. doi:Pii 931245010; doi:10.1080/01488376.2011.524531.
77. Washington HA. Burning love: big tobacco takes aim at LGBT youths. Am J Public Health. 2002;92(7):1086–95. doi:10.2105/Ajph.92.7.1086.

Part II
Screening for Cancer in LGBT Populations

Chapter 6
Cancer Screening in Lesbian and Bisexual Women and Trans Men

Melissa A. Clark, Ulrike Boehmer and Samantha Rosenthal

Abstract This chapter provides an overview of cancer screening among lesbian and bisexual women and trans men. Following a brief introduction to define terminology, the chapter is divided into four sections. The first section highlights recommendations for cancer screening for the most common cancer types and considerations for cancer screening specific to lesbian and bisexual women and trans men (LBT). The second section summarizes the available data about prevalence of cancer screenings among LBT populations. The third section describes barriers and facilitators to cancer screenings for LBT individuals as well as interventions that have been developed to improve screening rates among LBT communities. The fourth section provides recommendations for future research, policy, and practice for improving cancer screening within LBT communities.

Introduction

Lesbian and bisexual refer to sexual orientation designations and are terms often used to describe sexual minorities. Trans men refers to a gender identity designation and is often used to describe gender minorities. For the purposes of this chapter, lesbian refers to women who identify with the term lesbian and/or report being attracted to women, partnering exclusively with women, or having sex exclusively with other women. Bisexual refers to women who identify with the term bisexual and/or report being attracted to both women and men, partnering with both men and

M. A. Clark (✉)
Department of Epidemiology and Obstetrics & Gynecology, School of Public Health and Warren Alpert Medical School, Brown University, Providence, RI, USA
e-mail: melissa_clark@brown.edu

U. Boehmer
Department of Community Health Sciences, Boston University School of Public Health, Boston, MA, USA

S. Rosenthal
Department of Epidemiology, School of Public Health, Brown University, Providence, RI, USA

U. Boehmer, R. Elk (eds.), *Cancer and the LGBT Community*,
DOI 10.1007/978-3-319-15057-4_6

women, or having sex with both men and women. Trans men refers to individuals assigned at birth (natal) as female but who identify as male. This includes transsexual males who have undergone physical changes to align their appearance with their gender identity as well as transgender males who identify as male but have not necessarily undergone physical changes. FTM (female-to-male) has also been used to refer to trans men. The term trans men does not include "stud", which is a term that refers to African American lesbians who express masculinity through wearing men's clothes and adopting traditional male-identified mannerisms, roles, and behaviors [1].

Cancer Screening Recommendations

In the United States, both the American Cancer Society (ACS) [2] and the U.S. Preventive Services Task Force (USPSTF) [3] have issued guidelines for cancer screenings based on their respective interpretations of the scientific literature. Table 6.1 (columns 2 and 3) summarizes the recommendations from both organizations for average risk, asymptomatic individuals for the leading cancer sites relevant to females. While the recommended age at initiation, screening interval, and/or screening type differ slightly across organizations, both organizations recommend specific screening tests for cancers of the breast, cervix, colon-rectum, and lung. On the other hand, both organizations have concluded that there is insufficient evidence of the value of specific screening tests for cancers of the bladder, endometrial, oral cavity, ovary, skin, and thyroid. Rather, they recommend that individuals consult with a healthcare provider to determine the utility of screening for a particular cancer based on a personal and family history, and to seek immediate care if symptoms develop.

To date, there have been no recommendations for cancer screenings specific to lesbian and bisexual women. However, evidence suggests that sexual minority women should be screened based on their age, personal and family risk factors at intervals at least comparable to heterosexual women. Further, some individuals have suggested that cancer screening recommendations for lesbian and bisexual women should be more aggressive than for average-risk women in general because sexual minority women report more risk factors including lower levels of physical activity [4, 5] and diets low in fruits and vegetables [6], as well as higher rates of overweight/obesity [4–8], smoking [4, 5, 7–12], alcohol use [4–6, 9], and nulliparity [6].

Neither the ACS nor USPSTF have published recommendations for screening exams for trans men. However, organizations such as the American College of Obstetrics and Gynecology have provided opinions [13] and/or attempted to use limited available data to provide recommendations for cancer screenings for trans individuals [14, 15]. Table 6.1 (column 4) summarizes the recommendations compiled by the Center for Excellence in Transgender Health at the University of California, San Francisco [15] for trans men. In general, they recommend that screening

Table 6.1 Cancer screening guidelines for average risk asymptomatic individuals

	Natal women		Transgender men [15]
Cancer type	ACS [51]	USPSTF [3]	
Bladder	No recommended screening test	No recommended screening test	No recommendation made
Breast	*Age 20–39*: CBE every 3 years *Age ≥ 40*: CBE annually Mammogram annually as long as good health	*Age 40–49*: Individual decision about mammogram based on discussion with clinician *Age 50–74*: Mammogram every 2 years	Chest wall/axillary exam annually Mammography same as for natal women Mammogram not needed following chest reconstruction
Cervical	*Age 21–29*: Pap smear ever 3 years *Age 30–65*: Pap smear plus HPV test every 5 years; or Pap smear every 3 years	*Age 21–29*: Pap smear ever 3 years *Age 30–65*: Pap smear plus HPV test every 5 years; or Pap smear every 3 years	*Ovaries removed, uterus/cervix intact*: Same as natal women; may defer if no history of genital sexual activity; inform pathologist of current or prior testosterone use
Colon-Rectum	*Age ≥ 50*: Colonoscopy every 10 years; or Flexible sigmoidoscopy every 5 years; or Double-contrast barium enema every 5 years; or CT colonography every 5 year High-sensitivity fecal occult blood test annually	*Age ≥ 50*: Colonoscopy every 10 years; or Flexible sigmoidoscopy every 5 year with high sensitivity fecal occult blood tests; or High-sensitivity fecal occult blood test annually	No recommendation made
Endometrial (uterine)	No recommended screening test	No recommended screening test	No recommendation made
Lung	*Age 55–74 and fairly good health and ≥ 30 pack-year smoking history, and current smoker or quit smoking within last 15 years*: Low-dose computed tomography annually	Age 55–80 and asymptomatic and ≥ *30 pack-year smoking history, and current smoker or quit smoking within last 15 years*: Low-dose computed tomography annually; Screening should be discontinued after 15 years of no smoking	Same as for natal women
Oral Cavity	Clinical exam as part of routine dental or physical check-up	No recommended screening tests	No recommendation made
Ovary	No recommended screening test	No recommended screening test	No recommendation made

Table 6.1 (continued)

	Natal women		Transgender men [15]
Skin	Clinical exam as part of routine physical check-up	No recommended screening tests	No recommendation made
Thyroid	Clinical exam as part of routine physical check-up	Recommendations currently being updated	No recommendation made

ACS American Cancer Society, *USPSTF* United States Preventive Services Task Force, *CBE* Clinical Breast Exam, *FOBT* Fecal occult blood test.

should be conducted for the anatomy that is present regardless of an individual's self-description or identity. They also distinguish between those who have used cross-sex hormones or had gender-affirming surgery from those who have not. They recommend that for those who have not used hormones or had surgery the same criteria and risk parameters be used as for persons of their natal sex. Recommendations for those who have used hormones and/or had surgery vary depending on the type of surgery received and current and past hormone use.

Cancer Screening Prevalence

The majority of studies of cancer screening rates among lesbian and bisexual women have focused on screening for breast and/or cervical cancer with screening for colon-rectum cancers only included in more recent studies. To our knowledge, no study has explicitly included lesbian and bisexual individuals in any lung cancer screening studies.

We are also not aware of any studies of cancer screenings that have explicitly included trans men. However, studies have demonstrated that gender minorities often have many barriers to healthcare, including having no insurance [16, 17], being refused medical care [18], and experiencing uninformed, insensitive, biased, and even abusive providers [18, 19]. Therefore, it is hypothesized that screening rates for trans men may be even lower than those for sexual minorities, who have been documented to have more barriers to care than heterosexual individuals.

Breast Cancer There have been mixed results from studies comparing mammography screening behaviors among sexual minority and heterosexual women. Although two studies have documented higher mammography rates for lesbian compared to heterosexual women [5, 20], the majority of studies have reported that sexual minority women were less likely than heterosexual women to have had a recent mammogram [8, 21, 22] or there were no differences in mammography rates by sexual orientation [23–26]. Cross-sectional data from at least three large population- [21, 22] and community-based [8] samples suggest that sexual minority women may be less likely to be screened for breast cancer than heterosexual women. For example, in multi-lingual population-based surveys of more than 18,000 adults in New York City, Kerker et al. [21] found that women who had sex with women (WSW) were less likely to have had a mammogram in the past 2 years (53 vs. 73 %) than other women. Next, using a combined sample of almost 47,000 women from the 2000–2007 Behavioral Risk Factor Surveillance Surveys (BRFSS), Buchmueller and Carpenter [22] found that women in same-sex relationships were significantly less likely to have had recommended mammograms (adjusted odds ratio [AOR] = 0.75; 95 % CI = 0.61, 0.92) than women in different-sex relationships. Finally, Cochran et al. [8] found that 73 % of women aged 40–49 years and 83 % of women aged 50–75 years who described themselves as lesbian or bisexual in a combined sample of nearly 12,000 women from seven U.S. surveys of sexual minority women reported ever receiving a mammogram, compared to 87–90 % of women in U.S. general population surveys [8].

On the other hand, data from two cohort studies [6, 27] and one cross-sectional population-[28] and community-based sample [25] found no differences between lesbian and heterosexual women. For example, Valanis et al. [6] found that among a cohort sample of more than 93,000 women in the Women's Health Initiative (WHI), rates of having received a mammogram in the past 2 years among those aged 50–79 were comparable for lifetime lesbians (sex only with women ever; 82 %), adult lesbians (sex only with women after age 45 years; 84 %), and heterosexual women (84 %). Similarly, Austin et al. [27] compared prior 2 year mammography rates among 85,756 women in the Nurses' Health Study (NHS) II aged 40–60 years and found comparable rates for lesbian (82 %) and heterosexual women (84 %). Using a combined sample of more than 52,000 women from 10 states in the 2010 Behavioral Risk Factor Surveillance Surveys (BRFSS), Blosnich et al. [28] found no significant differences in ever having received a mammogram for lesbian (59 %), and heterosexual (65 %) women after controlling for differences in demographic characteristics. Finally, in a cross-sectional, community-based sample of more than 1600 women in Los Angeles, Mays et al. [25] reported that 2-year screening rates for women ≥40 years were comparable for Hispanic (62 %) and African American (88 %) lesbians compared to Hispanic (76 %) and African American (82 %) heterosexual women after accounting for age, education, and income.

Among studies that have explicitly reported screening rates for bisexual women, rates of mammography screening have generally been lower, although not always statistically significant, for bisexual compared to heterosexual women [6, 20, 24, 27, 28]. For example, in the WHI sample, Valanis et al. [6] found that bisexual women aged 50–79 years were slightly less likely to have received a mammogram in the past 2 years than same-aged heterosexuals (82 vs. 84 %). Similarly, Conron et al. [20] also reported slightly lower rates of ever having had a mammogram for bisexual compared to heterosexual women (56 vs. 59 %) in a sample of more than 27,000 women ≥40 years in the 2001–2008 Massachusetts BRFSS. Bisexual women also had slightly lower 2-year mammography rates than heterosexual women (79 vs. 84 %) in the Nurses' Health Study II reported by Austin et al. [27]. Finally, Blosnich et al. reported lower rates of ever having had a mammogram for bisexual compared to heterosexual (42 vs. 65 %) women in the combined 10-state BRFSS.

Cervical Cancer Similar to mammography screening, there have been mixed results from studies comparing gynecological screening behaviors among sexual minority and heterosexual women. Several cross-sectional studies using both population-[21, 22, 29, 30] and community-based [5, 8, 25, 31] samples as well as a cohort study [32], have documented lower rates of Pap testing among sexual minority compared to heterosexual women. For instance, Agenor et al. found lower odds of Pap test use in the past 12 months (OR=0.40, 95% CI=0.23, 0.68) among lesbians compared to heterosexual women in the 2006–2010 National Survey of Family Growth [30]. Combining 4 years of population-based data (2001, 2003, 2005, and 2007) from the California Health Interview Survey, Boehmer et al. found that lesbians (65%) were less likely than heterosexual (74%) and bisexual (77%) women to report having had a Pap test in the prior year [29]. Kerkeret al. [21] reported that women who had sex with women (WSW) were less likely to have had a Pap test in the past 3 years (66 vs. 88%) than other women in the New York City multi-lingual population-based surveys. In the combined BRFSS sample, Buchmueller and Carpenter [22] found that women in same-sex relationships were significantly less likely to have had a Pap test in the past 3 years (adjusted odds ratio [AOR]=0.74; 95% CI=0.57, 0.97) than women in different-sex relationships. Data were similar for some community-based samples. For example, using data from a multisite survey of women 20–86 years, Matthews et al. [31] found that lesbians were less likely to report annual Pap test screening (49 vs. 66%) and receipt of a Pap test every 3 years (81 vs. 90%) compared to heterosexual women. Mays et al. [25] also reported that 2-year Pap test rates were lower for Hispanic (70%) and African American (76%) lesbians compared to Hispanic (81%) and African American (81%) heterosexual women in their Los Angeles sample of racial and ethnic minority women. Finally in the cohort of women who were part of the Growing Up Today Study, Charlton et al. found lower odds of receipt of a Pap test in the past year among lesbian (AOR=0.25, 95% CI=0.12, 0.52) and mostly heterosexual/bisexual women (AOR=0.70, 95% CI=0.54, 0.92) compared to heterosexual women [32].

On the other hand, at least four studies, including cohort [6], population-based [20, 28], and community-based samples [26] have shown no differences in Pap test screening rates by sexual orientation. For instance, in the WHI sample, age adjusted rates of pap test in the prior 3 years were similar for lifetime lesbians (84%), adult lesbians (87%), bisexual women (82%), and heterosexual women (84%) [6]. Similarly, Conron et al. [20] found no differences in rates of Pap testing in the prior 3 years among lesbian (90%), bisexual (87%), and heterosexual women (90%) in the Massachusetts BRFSS. Blosnnich et al. [28] also reported no differences in ever having had a Pap test among lesbian (92%), bisexual (80%), and heterosexual (93%) women in the combined 10-state BRFSS survey. Finally, using a community sample of women 40–75 years, Clark et al. [26] reported that women who partner with women or both women and men (75%) were less likely than women who partner with men (84%) to be on-schedule for Pap testing according to ACS guidelines. However, there were no differences after controlling for demographic characteristics, health behaviors, cancer-related experiences, and participant recruitment source.

Colorectal Cancer To date, there have been few studies that have reported screening rates for cancer of the colon-rectum by sexual orientation, and these studies have generally found few differences. For example, in the WHI sample reported by Valanis et al. [6], receipt of a hemoccult screening within the prior 5 years among those 50–79 years was comparable for lifetime lesbians (59 %), adult lesbians (60 %), bisexual women (61 %), and heterosexual women (57 %). Similarly, among women 50 years and older in the Nurses' Health Study, Austin et al. [27] reported no differences in rates of ever having had a colonoscopy or sigmoidoscopy by sexual orientation (lesbians = 42 %; bisexual women = 39 %; heterosexual women = 39 %). In the Massachusetts BRFSS sample ≥ 50 years, Conron et al. [20] found no significant differences in ever having had a sigmoidoscopy or colonoscopy when they compared lesbian (58 %, AOR = 1.00, 95 % CI = 0.66, 1.51) and bisexual women (74 %, AOR = 2.16, 97 % CI = 0.96, 4.86) to heterosexual women (56 %). Blosnich et al. also found no differences in ever having had a colorectal cancer exam for lesbian (59 %), bisexual (64 %), and heterosexual (66 %) women in the combined BRFSS sample. Similarly, Boehmer et al. found no differences in ever having had a colorectal cancer exam for lesbian (74 %), bisexual (65 %), and heterosexual (68 %) women 50 years of age and older in the California population-based sample. Finally, in a community sample of 600 women, Clark et al. [26] reported that among women 50–75, 65 % of women who partnered with women or with both men and women and 67 % of women who partnered with men were on-schedule for colorectal cancer screening according to the American Cancer Society screening guidelines.

Summary Despite the number of large-scale cohort, population- and community-based studies, it is not possible to unequivocally conclude whether or not there are differences in the prevalence of cancer screenings by sexual orientation. The strongest evidence presented is for cervical screening where the majority of relevant studies have documented lower rates among sexual minority compared to heterosexual women. There are a number of possible explanations for the mixed results for the other types of cancer screenings. First, studies differed in measures of sexual orientation. Some used identity to classify women but differed as to whether they combined lesbian and bisexual women together or analyzed them separately. Other studies used behavior (e.g., women who have sex with women versus women who have sex with men) to identify sexual minority women. Second, data were collected in different geographic regions. These geographic regions may differ in their screening rates due to density of screening facilities [33] as well as the availability and accessibility of cancer screening programs, particularly for uninsured and underinsured women [34]. Third, studies differed with regard to the age eligibility of women included in the analyses of the respective screening exams. For example, some studies of mammographic screening included all women regardless of age despite the fact that it is not recommended by any professional organization before age 40 years. Fourth, studies differed in the proportion of racial and ethnic minority women included in the sample. For example, some studies were comprised of almost all white women whereas other studies included higher proportions of racial and ethnic minority women consistent with the populations from which the samples were drawn (e.g., New York City, Massachusetts, California). Finally, studies differed in the definition of the screening outcome. For example, intervals for on-schedule Pap testing included the past 12 months, past 2 years and past 3 years. Similarly, colon-cancer screening differed in interval as well as type of test (e.g., lifetime colonoscopy versus past 5-year fecal occult blood test).

Barriers and Facilitators to Cancer Screening

Barriers to Cancer Screening Among LBT Communities

Prior research has suggested that one of the largest barriers to sexual minority women seeking health care in general is fear of disclosing their sexual orientation to providers and the consequences that the disclosure may present. There is considerable data confirming that sexual minority women have had negative experiences with providers due to homophobic attitudes, inappropriate reactions and discrimination [35, 36]. In qualitative studies, sexual minority women report that these types of negative experiences as well as fear of discrimination due to sexual orientation are also barriers to cancer screenings [37, 38]. However, as shown in Table 6.2, there have been few empirical studies that have identified barriers and facilitators associated with breast and/or cervical cancer screenings among sexual minority women. Some of these studies have identified perceived or actual discrimination in health care settings, lack of trust in providers, and lack of provider knowledge about sexual minority health issues as barriers to screening. However, the majority of identified barriers and facilitators in studies of sexual minority women are common to women in general, such as lack of health insurance and/or a regular health care provider, competing life demands, body image, discomfort with the procedure, and fear of the outcome of the exam.

There have also been very few studies that have assessed the barriers and facilitators associated with screening of the colon-rectum among sexual minority women. In a qualitative study of barriers and facilitators of cancer screenings in general, both sexual minority and heterosexual women reported physical pain or discomfort and embarrassment associated with the screening tests and/or preparations as barriers to screening [37]. In addition, in a community sample of more than 600 sexual minority and heterosexual women, participants 50–75 years were less likely to be on-schedule for colorectal cancer screening if they reported they had put off or avoided screenings because of problems taking time off work and for reasons due to body image [26]. However, these barriers did not differ by sexual orientation.

To our knowledge, there have been no studies that have empirically documented the barriers and facilitators of cancer screenings for trans men. Given the high reported rates of no insurance [16, 17], provider insensitivity [19], and discrimination [18, 19] reported by trans individuals, it is likely that many of the barriers and facilitators to cancer screenings for sexual minorities are comparable for gender

Table 6.2 Barriers and facilitators to breast and cervical cancer screening among lesbian and bisexual women

Barriers and Facilitators	Breast screening	Cervical screening
Barriers		
Personal Factors		
Competing life demands such as taking time off from work	*Lauver et al. 1999* [38] Clark et al. 2009 [26]	
Fear and embarrassment	*Lauver et al. 1999* [38]	
Lack of perceived risk	*Lauver et al. 1999* [38] Hart and Bowen 2009 [52]	Price et al. 1996 [53] Matthews et al. 2004 [31]
Fear of outcome		Matthews et al. 2004 [31]
Body image	*Clark et al. 2003* [37]	*Clark et al. 2003* [37]
Less use of hormonal contraceptives		Charlton et al. 2014 [39]
Provider Factors		
Lack of trust in provider and/or health care system	*Lauver et al. 1999* [38] Hart and Bowen 2009 [52]	
Disclosure of sexual orientation; perceived or actual discrimination in health care settings	*Clark et al. 2003* [37]	Rankow and Tessaro 1998 [54] Diamant et al. 2000 [55] *Clark et al. 2003* [37]
Provider knowledge about sexual minority health issues	*Clark et al. 2003* [37]	Rankow and Tessaro 1998 [54] *Clark et al. 2003* [37]
System Factors		
Lack of insurance/cost	Rankow and Tessaro 1998 *Lauver et al. 1999* [38] Cochran et al. 2001 [8] *Clark et al. 2003* [37]	Price et al. 1996 [53] Rankow and Tessaro 1998 [54] Cochran et al. 2001 [8] *Clark et al. 2003* [37] Matthews et al. 2004 [31]
No regular health care provider		Diamant et al. 2000 [55]
Discomfort with procedure/ Don't like exam	*Lauver et al. 1999* [38] *Clark et al. 2003* [37]	*Clark et al. 2003* [37] Matthews et al. 2004 [31]
Difficulty in scheduling	*Lauver et al. 1999* [38]	
Facilitators		
Personal Factors		
Desire to take care of oneself	*Lauver et al. 1999* [38]	
Provider Factors		
Provider recommendation for exam	*Lauver et al. 1999* [38]	
System Factors		
Prior good experiences with screening		Fish and Anthony 2005 [56] Rankow and Tessaro 1998 [54]

References noted in italics were qualitative studies

minorities. However, there are likely other specific barriers to cancer screenings for gender minorities including the availability of only gender-specific facilities, lack of consensus about recommended screening guidelines for trans individuals, and unawareness by providers of gender-identity issues that contribute to non-adherence to cancer screenings. Finally, there may be unique cancer-specific screening barriers for trans men. For instance, in a recent study of Pap testing, FTM patients were more likely to have an inadequate test (10.8 vs. 1.3 % of tests) and had higher odds of having an inadequate test (AOR = 10.77, 95 % CI = 6.83, 16.83) compared to female patients, findings that are likely due to physical changes associated with testosterone therapy and patient/provider discomfort with the exam [39].

Interventions to Increase Cancer Screenings

There have been limited reports in the peer-reviewed literature about interventions to facilitate cancer screenings among lesbian and bisexual women and no studies that we are aware of that have included trans men. However, there are individual (i.e., patient)-, provider-, and system-level interventions that have been developed that may increase cancer screenings among sexual and gender minorities.

Individual-Level Interventions Two published studies found that tailoring interventions to sexual minority women increased adherence to mammography screening. Dibble et al. [40] demonstrated that two 1-hour lesbian-specific educational interventions led by a lesbian physician on cancer screening behaviors were able to increase breast and cervical screenings among lesbians within 6 months but had no impact on colorectal cancer screening. Bowen et al. [41] conducted a randomized trial of a breast cancer risk counseling intervention for sexual minority women. The intervention involved four weekly 2-hour group sessions led by a sexual minority woman health counselor and produced increases in breast screening rates at 24 months compared to the control arm. These data suggest that brief, low cost sexual minority specific interventions may improve adherence to cancer screenings among lesbian and bisexual women. Although there are no empirically tested interventions to increase cancer screenings among trans persons, there are current programs such as the "Get Screened" [42] and "Check it Out" [43] campaigns in Canada that specifically target the cancer screening needs of trans individuals through educational promotions. Data are needed about the efficacy and effectiveness of these types of educational campaigns as well as other individual-level intervention strategies for cancer screenings in LBT communities.

Provider-Level Interventions Because poor communication, including fear of discrimination if or when sexual orientation and/or gender identity is revealed, with health care providers has been documented as a barrier to screening, trainings directed toward providers about influences of sexual and gender minority status on health may improve patient-provider relationships and ultimately improve cancer screening rates. Examples of currently available programs include the Mautner

Project of Whitman-Walker Health's "Removing the Barriers" [44], the Gay and Lesbian Medical Association (GLMA) "Quality Healthcare for Lesbian, Gay, Bisexual & Transgender People" [45], The LGBT Aging Project's "Open Door Task Force" [46] as well as the educational resources available from the National LGBT Health Education Center of the Fenway Institute [47]. More research is needed to determine whether these programs improve patient outcomes, how to increase the numbers of providers exposed to these types of trainings, determine the best methods of delivering the information, and the most efficient and effective ways to encourage health systems to require competence of their providers in providing LBT compassionate and knowledgeable care.

System-Level Interventions There have been few system-level interventions specifically designed to increase cancer screenings among LBT individuals. One example of an intervention designed to improve health care in general is the annual Healthcare Equality Index (HEI) produced by the Human Rights Campaign [48]. The HEI enables inpatient and outpatient healthcare organizations to assess their policies and practices for Centers for Medicare and Medicaid Services (CMS) and Joint Commission requirements for LGBT patient-centered care, receive training and resources they may need to remedy gaps, and receive public recognition for their commitment to equity and inclusion. However, to date, it is not clear the extent to which facilities that have participated in the HEI differ from those that did not with regard to patient outcomes, including the extent to which their LBT patients are more likely to be on-schedule for recommended cancer screenings.

Recommendations for Future Research, Policy, and Practice for Improving Cancer Screening within LBT Communities

To achieve optimal cancer screening rates for lesbian and bisexual women and trans men, the following recommendations are made in the areas of research, policy, and practice.

Research

Both survey and intervention-based research is needed for improving cancer screening within LBT communities. First, given the mixed results regarding adherence to cancer screening guidelines among sexual minority women, large population-based studies are needed to identify specific subgroups of sexual minorities who are less likely to be screened at recommended intervals. Second, large scale studies are essential for determining the prevalence of cancer screening behaviors among trans individuals. In addition, research is needed to determine if cancer screening guidelines should be developed that are specific to trans individuals.

Population-based studies should be conducted to determine the barriers to and facilitators of screening for sexual and gender minorities. For sexual minorities, high priority areas include barriers and facilitators of screenings of the colon-rectum and lung. Given the dearth of available data, all cancer types should be considered when assessing barriers and facilitators of screening for trans persons. In addition, research should be conducted about unique issues facing communities within the LBT population, including studs, racial and ethnic minorities, individuals with disabilities, and those with limited English proficiency with regard to cancer screening behaviors. This research should include the assessment of the influence of the intersectionality of these identities on cancer screening behaviors. Finally, research is needed about the extent to which cancer screenings co-occur, the characteristics of individuals most likely to adhere to all endorsed screenings, and the factors that impede individuals from receiving all recommended screenings based on their age, family history, and personal risk factors.

In addition to studies focusing on sexual and gender minority individuals, additional data are also needed about the experiences of providers who care for LBT persons. For example, there is minimal data about cancer screening recommendations by providers to LBT individuals. Therefore, it is unclear the extent to which lower screening rates observed among sexual and gender minority persons are due to lack of provider recommendations or lack of patient adherence. Next, there are limited data about clinicians' reported barriers to providing high quality care to LBT individuals, including: lack of knowledge about sexual orientation and gender identity specific issues; lack of available equitable and inclusive facilities for which to refer LBT patients for cancer screenings; and perceptions that, given limited time with a patient, there are other health issues experienced by LBT individuals that are higher priority than cancer screenings (e.g., hormone use; smoking cessation).

In addition to survey research, individual-level interventions should be developed and tested to determine the factors that increase cancer screenings that are unique to sexual minority women relative to women in general. These interventions should be targeted to women most at risk due to prior low adherence to cancer screening behaviors. Next, given the dearth of available programs, individual-, provider- and system-level interventions should be developed and tested for decreasing barriers to cancer screenings among trans individuals. Next, evaluations should be conducted to determine the extent to which provider- and system-level interventions about providing LBT compassionate and knowledgeable care such as Whitman-Walker Health's "Removing the Barriers" [44] and the Human Rights Campaign Healthcare Equality Index (HEI) [48] have an impact on patient outcomes. Research is also needed to determine the most efficient and effective ways to increase the numbers of providers exposed to trainings, including methods of delivering the information.

Policy

Measures of sexual orientation and gender identity should be included in Surveillance, Epidemiology, and End Results (SEER) registries so that cancer incidence, prevalence, and mortality data are available. Without these data, the implications of differences by sexual orientation and gender identity in screening rates are unknown. Further, it is not possible to determine whether sexual and gender minorities are at higher risk for particular cancers. Therefore, the American Cancer Society, U.S. Preventive Services Task Force, and other relevant professional organizations do not have sufficient information to provide cancer screening guidelines that are specific to sexual and gender minorities. Measures of sexual orientation and gender identity should also be included as standard demographic questions in federally funded health surveillance and large-scale screening studies so population-based estimates are available for cancer screenings among sexual and gender minority communities.

Practice

The largest system-level barrier to care, lack of insurance coverage for cancer screenings, is likely to be reduced by mandates in the Patient Protection and Affordable Care Act [34]. In addition, insurance coverage may improve for individuals in same-sex relationships as there are increased federal and state benefits due to recognition of same-sex marriages. However, there will remain sexual and gender minority individuals who continue to be denied access to cancer screening services due to insurance coverage or intermittent or no relationship with a regular health care provider for which other system-wide interventions may be necessary. This could include increased marketing of the National Breast and Cervical Cancer Early Detection Program to underserved sexual and gender minorities. Another system-level intervention may involve the use of electronic medical records. Prior studies have documented that sexual minorities may hesitate or avoid responses to provider questions about sexual identity because of concerns about how and where the information will be retained. Therefore, with the increasing use of electronic records, protocols could be developed for providers to request permission from patients to chart their responses with systems in place to codify sexual and gender identity in medical records [49]. Next, some data suggest that sexual minority women who do not need birth control are not prompted for cervical screening, and that rates of cervical cancer for these sexual minority women will not increase until they reach an age when both mammography and Pap testing is recommended [50]. In addition, when asked in a qualitative study about factors that would increase cancer screenings, both sexual minority and heterosexual women reported being able to have more than one screening test on the same day or at the same time as a routine check-up [37]. Therefore, integrative programs could be considered to prompt individuals for adherence to comprehensive screening guidelines and to provide opportunities to obtain multiple cancer screenings during the same medical visit. Finally, regardless of whether screenings are organ specific or integrative, education should be routinely offered to service providers about how to increase the likelihood that sexual and gender minorities have high quality cancer screening experiences.

References

1. Lane-Steele L. Studs and protest-hypermasculinity: the tomboyism within black lesbian female masculinity. J Lesbian Stud. 2011;15:480–92.
2. Smith RA, Manassaram-Baptiste D, Brooks D, Cokkinides V, Doroshenk M, Saslow D, et al. Cancer screening in the United States, 2014: a review of current American cancer society guidelines and current issues in cancer screening. CA Cancer J Clin. 2014;64(1):30–51.
3. US Preventive Services Task Force. Recommendations for Adults. 2010 (15 January 2014). http://www.uspreventiveservicestaskforce.org/adultrec.htm#cancer. Accessed 15 January 2014.
4. Case P, Austin SB, Hunter DJ, Manson JE, Malspeis S, Willett WC, et al. Sexual orientation, health risk factors, and physical functioning in the Nurses' Health Study II. J Womens Health (Larchmt). 2004;13(9):1033–47.
5. Aaron DJ, Markovic N, Danielson ME, Honnold JA, Janosky JE, Schmidt NJ. Behavioral risk factors for disease and preventive health practices among lesbians. Am J Public Health. 2001;91(6):972–5.
6. Valanis BG, Bowen DJ, Bassford T, Whitlock E, Charney P, Carter RA. Sexual orientation and health: comparisons in the women's health initiative sample. Arch Fam Med. 2000;9(9):843–53.
7. Diamant AL, Wold C. Sexual orientation and variation in physical and mental health status among women. J Womens Health (Larchmt). 2003;12(1):41–9.
8. Cochran SD, Mays VM, Bowen D, Gage S, Bybee D, Roberts SJ, et al. Cancer-related risk indicators and preventive screening behaviors among lesbians and bisexual women. Am J Public Health. 2001;91(4):591–7.
9. Cochran SD, Keenan C, Schober C, Mays VM. Estimates of alcohol use and clinical treatment needs among homosexually active men and women in the U.S. population. J Consult Clin Psychol. 2000;68(6):1062–71.
10. Hughes TL, Jacobson KM. Sexual orientation and women's smoking. Curr Womens Health Rep. 2003;3(3):254–61.
11. Gruskin EP, Greenwood GL, Matevia M, Pollack LM, Bye LL. Disparities in smoking between the lesbian, gay, and bisexual population and the general population in California. Am J Public Health. 2007;97(8):1496–502.
12. Gruskin EP, Hart S, Gordon N, Ackerson L. Patterns of cigarette smoking and alcohol use among lesbians and bisexual women enrolled in a large health maintenance organization. Am J Public Health. 2001;91(6):976–9.
13. Committee on Health Care for Underserved Women. Committee opinion: health care for transgender individuals. American College of Obstetrics and Gynecologists; 2011.
14. Feldman J. Medical and surgical managment of the transgender patient: what the primary care clinician needs to know. United States of America: American College of Physicians; 2008.
15. University of California-San Francisco Center of Excellence for Transgender Health. General prevention and screening 2014 (15 January 2014). http://transhealth.ucsf.edu/trans?page=protocol-screening#S2X. Accessed 15 January 2014.
16. Conron KJ, Scott G, Stowell GS, Landers SJ. Transgender health in Massachusetts: results from a household probability sample of adults. Am J Public Health. 2012;102(1):118–22.
17. Nemoto T, Operario D, Keatley J, Nguyen H, Sugano E. Promoting health for transgender women: Transgender Resources and Neighborhood Space (TRANS) program in San Francisco. Am J Public Health. 2005;95(3):382–4.
18. Sperber J, Landers S, Lawrence S. Access to health care for transgendered persons: results of a needs assessment in Boston. Int J Transgenderism. 2005;10/11(8(2–3)):75–91.
19. Grant JM, Mottet LA, Tanis J, Harrison J, Herman JL, Keisling M. Injustice at every turn: a report of the national transgender discrimination survey; 2011.
20. Conron KJ, Mimiaga MJ, Landers SJ. A population-based study of sexual orientation identity and gender differences in adult health. Am J Public Health. 2010;100(10):1953–60.

21. Kerker BD, Mostashari F, Thorpe L. Health care access and utilization among women who have sex with women: sexual behavior and identity. J Urban Health. 2006;83(5):970–9.
22. Buchmueller T, Carpenter CS. Disparities in health insurance coverage, access, and outcomes for individuals in same-sex versus different-sex relationships, 2000–2007. Am J Public Health. 2010;100(3):489–95.
23. Brandenburg DL, Matthews AK, Johnson TP, Hughes TL. Breast cancer risk and screening: a comparison of lesbian and heterosexual women. Women Health. 2007;45(4):109–30.
24. Koh AS. Use of preventive health behaviors by lesbian, bisexual, and heterosexual women: questionnaire survey. Western J Med. 2000;172(6):379–84.
25. Mays VM, Yancey AK, Cochran SD, Weber M, Fielding JE. Heterogeneity of health disparities among African American, Hispanic, and Asian American women: unrecognized influences of sexual orientation. Am J Public Health. 2002;92(4):632–9.
26. Clark MA, Rogers ML, Armstrong GF, Rakowski W, Bowen DJ, Hughes T, et al. Comprehensive cancer screening among unmarried women aged 40–75 years: results from the cancer screening project for women. J Womens Health (Larchmt). 2009;18(4):451–9.
27. Austin SB, Pazaris MJ, Nichols LP, Bowen D, Wei EK, Spiegelman D. An examination of sexual orientation group patterns in mammographic and colorectal screening in a cohort of U.S. women. Cancer Causes Control. 2013;24(3):539–47.
28. Blosnich JR, Farmer GW, Lee JGL, Silenzio VMB, Bowen DJ. Health inequalities among sexual minority adults: evidence from ten U.S. states, 2010. Am J Prev Med. 2014;e-pub.
29. Boehmer U, Miao X, Linkletter C, Clark MA. Adult health behaviors over the life course by sexual orientation. Am J Public Health. 2012;102(2):292–300.
30. Agenor M, Krieger N, Austin SB, Haneuse S, Gottlieb BR. Sexual orientation disparities in Papanicolaou test use among US women: the role of sexual and reproductive health services. Am J Public Health. 2014;104(2):e68–73.
31. Matthews AK, Brandenburg DL, Johnson TP, Hughes TL. Correlates of underutilization of gynecological cancer screening among lesbian and heterosexual women. Prev Med. 2004;38(1):105–13.
32. Charlton BM, Corliss HL, Missmer SA, Frazier AL, Rosario M, Kahn JA, et al. Reproductive health screening disparities and sexual orientation in a cohort study of U.S. adolescent and young adult females. J Adolesc Health. 2011;49(5):505–10.
33. Elkin EB, Atoria CL, Leoce N, Bach PB, Schrag D. Changes in the availability of screening mammography, 2000–2010. Cancer. 2013;119(21):3847–53.
34. Levy AR, Bruen BK, Ku L. Health care reform and women's insurance coverage for breast and cervical cancer screening. Prev Chronic Dis. 2012;9:E159.
35. Bowen DJ, Bradford JB, Powers D, McMorrow P, Linde R, Murphy BC, et al. Comparing women of differing sexual orientations using population-based sampling. Women Health. 2004;40(3):19–34.
36. Brotman S, Ryan B, Cormier R. The health and social service needs of gay and lesbian elders and their families in Canada. Gerontologist. 2003;43(2):192–202.
37. Clark MA, Bonacore L, Wright SJ, Armstrong G, Rakowski W. The cancer screening project for women: experiences of women who partner with women and women who partner with men. Women Health. 2003;38(2):19–33.
38. Lauver DR, Karon SL, Egan J, Jacobson M, Nugent J, Settersten L, et al. Understanding lesbians' mammography utilization. Womens Health Issues. 1999;9(5):264–74.
39. Peitzmeier SM, Reisner SL, Harigopal P, Potter J. Female-to-male patients have high prevalence of unsatisfactory Paps compared to non-transgender females: implications for cervical cancer screening. J Gen Intern Med. 2014;29(5):778–84.
40. Dibble SL, Roberts SA. Improving cancer screening among lesbians over 50: results of a pilot study. Oncol Nurs Forum. 2003;30(4):E71–9.
41. Bowen DJ, Powers D, Greenlee H. Effects of breast cancer risk counseling for sexual minority women. Health Care Women Int. 2006;27(1):59–74.
42. Canadian Cancer Society. The Get Screened Campaign 2014 (20 February 2014). http://convio.cancer.ca/site/PageServer?pagename=SSL_ON_GEN_About#.Uwod4IX_L3U. Accessed 20 February 2014.

43. Queer Women's Health Initiative. Check it Out Guys. 2014 (20 February 2014). http://www.checkitoutguys.ca/. Accessed 20 February 2014.
44. Mautner Project. Removing the barriers: providing culturally competent care to lesbians and women who partner with women (20 February 2014). http://www.corexcel.com/rtb/. Accessed 20 February 2014.
45. GLMA. Cultural competence webinar series: quality healthcare for lesbian, gay, bisexual & transgender people 2014. (20 February 2014). http://www.glma.org/index.cfm?fuseaction=Page.viewPagepageId=1025grandparentID=534parentID=940nodeID=1. Accessed 20 February 2014.
46. LGBT Aging Project. Open Door Task Force. 2014 (20 February 2014). http://www.lgbtagingproject.org/our-programs-and-services/cultural-competency-training/open-door-task-force/. Accessed 20 February 2014.
47. The Fenway Institute. The National LGBT Health Education Center. 20 February 2014. http://www.lgbthealtheducation.org/. Accessed 20 February 2014.
48. Human Rights Campaign. Healthcare Equality Index. 2014 (1 March 2014). http://www.hrc.org/hei/#.UxJjpIX_L3U. Accessed 1 March 2014.
49. van Dam MA, Koh AS, Dibble SL. Lesbian disclosure to health care providers and delay of care. J Gay Lesbian Med Assoc. 2001;5(1):11–9.
50. Tracy JK, Lydecker AD, Ireland L. Barriers to cervical cancer screening among lesbians. J Womens Health (Larchmt). 2010;19(2):229–37.
51. Smith RA, Brooks D, Cokkinides V, Saslow D, Brawley OW. Cancer screening in the United States, 2013: a review of current American Cancer Society guidelines, current issues in cancer screening, and new guidance on cervical cancer screening and lung cancer screening. CA Cancer J Clin. 2013;63(2):88–105.
52. Hart SL, Bowen DJ. Sexual orientation and intentions to obtain breast cancer screening. J Womens Health (Larchmt). 2009;18(2):177–85.
53. Price JH, Easton AN, Telljohann SK, Wallace PB. Perceptions of cervical cancer and Pap smear screening behavior by women's sexual orientation. J Community Health. 1996;21(2):89–105.
54. Rankow EJ, Tessaro I. Cervical cancer risk and Papanicolaou screening in a sample of lesbian and bisexual women. J Family Pract. 1998;47(2):139–43.
55. Diamant AL, Wold C, Spritzer K, Gelberg L. Health behaviors, health status, and access to and use of health care: a population-based study of lesbian, bisexual, and heterosexual women. Arch Fam Med. 2000;9(10):1043–51.
56. Fish J, Anthony D. UK national lesbians and health care survey. Women Health. 2005;41(3):27–45.

Chapter 7
Cancer Screening in Gay and Bisexual Men and Transgender People

Thomas O. Blank, Lara Descartes and Marysol Asencio

Abstract This chapter summarizes what is currently known about cancer screening needs and behaviors among gay and bisexual men and transgender people, as well as the services available to them. Two issues are of importance: (1) Whether or not screening rates in these populations differ from screening rates of heterosexual men, and (2) Whether there are specific factors related to these populations that may merit screening guidelines being different. We begin by addressing the various nomenclatures and categories used across the cancer screening literature when referring to gay and bisexual men and transgender people. Then we cover overall screening guidelines for men and their applicability to men who have sex with men (MSM), whether they identify as gay or bisexual (GB) or not, as well as transgender people (T). We then focus on the literature specifically addressing GB populations and cancer screening. This section includes differential screening patterns related to particular cancers and specific sub-groups that may merit enhanced levels of screening due to varying risk factors. This is followed by an examination of these topics as they relate to transgender people. At the end, we discuss implications and provide recommendations for future research, practice and policy.

Overview

This chapter summarizes what is currently known about cancer screening needs and behaviors among gay and bisexual men and transgender people, as well as the services available to them. Two issues are of importance: (1) Whether or not screening rates in these populations differ from screening rates of heterosexual men, and (2) Whether there are specific factors related to these populations that may merit screening guidelines being different. We begin by addressing the vari-

T. O. Blank (✉) · M. Asencio
University of Connecticut, Storrs, CT, USA
e-mail: Thomas.blank@uconn.edu

L. Descartes
Brescia University College, London, ON, Canada

U. Boehmer, R. Elk (eds.), *Cancer and the LGBT Community*,
DOI 10.1007/978-3-319-15057-4_7

ous nomenclatures and categories used across the cancer screening literature when referring to gay and bisexual men and transgender people. Then we cover overall screening guidelines for men and their applicability to men who have sex with men (MSM), whether they identify as gay or bisexual (GB) or not, as well as transgender people (T). We then focus on the literature specifically addressing GB populations and cancer screening. This section includes differential screening patterns related to particular cancers and specific sub-groups that may merit enhanced levels of screening due to varying risk factors. This is followed by an examination of these topics as they relate to transgender peopleAt the end, we discuss implications and provide recommendations for future research, practice and policy.

MSM, G, B, T: Nomenclature and Categories

Before addressing cancer screening in gay and bisexual men and transgender people, it is important to point out that these populations are referred to across studies with a variety of nomenclatures that may represent distinct populations, identities, and sexual behaviors. The term MSM (men who have sex with men), used widely in behavioral research, includes any man who has sex with another man, regardless of the particular sexual activity or if he identifies as gay, bisexual or transgender [1]. It obfuscates the implications of the various behaviors and identities, such as gay, which are rooted in particular histories and communities [2]. The term "sexual minorities" also has been used to refer to gay and bisexual men as well as transgender people. But the term also can be used to refer to heterosexuals who engage in minority sexual practices such as bondage and discipline. Even if one uses the general categorical terms of gay and bisexual men and transgender people, as we do, or the acronym "GBT," it is not always clear whether the sub-groups are equally represented or if each sub-group is facing the same (or even compatible) issues.

As we review what is known about cancer screening among men in general and these populations in particular, it should be kept in mind that what nomenclature or classifying set of categories is used in the research matters, because different studies may conclude different things depending on who is included under each terminology; that may influence what we know (and don't know) about gay men, bisexual men and transgender people and their particular needs for cancer screening or access to cancer screening.

Introduction to Cancer Screening and Gay, Bisexual Men and Transgender People

Cancer is the second leading cause of death for men in the U. S. [3]. Among men across all racial/ethnic categories, the highest death rates result from, in decreasing order: lung, prostate (PCa), colorectal, pancreatic, and leukemia [4]. In general, it is assumed that the earlier a cancer is detected and identified, the better, as treatment can begin during earlier stages of the disease. Effective cancer screening depends in part on; (1) health providers' overall knowledge of risk factors, ideal types of screening, and appropriate screening intervals, so that they can advise their patient population appropriately, (2) their awareness of their patients' identity- and behavior-based risk factors, (3) patients' awareness of what is important to monitor about themselves and communicate to their physicians, and (4) patients' willingness and likelihood to comply with screening recommendations.

Based on the assumption that organized and effective screening maximizes early detection, major organizations, including the American Cancer Society, the United States Preventive Services Task Force (USPSTF), and professional associations for specific specializations have developed screening recommendations or guidelines (see Table 7.1). It should be noted that the clinical use of guidelines for some cancers is particularly complex. Recent discussions of screening for several cancers have noted that aggressive treatment may not always be warranted. As in the case of prostate cancer, some diseases are unlikely to progress to mortality before the person's expected life span is reached. Moreover, there are side-effects of treatment

Table 7.1 Cancer screening guidelines

Cancer type	American Cancer Society (ACS) from http://www.cancer.org/healthy/findcancerearly/cancer-screeningguidelines/american-cancer-society-guidelines-for-the-early-detection-of-cancer	United States Preventive Services Task Force (USP-STF) from www.preventiveservices-taskforce.org	Specialization-specific Medical Associations
Prostate cancer	Average risk: 50 years old expecting to live more than 10 years should discuss with healthcare provider if testing is appropriate High risk: Men≥45 if African-American or if first-degree relative (father, brother, son) diagnosed with PCa before age 65, should receive a PSA test (if testing is decided) with or without DRE. PSA level determines frequency of testing PSA 2.5 ng/mL should be retested biyearly PSA≥2.5 ng/mL should be retested yearly	Screening is harmful. Recommends against screening until better testing options are available	American Urological Association (AUA) from http://www.auanet.org/education/guidelines/prostate-cancer-detection 40: No screening. 40–54 at average risk: Routine screening not recommended (unless African-American or family history of PCa). 55–69: shared decision-making recommended. 70+: If 10–15 year life expectancy, screening should not be done

Table 7.1 (continued)

Testicular cancer	Testicular exam recommended when having a routine cancer-related checkup No recommendation on regular testicular self-exams	Screening not recommended	NCI (National Cancer Institute): No recommended screening
Colorectal	50 at average risk should have one of the following Colonoscopy every 10 years Flexible sigmoidoscopy every 5 years Double-contrast barium enema every 5 years CT colonography (virtual colonoscopy) every 5 years	50–75, either Annual screening with high-sensitivity fecal occult blood testing; or Sigmoidoscopy every 5 years, with high-sensitivity fecal occult blood testing every 3 years; or Screening colonoscopy every 10 years	American College of Gastroenterology ACG from http://www.gi.org/guideline/colorectal-cancer-screening/ ≥50: Colonoscopy every 10 years beginning at age 50 preferred (age 45 for African-Americans) Alternatives to this Flexible sigmoidoscopy every 5–10 years; or Computed tomography (CT) colonography every 5 years; or Fecal immunochemical test for blood (Cancer detection test)
Anal	No screening recommendations. (Stated on ACS website: some experts recommend yearly anal Pap tests in HIV+ men who have sex with men, and every 2–3 years if HIV−.)	No screening recommendations	
Lung	55–74 in fairly good health: Annual low dose chest CT scan (if screening chosen) for current smokers with ≥30 pack-year smoking history or quit within past 15 years	50–80: Annual low-dose CT scan for current smokers with 30 pack-year smoking history or have quit within the past 15 years. Screening should terminate after 15 years no smoking	

that may be deleterious to quality of life. In those cases, it may be better *not* to have general screening [5, 6]. This is what has been recommended for prostate cancer, for example, especially by the USPSTF reviews. In other cases, there are simply no available screening tools. But in general, screening men for cancers for which they may be at risk is desirable, especially as not all cancers have clear (or any) symptoms even though the cancer may be aggressive. As a result, some experts believe that emphasis often should be on *targeted* screening of persons who are at risk of developing a specific cancer. An example is advising screening for men who smoke to be screened for lung cancer (see Table 7.1).

To be able to target sub-populations effectively, clinicians need to know who may be at higher risk for various cancers. Currently, however, data on if and how sexual and gender identity impacts risk and screening for male cancers is sparse, and even where these factors are examined (e.g., in work by Boehmer and her colleagues [7–9]) results differ from data set to data set. Inconsistencies may arise from the ways that samples are drawn and included under the pan-labels "sexual minorities" and "MSM," which can obscure information, as noted earlier. Some data are known: for example, that anal cancer rates are higher in populations of MSM [10], but that is different than simply stating that self-identified gay men are at risk. Also, the risk is related to anoreceptivity, rather than simply participating in anal sex, thus indicating the need for information about individual sexual histories and behaviors. Being HIV positive also increases the likelihood to contract certain types of cancers that are clearly related to that status [11–13]. In another HIV-related finding, Shiels, Goedert, Moore, Platz, & Engels [14] reported a lower rate of prostate cancer among men with AIDS compared to the general population. These thus are some behavior-based and concomitant risk factors of importance in focusing screening efforts. Other potentially important behavior-related risk factors are higher levels of tobacco smoking, drug use, obesity, and/or hormonal use. Some of these behaviors are found to be more prevalent among some sub-segments of the GBT populations, but not all [15, 16].

In addition to considering whether GBT people have higher rates of specific risk factors, in order to screen for cancers effectively, it is important to know whether or not they are recipients of general screening at comparable levels to the general heterosexual (or presumptively heterosexual) male population. We begin by addressing the overall screening guidelines for men, with the question of whether GB men follow the screening guidelines or recommendations differently than heterosexual men. Ulrike Boehmer and her colleagues [17, 18] point out that there is very little known about sexual minorities and cancer overall, as do Heslin, Gore, King, and Fox [19], speaking specifically to prostate and colorectal cancer. That general situation is even more evident specifically relating to screening. Although Boehmer and her co-authors' publications (and others such as Heslin et al.) take much-needed steps toward addressing the gap and gathering basic information on health behaviors, there is still much left to discover.

Thus, an emphasis on screening, at least for specific cancers, is called for, based on evidence of higher risk for at least some sexual minority male populations for several cancers. (Sometimes the risk can be traced to specific behaviors or the presence of viruses related to behaviors, sometimes not). At the same time, there does not appear to be any information about whether or not there are differential rates of cancers other than prostate, colorectal, and anal, including at least one that is very much a male cancer—testicular. If we know that there may be differential risks for at least some cancers, to what degree do those risks produce higher screening rates in vulnerable populations?

As we earlier noted, effective screening depends on both health provider and patient factors. Both are dependent on knowledge of and dissemination of that knowledge about risk factors. Some is known about both risks and screening related to HIV-defining cancers [12, 13] and quite a bit about HPV and anal cancer [20–22]. There is likely much more to know, however, about GB men who live long-term with HIV/AIDS and their risk for both HIV- and non-HIV-related cancers and the influence of HPV on other cancers. But for many cancers we do not have a knowledge base about whether more aggressive screening is appropriate or not.

A critical element in screening depends upon men getting to health care providers in the first place. California Health Interview Survey data show that gay men were much more likely than heterosexual men to have seen a physician in the past year [23], which is positive in terms of making sure their health needs are met. Unfortunately, Durso and Meyer [24] found that 40 % of bisexual men in their New York City sample and 10 % of gay men did not disclose sexual identity to their health care providers. Not disclosing such information may cause potentially pertinent screening questions to be omitted even when there is knowledge that persons with certain characteristics should be screened.

Moreover, there are the issues of GBT men's and MSM's own knowledge of screening procedures and their willingness and likelihood to undergo screening procedures. This has been addressed most fully in research on HPV and anal, colorectal, and prostate cancer. Concerning anal cancer, Newman, Roberts, Masongsong, & Wiley [25], working with Los Angeles focus groups of community health advocates, identified a number of barriers to anal cancer screening: perceived stigma with having an anal Pap smear, unease about the procedure and revealing the anus, concern over clinicians' discomfort with the process, lack of concern for anal cancer relative to concern over HIV, general reluctance to seek out health care, and lack of awareness about HPV as problematic. Blackwell and Eden [26] and Seay, Sadiq, Roytburd, Menezes, & Quinlivan [27] found very poor knowledge about both HPV and anal cancer in their sample of MSM, both with and without HIV. Despite this lack of knowledge, Seay, Sadiq, Roytburd, Menezes, & Quinlivan [27] found nearly full acceptance of anal Pap smears (a swab screening method for HPV) among their sample of men with HIV. This level of acceptance may have to do with the men's seropositive status, whether that be related to heightened concerns about health or greater familiarity with invasive testing. In a national-level study of HIV+ and HIV− MSM, conducted by D'Souza, Cook, Ostrow, Johnson-Hill, Wiley, & Silvestre [28], HIV+ men were more likely to have had an anal Pap. The work of Reed, Reiter, Smith, Palefsky, & Brewer [29] found that gay men were more likely to both get screened and to pay for the test if need be than bisexual men, highlighting the importance of identity on screening—and the need to focus attention more directly on bisexual men than has been the case.

Some aspects of the results of D'Souza et al.'s research [28], however, are of concern: 47 % of HIV+ men and 32 % of non-HIV+ men had a history of anal warts (which can be HPV- or non-HPV-related), but only 16 and 7 % respectively had ever had an anal Pap test. Factors enabling screening were awareness of available screening in the community and having health insurance [28]. Health insurance obviously matters in men's likelihood to be screened for anal cancer: Reed, Reiter, Smith, Palefsky, & Brewer [29] conducted a survey of GB men (over 80 % of whom were HIV−) to ask about their willingness to receive anal Pap screening. Less than one-third of the sample was willing to get the test if it would cost them $150, but over 80 % were willing if it were free.

Given this, we can identify some information about whether or not GBT men are more or less likely to get standard screening. Several researchers have looked at rates of participation in screening for prostate cancer. For example, using the large-scale California Health Interview Survey (CHIS), Heslin et al. [19] found no difference between GB and heterosexual men in likelihood to undergo screening for prostate cancer. However, GB black men were less likely to have such testing than heterosexual black men or GB white men. On the other hand, GB men living alone were more likely to have the PSA (prostate-specific antigen) test than those not living alone. They also found that smokers were less likely to be tested for prostate or colorectal cancer than non-smokers, a problem as Heslin et al. note that smokers are at higher risk for both. Of concern in these findings is that the GB men who are less likely to get screening appear to be those who are at higher risk due to lifestyle or ethnicity factors and thus should be screened. This illustrates the inadequacy of paying attention only to sexual minority or racial/ethnic minority status and the need to consider the intersections of multiple identities (and the behaviors that may be related to those). Blank et al. [30] found both a high level of misinformation about prostate cancer but a high level of having been screened (PSA and digital exam) among gay men in their 40's and 50's. Given their lack of knowledge, the reason they were tested had to do with access to general health care (this was in a time before recommendations against general screening by the USPSTF). Thus, a key factor is access to health care, and any reduction in access will result in reduced screening efforts, not just with prostate cancer, but generally. Heslin, Gore, King, and Fox [19] and Boehmer, Miao, Linkletter, & Clark [23], using the CHIS, found a higher rate of screening for colorectal cancer among GB men than heterosexual men. Heslin et al. speculated that the rates may be related to higher likelihood to have HIV, and concomitant HIV-related health care.

Thus, overall it seems that there is scant evidence suggesting different screening levels for prostate and colorectal cancer when comparing GB men as a group to heterosexual men. Most results show little or no difference with an overall comparison of all GB men (or MSM, depending on the study) and the general population, and indeed some situations in which GB men may be better screened than general populations. At the same time, there are several indications that there appear to be problems with various specific sub-groups' likelihood to access and receive screening, and these are the ones who are men most likely to merit aggressive screening due to specific risk factors.

Cancer Screening of Transgender and Gender Variant People

Transgender is a term usually applied to people who live their lives fully or partially in another gender than the one assigned based on anatomy at birth (natal). The term includes those who have undergone significant hormonal therapy and/or surgical procedures (transsexuals) as well as others who have had little to no physical alteration of their bodies. The latter populations, however, may be affected by how they are perceived, addressed or treated due to their gender non-conformity. Gender variant or gender non-conforming are terms used for a range of gender identifications and/or characteristics seen by society as incongruent to their natal anatomy. For a more comprehensive list of gender identities, see the information from the National Center for Transgender Equality [31].

The concerns of male to female (MtF) transgender or transsexual individuals may be different than those of female to male (FtM) transgender or transsexual people and are further complicated by issues of race, ethnicity, and socioeconomic status [32, 33]. Moreover, not all transgender, transsexual or gender variant people are gay or lesbian identified; they can also be heterosexual, bisexual, asexual, and pansexual [34] (see their Table I, p. 290). Outside of western notions of gender and sexual identity, there also exist people who are recognized within their society as third genders, such as the muxe of Oaxaca, Mexico [35], the hijras of India [36] and the bakla of the Philippines [37] and Native Americans who are reclaiming the gender identities and traditions of the two-spirit peoples of the past [36]. Therefore, gender variant populations also may be encountered as immigrant populations are located within certain geographical locations.

This range of gender identities, including transsexual identities, has major implications for receiving appropriate cancer care, including screening. It is important to stress that most surgical procedures a transsexual person may undergo do *not* remove natal internal organs; thus, MtF women are likely to still have prostates and FtM men to have ovaries. It is also very important to note that the massive use of hormonal alterations to suppress the sex hormones of the natal biology and to greatly increase the complementary other-sex hormones may have major effects not only on sex-related cancers such as prostate, testicular, ovarian, etc., but also on other cancers. Very little is known about the potential physical impacts of hormonal treatments [38].

There is a dearth of empirical research on specific cancer screenings with the various populations of gender variant people, with only a few articles readily found (as well as some case studies of a specific transgender or transsexual person who presented with a cancer related to natal anatomy—a good source referencing these case studies is Gooren & Asscheman, [38], pp. 287–289). Weyers, Decaestecker, Verstraelen, Monstrey, et al.'s ([39], p. 192) study of gynecological exams in Dutch transsexual women (MtF) revealed that most had not had a speculum exam, nor a vaginal ultrasound, and that none had had a vaginal digital exam. The study also showed that it was possible to use the vaginal exam for palpation of the prostate and a trans-vaginal ultra-sound to examine the prostate for cancer. This study recommended particular techniques that can assist with prostate screening in transsexual women with minimal discomfort. In another article focusing on mammography screening of Dutch transsexual women, it was noted that while there is little research on whether there is elevated breast cancer risk among transsexual women, there is no reason for not following the general guidelines with them regarding screening for all women [40]. Note that both the specific studies and general information about transgender populations [41], edited by Kreukels, Steensma, & de Vries, (which includes the Gooren & Asscheman chapter noted above) are all by Dutch researchers and clinicians, i.e., are not studies conducted with U.S. populations. There were no studies found regarding cancer screening for transsexual (FtM) or transgender men. *The Transgender Discrimination Survey: Report on Health and Health Care* by the National Center for Transgender Equality and the National Gay and Lesbian Task Force [42], drawing on a sample of over 7000 transgender and gender variant respondents, reported several key findings that are of relevance to cancer screening: a high percentage of those interviewed postponed medical care due to discrimination or cost; a significant number reported outright refusal of care, with gender variant people of color more likely to report refusal of care; and more upsettingly, a significant number of participants reported experiencing harassment, including violence, in the clinical setting. This report found that only 28 % of the respondents "were out to all their medical providers" [42, p. 3]. Moreover, the report also found that providers lacked sufficient knowledge about transgender people. It should be noted that the American College of Obstetricians and Gynecologists have been proactive in providing information on screening to their members [43]. Their essential point is that clinicians must treat all transgender persons with respect and should provide screening appropriate to their anatomy, and we would include, their gender.

Recommendations for Future Research, Practice and Policy

Research

In 2002, Boehmer noted that LGBT populations were vastly underrepresented in medical literature, and what was there was largely STD-related. Our review of the research related to GBT men and MSM and cancer shows that while there is certainly now some research, including on screening, that is not specifically STD-related, much of the cancer research does still focus on STD connections. The preceding discussions reveal areas that continue to need more research. The HIV-associated cancers need attention, but the cancers not related to HIV and other sexually transmitted diseases also need attention, both for the minority of GB men and T persons who are HIV+ and the majority who are not. The general question of how sexual and gender identity, and sexual practices, affect or don't affect men's likelihoods to develop these diverse cancers remains largely unaddressed. Until that is better known, it is difficult to assess whether and, if so, how to direct screening specifically to GB men and T people.

Non-standardized nomenclature and language is one area researchers need to address in order to gather information that will be useful for practice and policy. This is sometimes but not always related to how the sample is obtained and the range of persons included in a particular study. Some studies use GB and T, some use MSM, some use "sexual minority men." Further, the common approach of making comparisons of GBT to presumably or definitively heterosexual samples continues heteronormative hegemony. In fact, most comparative studies compare their findings to samples that are only presumptively heterosexual and, indeed, likely include a subset of G and/or B men. Related to that, there is virtually no data base *specifically* on bisexual men, despite potentially different ranges of sexual behavior, from either exclusively same-sex to exclusively other-sex behaviors.

There is a need to specifically include transgender populations in cancer screening research and recommendations. Not only is more study needed on every aspect of cancer screening among transgender and gender variant people, but "[r]esearchers should make note of all gender categories that exist in a given social formation and avoid the tendency to see gender as a binary system anchored to the categories 'men' and 'women'" ([1], p. 241). In other words, researchers need to be more sophisticated in capturing the various ways that gender variance may affect cancer screening.

One specific problem with work on screening is that much of the research cited above is based on the California Health Interview Survey, which has its own issues of bias (cross-sectional design, limited to California's unique population) and may not be fully generalizable to other geographic areas. Other work is based in New York City, and like California, this region likely has differences from the rest of the country. D'Souza, Cook, Ostrow, Johnson-Hill, Wiley, & Silvestre [28], for example, noted that in just four major metropolitan areas (Los Angeles, Pittsburgh, Chicago, Baltimore) there was a great deal of variation in awareness about screening for anal cancer and the likelihood of being screened. Such differences are probably even larger scale between urban and rural regions, the South and North, the East and West, etc.

Studies sometimes include diversity factors in their sample, whether obvious ones such as age, HIV status, and race, or less obvious ones, such as likelihood to engage in anoreceptive sex [28], access to health insurance [18] and living situation [23]. Yet, in many studies, such factors often are omitted. More attention to different types of diversity in identity and practices is needed. One example may be the question of whether age is related to screening behaviors. Age is inextricably linked with a cohort divide between those GBT men who grew up before both the Stonewall Rebellion and subsequent gay rights movements (and, thus, were criminals just for having sex with men) *and* the rise of HIV/AIDS, especially among gay men, and those who grew up after those events [44]. Current age as related to cohort thus affects a wide range of factors having to do with vast differences in likelihood of outness, relationship to doctors, and the degree to which HIV/AIDS dominates GBT individuals' view of health care. Also relevant is whether health care providers may make *a priori* assumptions that if a patient self-identifies as gay, then AIDS is a major concern. These factors will affect whether or not the men are referred for and can access appropriate screening.

The nature of different men's diverse needs for screening is an area of needed research. An example that is relevant to at least a subset of GB men more than to the general population concerns anal cancer. Questions have been raised as to whether repeat screening is called for [45], and if so, the best interval times for repeat screenings [6, 22]. More research needs to be conducted on effective screening practices, highlighted by the fairly low accuracy rate of the anal Pap smear [46]. These authors state that screening for anal cancer increases longevity and quality of life, but Oon and Winter [47] contest this assumption. Their review of anal screening and cancer treatment led them to conclude that treating anal cancer at all is problematic due to quite negative side effects and a high recurrence rate. Obviously such questions need further research. This is similar to the USPSTF [5] logic related to prostate cancer screening and their decision to recommend against it in any mass screening way.

Finally, although, as noted, the anal Pap smear seems to have comparatively low accuracy, and the anal cancer it helps identify may not be easily treatable, it is one method that can actually be done by men at home. Lampinen et al. [45] performed an evaluation of the efficacy of the self-swab, comparing them to physician-taken swabs. They noted that physician Paps (92 % usable) were higher quality, but self-swabs were reasonably comparable (83 %). Any kind of screening, especially of the anogenital region, that men can do in privacy and/or more cheaply than in a clinical setting is worth researching and developing further.

Practice

In general, clinicians must be well-trained in risk factors and screening practices in order to effectively care for their patients. Yet not all clinicians have sufficient knowledge of GB men's or T people's health needs or comfort levels with the types of screening practices required. For example, Oon and Winter note the lack of clinicians trained to do anal screening (in Ireland), as do Newman, Roberts, Masongsong, & Wiley [25] and Goldstone & Moshier [22] (in the U.S.). Pitts, Couch, & Smith [48] make the very good point that clinicians cannot assume that men, even men with wives and children, do not or have not had sex with men. They advocate asking about past and present practices rather than identity in order to determine risk and screening needs. As with the example of anal screening, some of the implications for practice are specifically related to cancer screening, although much is simply related to better practice with GBT men, specifically, or even more generally with LGBT populations [16, 42].

Related to practice, many theorists have discussed—and developed models about—why people do or do not practice healthy behaviors, see doctors, and adhere to medications (see [49] for an overview and [50–52] for examples of such models). Most of these include an individual component of some sort—such as attitudes toward health care, trust, appraisals of threat, illness models, general personal approach to life, etc.—and contextual or external ones, many of which are structural. One of the foremost of the latter is access, which includes both availability of insurance and availability of providers who are sensitive and welcoming, and the ability to pay for those providers. Lack of positive individual or external factors (such as social support, welcoming providers) and/or presence of negative ones (such as stigma) will lead to lower compliance with screening, as with other medical advice and recommendations for self-health. Importantly, the impact of negative factors related to people's likelihood to receive quality health care is likely to be exacerbated among LGBT persons [15, 16].

Advocating with insurers to provide adequate coverage for recommended practices would be ideal. Lindsey, DeCristofaro, & James [46], for example, discussing whether or not to screen for anal cancer, observe that the Pap smear is less accurate than biopsies. The authors note, however, that many insurers will not pay for DNA testing for HPV should a man's swab turn up positive, as the procedure is not FDA-approved for men [53], as it is for women's cervical Paps. Clinicians can do more to reach out to populations at risk. Newman, Roberts, Masongsong, & Wiley [25] asked their sample of community health professionals for recommendations about the anal Pap and they were: public awareness campaigns among men of diverse backgrounds, enhanced medical training, and non-clinical sites for screening, including bars, at home, or even in clinical settings, but as routine parts of check-ups.

Speaking specifically to anal cancer, given concerns with masculinity, including in GBT populations (see [25] for discussion of masculinity), any test that seems feminized is likely to be unpopular. Calling the anal Pap smear a "Pap smear," linked as the phrase is with women's health, may challenge men's comfort levels. Even the word 'smear' may trigger fears about hygiene (see [25] for a discussion of such concerns). We recommend paying attention to language as much as possible. Interestingly, also related to concerns about perceptions of masculinity, a number of gay men in our study [30, 54] expressed specific discomfort about the penetration required during the DRE (digital rectal exam) for prostate cancer. Their concerns primarily centered around the clinicians' potential perceptions of them as gay men "enjoying" the exam too much.

Also, it is important to note that those who have undergone significant surgical procedures to alter their anatomical sex may be unaware that their bodies as women possess a prostate or their bodies as men possess ovaries and a uterus. Thus, prostate screening for transsexual women and gynecological cancer screening for transsexual men is needed: if the organ is there, it should be screened [55]. While these types of cancer screenings are anatomy-specific, they can be unsettling or disruptive to the patient's gender identity [56]. These screenings can be performed in a manner that is sensitive and affirming to the patient's gender identity within the wide range of gender identities and gender and sexual expression [39, 40, 55]. This also may hold for those who may not have had any significant surgery but feel uncomfortable with getting genital and reproductive cancer screening due to their preferred gender presentation and feelings about their gender identity.

Health practitioners, due either to their bias, discomfort, or simply to their lack of knowledge of how to approach these types of screening exams, may not be able or willing to provide appropriate services. While in the last few decades the medical and health care system has recognized the need for cultural competence in screening and treatment of diverse racial/ethnic groups, a similar campaign is needed to address the variety of sexual identities, gender identities, gender performances and their relationships to cancer screening.

Seeking or accessing screening can be obstructed by common gender assumptions. Practitioners and staff need to be aware of how the physical environment, the forms to be filled out, and the language used can obstruct cancer screening in gender and sexual minorities. Cancer screenings that: are unigender-focused (i.e., screening materials/outreach aimed at "men"); involve unigender environments such as waiting rooms with only depictions of men dealing with that cancer and materials assuming and portraying only males in heteronormative relationships; are in sites with no unisex bathrooms available; and/or employ clinical staff who use language and behavior reinforcing conventional ideas of gender, regardless of patient/client preferences, will all inhibit many individuals' interest in disclosing their sexual and gender identities and their likelihood to follow through on screening at such sites. Instead, screening sites and all clinical settings need to actively create an environment that is inclusive. It also must be physically safe and secure, particularly for transgender and gender variant people, who suffer aggravated rates of violence [57], to enter and use. This includes staff being prepared to address inappropriate comments, behaviors, and/or abuse by other patients.

There is also a danger in only seeing specific cancers, such as anal cancer, as relevant for screening MSM or trans people or a sub-segment of those populations, while ignoring all other cancer screenings or cancer risks. Therefore, people in these populations need to be addressed as whole human beings with a range of cancer screening needs. Fundamentally, improving cancer screening among sexual and gender minority populations involves addressing general assumptions about gender and sexuality and the heteronormativity still embedded in health research, medical practices and clinical settings [16, 42].

Policy

The Institute of Medicine [16] recently focused attention on health issues related to LGBT populations, and in the process highlighted a number of policy areas that address specific lacks of inclusion in research, lack of sensitivity in communication between doctors and LGBT patients, and problems with access to quality care. Even more recently, a National Summit on Cancer in LGBT Communities convened in New York City in early 2014. One of the foci of the Summit was policy, and a number of policy issues were identified. While proceedings of the conference have not yet been distributed, discussion of policy, specifically related to screening, identified issues similar to those we have included in this review. As was the case with implications for practice, suggestions from the Institute of Medicine [16], other commentators and from our review range across alterations in policy that concern broad changes in research and practice, encompassing the health of populations such as gay and bisexual men and transgender people [16, 42], while others are more specific to cancer, specific cancers, and/or GBT men.

After reviewing the literature we call for funding for more research on effective screening, screening intervals, relative benefits and risks of screening, and screening training, especially how to direct appropriate screening messages to GB men, MSM, and transgender people. This can be accomplished by inclusion of these groups in studies on ways to evaluate the value of screening for different cancers and on ways to develop interventions that either encourage the use of standard screening practices or more aggressively target specific sub-groups for screening who may have specific behavioral risk factors. Campaigns on prevention, such as male vaccination for HPV, should be developed and presented in a systematic way.

It is important to reiterate that the discussion of cancer screening in the context of MSM and GBT people quickly becomes part of a broader discussion—of the value of screening in general and its applicability to all men; of the relationship of screening to risk factors that include biological, life style, and institutional aspects; of barriers to access to health care generally and in the specific circumstances of having a non-majority sexual or gender identity; and of the relationships among all persons and their health care providers. The challenge remains to integrate appropriate cancer screening activities and interventions directed specifically to gay men, bisexual men, and transgender and gender variant persons.

Acknowledgements The authors express appreciation for the assistance of Besnik Qeriqi in the preparation of this chapter.

References

1. Ochoa M. Latina/o transpopulations. In: Asencio M, Editor. Latina/o sexualities: probing powers, passions, practices, and policies. New Brunswick: Rutgers University Press; 2010. pp. 230–42.
2. Young RM, Meyer IH. The trouble with "MSM" and "WSW": erasure of the sexual-minority person in public health discourse. Am J Public Health. 2005;95(7):1144–9.
3. Centers for disease control and prevention. Age-adjusted cancer death rates for the 10 primary sites with the highest rates within race- and ethnic-specific categories. http://apps.nccd.cdc.gov/uscs/toptencancers.aspx. Accessed 2 November 2013.
4. Centers for disease control and prevention. Leading causes of death in males United States. 2009. http://www.cdc.gov/men/lcod/2009/index.htm. Accessed 2 November 2013.
5. Moyer VA. Screening for prostate cancer: US preventive services task force recommendation statement. Ann Intern Med. 2012;157(2):120–34.
6. Mani D, Aboulafia DM. Screening guidelines for non-AIDS defining cancers in HIV-infected individuals. Curr Opin Oncol. 2013;25(5):518–25.
7. Boehmer U, Ozonoff A, Miao X. An ecological analysis of colorectal cancer incidence and mortality: differences by sexual orientation. BMC Cancer. 2011;11:400.
8. Boehmer U, Cooley TP, Clark MA. Cancer and men who have sex with men: a systematic review. Lancet Oncol. 2012;13(12):e545–53.

9. Boehmer U, Ozonoff A, Miao X. An ecological approach to examine lung cancer disparities due to sexual orientation. Public Health. 2012;126(7):605–12.
10. Chin-Hong PV, Vittinghoff E, Cranston RD, Browne L, Buchbinder S, Colfax G, et al. Age-related prevalence of anal cancer precursors in homosexual men: the EXPLORE study. J Natl Cancer Inst. 2005;97(12):896–905.
11. National Cancer Institute. HIV infection and cancer risk. http://www.cancer.gov/cancertopics/factsheet/risk/hiv-infection. Accessed 2 November 2013.
12. Shiels MS, Pfeiffer RM, Gail MH, Hall HI, Li J, Chaturvedi AK, et al. Cancer burden in the HIV-infected population in the United States. J Natl Cancer Inst. 2011;103(9):753–62.
13. Simard EP, Pfeiffer RM, Engels EA. Cumulative incidence of cancer among individuals with acquired immunodeficiency syndrome in the United States. Cancer. 2011;117(5):1089–96.
14. Shiels MS, Goedert JJ, Moore RD, Platz EA, Engels EA. Reduced risk of prostate cancer in U.S. men with AIDS. Cancer Epidemiol Biomark Prev. 2010;19(11):2910–5.
15. Fredriksen-Goldsen KI. Resilience and disparities among lesbian, gay, bisexual, and transgender older adults. Public Policy Aging Rep 2011;21(3):3–7.
16. Institute of Medicine. Health of lesbian, gay, bisexual, and transgender people: building a foundation for better understanding. Washington, D. C.: National Academies Press; 2011.
17. Boehmer U. Twenty years of public health research: inclusion of lesbian, gay, bisexual, and transgender populations. Am J Public Health. 2002;92(7):1125–30.
18. Boehmer U, Miao X, Ozonoff A. Cancer survivorship and sexual orientation. Cancer. 2011;117(16):3796–804.
19. Heslin KC, Gore JL, King WD, Fox SA. Sexual orientation and testing for prostate and colorectal cancers among men in California. Med Care. 2008;46(12):1240–8.
20. Frisch M, Fenger C, van den Brule AJ, Sorensen P, Meijer CJ, Walboomers JM, et al. Variants of squamous cell carcinoma of the anal canal and perianal skin and their relation to human papillomaviruses. Cancer Res. 1999;59(3):753–7.
21. Frisch M, Glimelius B, van den Brule AJ, Wohlfahrt J, Meijer CJ, Walboomers JM, et al. Sexually transmitted infection as a cause of anal cancer. N Engl J Med. 1997;337(19):1350–8.
22. Goldstone SE, Moshier E. Detection of oncogenic human papillomavirus impacts anal screening guidelines in men who have sex with men. Dis Colon Rectum. 2010;53(8):1135–42.
23. Boehmer U, Miao X, Linkletter C, Clark MA. Adult health behaviors over the life course by sexual orientation. Am J Public Health. 2012;102(2):292–300.
24. Durso LE, Meyer IH. Patterns and predictors of disclosure of sexual orientation to healthcare providers among lesbians, gay men, and bisexuals. Sex Res Soc Policy. 2013;10(1):35–42.
25. Newman PA, Roberts KJ, Masongsong E, Wiley DJ. Anal cancer screening: barriers and facilitators among ethnically diverse gay, bisexual, transgender, and other men who have sex with men. J Gay Lesbian Soc Serv. 2008;20(4):328–53.
26. Blackwell CW, Eden C. Human papillomavirus and anorectal carcinoma knowledge in men who have sex with men. J Assoc Nurses AIDS Care. 2011;22(6):444–53.
27. Seay J, Sadiq T, Roytburd K, Menezes P, Quinlivan EB. High acceptance rate of anal pap screening despite limited knowledge about anal dysplasia among HIV MSM. Infect Agents Cancer. 2010;5(Suppl 1):A31.
28. D'Souza G, Cook RL, Ostrow D, Johnson-Hill LM, Wiley D, Silvestre T. Anal cancer screening behaviors and intentions in men who have sex with men. J Gen Intern Med. 2008;23(9):1452–7.
29. Reed AC, Reiter PL, Smith JS, Palefsky JM, Brewer NT. Gay and bisexual men's willingness to receive anal Papanicolaou testing. Am J Public Health. 2010;100(6):1123–9.
30. Blank TO, Asencio M, Descartes L, Griggs J. Aging, health, and GLBTQ family and community life. J GLBT Fam Stud. 2009;5(1–2):9–34.
31. National Center for Transgender Equality. Transgender terminology. 2014. http://transequality.org/Resources/TransTerminology_2014.pdf. Accessed 2 April 2014.
32. Dozier R. Beards, breasts, and bodies doing sex in a gendered world. Gend Soc. 2005;19(3):297–316.
33. Rosser BS, Oakes JM, Bockting WO, Miner M. Capturing the social demographics of hidden sexual minorities: an internet study of the transgender population in the United States. Sex Res Soc Policy. 2007;4(2):50–64.

34. Bockting WO, Robinson BE, Forberg J, Scheltema K. Evaluation of a sexual health approach to reducing HIV/STD risk in the transgender community. AIDS Care. 2005;17(3):289–303.
35. Stephen L. Sexualities and genders in Zapotec Oaxaca. Lat Am Perspect. 2002;29(2):41–59.
36. Herdt G. Same sex, different cultures: exploring gay and lesbian lives. Boulder: Westview Press; 1997.
37. Tan ML. Survival through pluralism: emerging gay communities in the Philippines. J Homosex. 2001;40(3–4):117–42.
38. Gooren L, Asscheman H. Sex reassignment: endocrinological interventions in adults with gender dysphoria. In: Kreukels BPC, Steesma T., deVries ALC, Editors. Gender dysphoria and disorders of sex development. New York: Springer; 2014. pp. 277–97.
39. Weyers S, Decaestecker K, Verstraelen H, Monstrey S, T'Sjoen G, Gerris J, et al. Clinical and transvaginal sonographic evaluation of the prostate in transsexual women. Urology. 2009;74(1):191–6.
40. Weyers S, Villeirs G, Vanherreweghe E, Verstraelen H, Monstrey S, Van den Broecke R, et al. Mammography and breast sonography in transsexual women. Eur J Radiol. 2010;74(3):508–13.
41. Kreukels BPC, Steensma T, de Vries ALC. Gender dysphoria and disorders of sex development. New York: Springer; 2014.
42. National Center for Transgender Equality and National Gay and Lesbian Task Force. National transgender discrimination survey report on health and health care. http://www.thetaskforce.org/static_html/downloads/reports/reports/ntds_report_on_health.pdf. Accessed 6 November 2013.
43. American Council of Obstetricians and Gynecologists (ACOG). Ob-gyns prepare to treat transgender patients. 2011. http://www.acog.org/About_ACOG/News_Room/News_Releases/2011/Ob-Gyns_Prepare_to_Treat_Transgender_Patients. Accessed 28 March 2014.
44. de Vries B. LG (BT) persons in the second half of life: the intersectional influences of stigma and cohort. LGBT Health. 2014;1(1):18–23.
45. Lampinen TM, Miller ML, Chan K, Anema A, van Niekerk D, Schilder AJ, et al. Randomized clinical evaluation of self-screening for anal cancer precursors in men who have sex with men. Cytojournal. 2006;3:4.
46. Lindsey K, DeCristofaro C, James J. Anal pap smears: should we be doing them? J Am Acad Nurse Pract. 2009;21(8):437–43.
47. Oon SF, Winter DC. Perianal condylomas, anal squamous intraepithelial neoplasms and screening: a review of the literature. J Med Screen. 2010;17(1):44–9.
48. Pitts MK, Couch MA, Smith AM. Men who have sex with men (MSM): how much to assume and what to ask? Med J Aust. 2006;185(8):450–2.
49. Dunbar-Jacob JM, Berg, J, Evangelista LS, Carruthers D. Adherence. In: Lubkin IM, Larsen PD Editors. Chronic illness: impact and intervention 8 ed. Sudbury MA: Jones and Bartlett Learning; 2011. pp 207–241.
50. Andersen R, Newman JF. Societal and individual determinants of medical care utilization in the United States. Milbank Mem Fund Q Health Soc. 1973;51(1):95–124.
51. Leventhal H, Brissette I, Leventhal EA. The common sense model of self-regulation of health and illness. In: Cameron L, Leventhal H, Editors. The self-regulation of health and illness behavior. New York: Routledge; 2003. pp 42–65.
52. Prochaska JO, Velicer WF. The transtheoretical model of health behavior change. Am J Health Promot. 1997;12(1):38–48.
53. Labcorp. Anal (rectal) cytology, liquid-based preparation. 2007. http://www.labcorp.com/dos/index.html. Accessed 4 Dec 2007.
54. Asencio M, Blank T, Descartes L, Crawford A. The prospect of prostate cancer: a challenge for gay men's sexualities as they age. Sex Res Soc Policy J NSRC. 2009;6(4):38–51.
55. Sobralske M. Primary care needs of patients who have undergone gender reassignment. J Am Acad Nurse Pract. 2005;17(4):133–8.
56. Robinson F. Raising awareness of cervical cancer. Pract Nurse. 2010;40(6):10–1.
57. Kenagy GP. Transgender health: findings from two needs assessment studies in Philadelphia. Health Soc Work. 2005;30(1):19–26.

Part III
Cancer Survivorship

Chapter 8
What Are the Numbers? The Epidemiology of Cancer by Sexual Orientation and Gender Identity

Madina Agénor

Abstract The lack of information on sexual orientation and gender identity in cancer registries has prevented epidemiologists from assessing cancer disparities related to these dimensions of social inequality at the individual level. Nonetheless, researchers in North America and Europe have conducted studies to estimate sexual orientation and gender identity disparities in the risk of developing or dying of certain cancers, some of which provide evidence of a higher burden of cancer among lesbian, gay, bisexual, and transgender (LGBT) populations. Specifically, U.S. investigators have found a positive association between same-sex partner household density and the incidence of breast (among women), colorectal (among women and men), and lung (among men only) cancers at the county level. At the individual level, research shows that breast cancer incidence may be slightly higher among lesbian and bisexual women relative to heterosexual women, and that the incidence of anal cancer may be higher among men who have sex with men compared to men in general. Some studies have also suggested that transgender women receiving hormone therapy may be at higher risk than the population in general of dying of lung and blood cancers. Additional research is needed to identify the long-term effect of estrogen and testosterone on the risk of developing hormone-related tumors among transgender women and men receiving hormone therapy. Further, studies that consider the influence of the lifecourse and contextual factors on outcomes along the full cancer continuum, include LGBT people of color and low-income LGBT individuals, and focus on populations in developing countries are needed.

Introduction

Given the absence of information on sexual orientation and gender identity in cancer registries [1, 2], epidemiologic research on the prevalence, incidence, and mortality of cancer among lesbian, gay, bisexual, and transgender (LGBT) populations

M. Agénor (✉)
Department of Social and Behavioral Sciences,
Harvard T.H. Chan School of Public Health, Boston, MA, USA
e-mail: magenor@mail.harvard.edu

U. Boehmer, R. Elk (eds.), *Cancer and the LGBT Community*,
DOI 10.1007/978-3-319-15057-4_8

is limited. However, studies suggest that sexual (i.e., lesbian, gay, and bisexual individuals) and gender (i.e., transgender individuals) minorities may be at increased risk of developing or dying of certain malignancies compared to the population in general and their heterosexual and cisgender counterparts in particular. Cancer risk factors that disproportionately affect LGBT individuals throughout the lifecourse include cigarette smoking, alcohol use, overweight and obesity (among women and girls only), sexual risk behaviors, and low levels of cancer screening services use [3–7]. The vast majority of research on cancer and the LGBT community pertains to these risk factors, on which, unlike cancer outcomes, high-quality, individual-level data exist. Studies examining sexual orientation and gender identity disparities in cancer risk factors are reviewed in Chaps. 2, 3, 4, and 5 of this book.

While cancer risk factors do not necessarily translate into cancer outcomes, several investigators have hypothesized that, based on the elevated level of cancer-related indicators among sexual and gender minorities, LGBT individuals may be at higher risk than their heterosexual counterparts of developing cancer, including breast tumors [3–5, 8–12]. In recent years, several researchers have assessed sexual orientation disparities in observed and predicted breast cancer risk and many have found some evidence of a higher risk of developing the malignancy among lesbians relative to their heterosexual counterparts [11, 13–17]. Moreover, research findings show that men who have sex with men (MSM), especially those living with human immunodeficiency virus (HIV) infection [18], have an excess incidence of anal cancer relative to men in general [13, 19–22] and a higher risk of developing the disease compared to non-MSM [23, 24]. Further, scientists have posited that transgender individuals who obtain hormone therapy may be more likely than cisgender persons to develop hormone-related tumors, including breast, prostate, and endometrial cancers [25–27]. Research on the relationship between gender identity and cancer outcomes is in its infancy, and existing studies present methodological limitations that make it difficult to ascertain the long-term effect of exposure to estrogen and testosterone on cancer incidence among transgender populations receiving hormone therapy [25–27].

In this chapter, I review the available evidence on the burden of cancer—namely, breast, anal, colorectal, lung, and reproductive cancers—among LGBT populations and highlight who and what is missing from this literature. I conclude by identifying the implications of these findings for population health research, healthcare policy, and clinical and public health practice.

What Do We Know about the Epidemiology of Cancer by Sexual Orientation?

Sexual Orientation and Breast Cancer

Breast cancer is the most common cancer (other than skin cancer) and second leading cause of cancer death among U.S. women [28], with age-adjusted incidence and mortality rates of 123.8 and 22.6 per 100,000 women per year, respectively, between 2006 and 2010 [29]. The American Cancer Society estimated that, in 2014, approximately 232,670 new cases of invasive breast cancer would be diagnosed in the United States and about 40,000 U.S. women would die of the disease [28]. Studies show that, among U.S. women, pronounced inequities exist in breast cancer incidence and mortality by race/ethnicity, socioeconomic position (SEP), and geographic location [30, 31]. Several investigators have hypothesized that lesbian and bisexual women may be at greater risk of developing breast cancer compared to heterosexual women as a result of a higher prevalence of breast cancer risk factors, including nulliparity, alcohol use, and obesity [3–5, 8–12]. However, given the lack of information on sexual orientation in cancer registries [1, 2], epidemiologic research on sexual orientation disparities in breast cancer remains scarce [8]. Nonetheless, scientists have employed novel strategies to ascertain the relationship between sexual orientation and breast cancer prevalence, incidence, and mortality among women [32].

Breast Cancer Prevalence

In a U.S. study of predominately white women aged 50–79 years, Valanis et al. [3] found that "lifetime" lesbians (defined as women with only female sexual partners in their lifetime; prevalence [pr] = 5.8 %), "adult" lesbians (defined as women with only female sexual partners after age 45 years; pr = 7.0 %), and bisexual women (defined as women with both male and female sexual partners in their lifetime; pr = 8.4 %) each had a higher self-reported prevalence of breast cancer than heterosexual women (defined as women with only male sexual partners in their lifetime; pr = 4.9 %). In contrast, using pooled data from the 2001, 2003, and 2005 California Health Interview Survey (CHIS), Boehmer and colleagues [33] found no statistically significant sexual orientation differences in the self-reported prevalence of breast cancer among California women aged 18–85 years ($p = 0.28$). Similarly, analyses by Cochran and colleagues [4] showed that the self-reported prevalence of breast cancer derived from seven independently conducted surveys of predominately white (86 %) lesbian and bisexual women aged 18–75 years (pr = 0.9 %; 95 % confidence interval [CI]: 0.8 %, 1.1 %) did not differ from the standardized self-reported prevalence of breast cancer among U.S. women in general, estimated using National Health and Nutrition Examination Survey III data (pr = 0.9 %; 95 % CI: 0.4 %, 1.3 %). However, the authors cautioned that their study may have underestimated lesbian and bisexual women's prevalence of breast cancer, for which the median age at diagnosis between 2006 and 2010 was 61 years [29], as a result of the sample's relatively young mean age (36 years) [4].

Breast Cancer Incidence

Because prevalence only captures existing cases of disease at a given point in time [34], this measure may underestimate the burden of breast cancer among lesbian and bisexual women if they have a higher breast cancer mortality rate than heterosexual women [4]. Thus, incidence, which reflects the development of new cases of disease over a specified period of time [34], provides more accurate information about how sexual orientation shapes the population distribution of breast cancer independently of survival. Using standardized incidence ratios, Frisch et al. [13] found that, in Denmark, breast cancer incidence among women aged 18–80 years (median age: 37 years) in a registered same-sex partnership between 1989 and 1997 was similar to that of women in general (standardized incidence ratio [SIR]=0.9; 95 % CI: 0.4, 1.9). In the United States, the Surveillance, Epidemiology, and End Results (SEER) Program of the National Cancer Institute, which collects surveillance data on cancer incidence from population-based cancer registries that capture approximately 28 % of the U.S. population [35], does not provide information on sexual orientation [1, 2]. As a result, researchers are unable to assess sexual orientation disparities in breast cancer incidence among U.S. women using information from the SEER Program alone. In order to address this gap in knowledge, Boehmer and colleagues [14] linked 1996 to 2004 SEER data on the incidence of breast cancer and 2000 U.S. Census data on the density of female same-sex partner households, which they used as a surrogate for lesbian population density. This study showed that, at the county level, a one-unit increase in the density of adult women living with a same-sex partner was associated with a 13 % higher age-adjusted breast cancer incidence rate, accounting for county-level race/ethnicity and federal poverty level (incidence rate ratio [IRR]=1.13; 95 % CI: 1.11, 1.16) [14].

In recent years, researchers have used mathematical prediction models to estimate sexual orientation group differences in a woman's probability of developing breast cancer during a specified period of time based on her age and other known risk factors [17, 36]. Applying the National Surgical Adjuvant Breast and Bowel Project (NSABP)-modified Gail breast cancer risk model [37] to cross-sectional data, Dibble et al. [15] found that predominately white self-identified lesbians aged 40 years and over living in California between 1999 and 2002 had a slightly higher five-year (1.2 % vs. 1.07 %, $p<0.001$) and lifetime (11.1 % vs. 10.4 %, $p=0.001$) risk of developing breast cancer than their heterosexual sisters. Using survey data collected between 1994 and 1996 among predominately white adult (mean age: 43 years) women living in Chicago, New York, and Minneapolis, Brandenburg et al. [16] found that the five-year (0.96 % vs. 0.85 %, $p<0.05$) and lifetime (11.6 % vs. 10.7 %, $p<0.05$) predicted risk of developing breast cancer, which they calculated using the Gail model, was significantly higher for lesbians (defined as women who were only or mostly attracted to and sexually active with women or not sexually active in the past year) relative to heterosexual women (defined as women who were only or mostly attracted to and sexually active with men or not sexually active in the past year). The direction and statistical significance of these associations persisted in linear regression models adjusting for education, race/ethnicity, and study site [16]. In 2012, Austin and colleagues [17] published the first study to estimate sexual orientation group differences in a woman's predicted risk of developing breast cancer using longitudinal data. Applying a modified version of the Rosner-Colditz risk prediction model, which accounts for risk factors that vary by age and reproductive history, the researchers found that, among predominately white (94 %) premenopausal women aged 25–58 years who participated in the Nurses' Health Study II between 1989 and 2005, the predicted breast cancer incidence rate was slightly higher among lesbian (IRR = 1.06; 95% CI: 1.06, 1.06) and bisexual women (IRR = 1.10; 95% CI: 1.10, 1.10) relative to heterosexual women [17].

In contrast, other studies have found no statistically significant association between sexual orientation and breast cancer risk. Using data from a population-based case-control study of women aged 21–45 years living in the state of Washington, Kavanaugh-Lynch et al. [11] found no significant difference in the odds, which approximate risk when the outcome is rare [34], of breast cancer between lesbians (defined as women who never had a male sexual partner) and women with male lifetime sexual partners (odds ratio [OR] = 1.74; 95% CI: 0.62, 4.91). However, the number of lesbians in this study was small (sample size [n] = 18, 10 cases and 8 controls) and results may not be precise. Further, adjusting for age, race/ethnicity, employment, and disability status, Roberts et al. [38] found similar odds of having ever received a breast cancer diagnosis (OR = 1.00; 95% CI: 0.21–4.80) between predominately white (70%) self-identified lesbian and heterosexual women aged 35–75 years (mean age: 43 years) who received care at Lyon-Martin Women's Health Services in San Francisco, CA between 1995 and 1997. Using the NSABP-modified Gail model, McTiernan and colleagues [36] assessed sexual orientation disparities in predicted breast cancer risk in a Seattle-based sample of 491 women aged 18–74 years with a family history of breast cancer. In this cross-sectional study, the authors did not find self-identified lesbians (n = 65, mean Gail risk to age 79 years: 13.2) to be at higher risk of developing breast cancer than women in general (n = 317, mean Gail risk to age 79 years: 14.2) [36].

Breast Cancer Mortality

In a recent study, Cochran and Mays [39] used 1997 to 2003 National Health Interview Survey and National Death Index data to investigate possible sexual orientation differences in breast cancer mortality risk among U.S. women aged 18–80 years, the majority of whom were between 18 and 44 years of age. Adjusting for age, the researchers found some evidence of a greater risk of dying of breast cancer among women married to or cohabitating with a same-sex partner, who were presumed to be lesbian or bisexual, relative to women married to or cohabitating with a different-sex partner, who were presumed to be heterosexual (Cox proportional hazard ratio [HR] = 3.2; 95% CI: 1.01, 10.21) [39].

Sexual Orientation and Anal Cancer

Between 2006 and 2010, the age-adjusted anal cancer incidence rate was 1.5 per 100,000 persons per year among U.S. men in general, with an estimated 7,060 new cases and 880 deaths in 2013 [40, 41]. However, research shows that the population distribution of anal cancer incidence varies by sexual orientation, with MSM, especially those living with HIV infection [18], at elevated risk of developing the disease [19]. In a 2012 meta-analysis, which included nine studies of anal cancer incidence among MSM (two of which provided data on HIV-negative MSM), Machalek and colleagues [19] found a pooled anal cancer incidence rate of 5.1 per 100,000 men per year (95% CI: 0.0, 11.5 per 100,000 person-years, n=48,881) among HIV-negative MSM; the rate among HIV-positive MSM was considerably higher at 45.9 per 100,000 men per year (95% CI: 31.2, 60.3 per 100,000 person-years, n=956,095). In a study of 6972 MSM who participated in the U.S. Multicenter AIDS Cohort Study between 1984 and 2006, D'Souza et al. [18] found an overall anal cancer incidence rate of 37 per 100,000 men per year (95% CI: 25, 53 per 100,000 person-years) among MSM in general—with an incidence rate of 14 per 100,000 men per year (95% CI: 6, 30 per 100,000 person-years) among HIV-negative MSM and 69 per 100,000 men per year (95% CI: 46, 105 per 100,000 person-years) among HIV-positive MSM in particular. Among HIV-infected men who participated in cohort studies from the United States and Canada between 1996 and 2007, Silverberg and colleagues [42] found that the incidence rate of anal cancer was significantly higher among MSM (incidence rate [IR]=131; 95% CI: 109, 157 per 100,000 person-years) relative to other men (namely, heterosexual men, men who use intravenous drugs, and men with another HIV risk factor) (IRR=3.3; 95% CI: 1.8, 6.0 per 100,000 person-years).

Given the absence of data on sexual orientation in cancer registries [1, 2], no study has directly assessed disparities in anal cancer incidence among MSM among men overall relative to men who have sex with women only. In order to address this gap in the literature, Piketty et al. [23] examined sexual orientation disparities in anal cancer risk among HIV-positive men using data from the French Hospital Database on HIV. The researchers found that, between 1992 and 2004, the anal cancer risk among HIV-positive men was significantly higher among HIV-positive MSM compared to HIV-positive non-MSM (HR=3.0; 95% CI: 2.0, 4.5). Estimating risk using odds [34], Daling and colleagues [24] found that, among men aged less than 75 years living in the Seattle area between 1986 and 1998, MSM had a significantly higher risk of anal cancer than men who reported having sex with women only (OR=17.3; 95% CI: 8.2, 36.1). Providing evidence about the mechanism driving the elevated risk of anal cancer among MSM relative to non-MSM, Daling et al. [24] found that, receptive anal intercourse—during which human papillomavirus (HPV) types that have been linked to anal cancer can be transmitted [43]—was positively related to the risk of anal cancer among both men (OR=6.8; 95% CI: 1.4, 33.8) and women (OR=2.2; 95% CI: 1.4, 3.3).

Given the lack of population-based data on anal cancer incidence by sexual orientation, several investigators have compared the risk of developing anal cancer among MSM to that of men in general. Using standardized incidence ratios, Koblin and colleagues [20] found that the age-adjusted anal cancer incidence among predominately white MSM living in New York City and San Francisco between 1978 and 1990 (mean age: 29.6 years) was significantly higher than that of adult U.S. men in general, which the authors estimated using 1984 to 1988 SEER data (SIR=24.2, 95% CI: 13.5, 39.9). Similarly, Chaturvedi et al.'s [21] findings showed that, in nine U.S. states and six U.S. metropolitan regions, the incidence of invasive anal cancer was significantly higher among MSM aged 15 years and older who were diagnosed with HIV between 1980 and 2004 relative to men in general (SIR=51.8, 95% CI: 45.3, 59.0). Further, in Denmark, Frisch et al. [13] found that, overall, men aged 18–87 years (median age: 38 years) in a registered same-sex partnership between 1989 and 1997 (n=3,391) had a 31 times greater incidence of anal cancer than men in general (SIR=31.2; 95% CI: 8.4, 79.8). For HIV-negative men with a same-sex registered partner in particular (n=3,054) relative to men in general, the standardized incidence ratio was 16.7 (95% CI: 1.9, 60.2) [13]. In Italy, Dal Maso and colleagues [22] found that HIV-positive MSM had a 47 times greater risk of developing anal cancer between 1997 and 2004 compared to men in general (SIR=47.0; 95% CI: 8.9, 139).

Sexual Orientation and Colorectal Cancer

Colorectal Cancer Prevalence

Colorectal cancer is the third most common cancer among U.S. women and men [44], with an age-adjusted incidence rate of 45 per 100,000 persons per year between 2006 and 2010 [45]. The American Cancer Society estimates that, in 2014, approximately 136,830 cases of colorectal cancer will be diagnosed in the United States and 50,310 U.S. individuals will die of the disease [44]. U.S. studies have identified racial/ethnic and geographic disparities in colorectal cancer incidence and mortality rates [46], and some researchers have investigated whether the prevalence, incidence, and mortality of the disease also differ by sexual orientation. In a multisite study of postmenopausal U.S. women aged 50–79 years, Valanis et al. [3] found that a higher proportion of "lifetime" lesbians (defined as women with only female sexual partners during their adult lifetime; pr=2.1%) reported a history of colorectal cancer relative to heterosexual (defined as women with only male sexual partners during their adult lifetime; pr=0.8%) and bisexual (defined as women with both male and female sexual partners during their adult lifetime; pr=0.8%) women.

Colorectal Cancer Incidence

In a Danish study, Frisch and colleagues [13] found no excess incidence of gastrointestinal cancer, which includes cancers of the colon and rectum, among women in a registered same-sex partnership between 1989 and 1997 relative to women in general (SIR=1.1; 95% CI: 0.2, 3.2). Similarly, the researchers found no difference in the risk of developing cancers of the colon (SIR=0.7; 95% CI: 0.2, 2.1) and rectum (SIR=0.7; 95% CI: 0.1, 2.7) among Danish men in a registered same-sex partnership between 1989 and 1997 and Danish men in general [13]. In a large cohort of predominately (94%) white U.S. women aged 25–64 years, Austin et al. used the Rosner-Wei risk-prediction model to estimate colorectal cancer incidence rate ratios comparing lesbians and bisexual women to their heterosexual counterparts, based on each woman's individual risk factor profile [47]. Adjusting for age, they found no statistically significant relationship between sexual orientation identity and colorectal cancer incidence in this population during the 20-year study period (IRR for lesbian versus heterosexual women = 1.01, 95% CI: 0.99, 1.04; IRR for bisexual versus heterosexual women = 1.01, 95% CI: 0.98, 1.04) [47].

Given that, in the U.S., the SEER Program does not collect information on individuals' sexual orientation, Boehmer et al. [48] conducted an ecological study investigating the county-level association between the density of same-sex partner households using 2000 U.S. Census data, and age-adjusted colorectal cancer incidence using 1996 to 2004 SEER data on 215 U.S. counties. Adjusting for county-level race/ethnicity and federal poverty level, the investigators found a positive relationship between same-sex partner household density, which they used as a surrogate for gay or lesbian population density, and colorectal cancer incidence among U.S. men (IRR = 1.04; 95% CI: 1.02,1.06) and women (IRR = 1.06; 95% CI: 1.01,1.12) at the county level [48].

Colorectal Cancer Mortality

Among U.S. men, Boehmer and colleagues [48] also found that a one unit increase in same-sex partner household density was associated with a 4% higher colorectal cancer mortality rate at the county level (mortality rate ratio [MRR]= 1.04; 95% CI: 1.01,1.08), adjusting for county-level race/ethnicity and federal poverty level. No statistically significant county-level relationship between same-sex partner household density and colorectal cancer mortality was observed among U.S. women (MRR = 1.06; 95% CI: 0.97, 1.15) [48].

Sexual Orientation and Lung Cancer

In the United States, lung cancer is the second most common cancer and leading cause of cancer death among both men and women, with age-adjusted lung cancer incidence and mortality rates of 61.4 and 49.5 per 100,000 persons per year, respectively, between 2006 and 2010 [49]. In 2014, an estimated 224,210 new lung cancer cases will be diagnosed and 159,260 U.S. individuals will die of the disease [50]. U.S. studies show that the population distribution of lung cancer incidence and mortality varies by race/ethnicity and geography [46], and some researchers have investigated whether the risk of developing lung cancer also differs by sexual orientation. In a U.S. ecological study, Boehmer and colleagues [51] found that, at the county level, the density of male same-sex partner households, which they used as a surrogate for gay population density, was positively associated with age-adjusted lung cancer incidence (IRR = 1.05; 95% CI: 1.04, 1.07) and mortality (MRR = 1.03; 95% CI: 1.01, 1.05), controlling for county-level race/ethnicity, federal poverty level, and education.

On the contrary, female same-sex partner household density, which the researchers used as a surrogate for lesbian population density, was inversely related to age-adjusted lung cancer incidence (IRR=0.83; 95 % CI: 0.79, 0.88) and mortality (IRR=0.87; 95 % CI: 0.82, 0.92) at the county level [51]. This finding is contrary to what the investigators expected given that the prevalence of cigarette smoking, the primary cause of lung cancer [52], is higher among both gay/lesbian and bisexual men and women relative to their heterosexual counterparts [53]. However, the authors suggested that the absence of a positive association between the density of female same-sex partner households and lung cancer may be due to the later uptake of smoking among women compared to men [51]. Similarly, in a Danish study, Frisch et al. [13] found no statistically significant difference in lung cancer incidence between women living in a registered same-sex partnership between 1989 and 1997 and women in general (SIR=2.1; 95 % CI: 0.6, 5.4); the researchers found similar results among Danish men (SIR=0.6; 95 % CI: 0.2, 1.4).

Sexual Orientation and Female Reproductive Cancers

In a sample of predominately white U.S. women aged 50–79 years, Valanis and colleagues [3] found a slightly higher self-reported prevalence of cervical cancer among bisexual women (defined as women with both male and female sexual partners in their lifetime; pr=2.1 %) and "lifetime" lesbians (defined as women with only female sexual partners in their lifetime; pr=2.2 %) relative to heterosexual women (defined as women with only male sexual partners in their lifetime; pr=1.3 %). Moreover, using pooled data from the 2001, 2003, and 2005 CHIS, Boehmer et al. [33] found a significantly higher self-reported prevalence of cervical cancer among adult self-identified bisexual women (pr=41.24 %) compared to adult self-identified heterosexual (pr=14.00 %) and lesbian (pr=16.52 %) women ($p<0.0001$) and a significantly higher self-reported prevalence of uterine cancer among self-identified lesbians (pr=11.66 %) relative to self-identified heterosexual (pr=6.45 %) and bisexual (pr=0.45 %) women ($p=0.03$).

In contrast, Frisch and colleagues [13] found no statistically significant difference in the risk of developing cervical (SIR=1.8; 95 % CI: 0.4, 5.2) and uterine (SIR=3.4; 95 % CI: 0.7, 10.0) cancer between Danish women in a registered same-sex partnership between 1989 and 1997 and Danish women in general. Additionally, the investigators' results showed no difference in the incidence of ovarian cancer (SIR=0.9; 95 % CI: 0.0, 4.8) between Danish women in a registered same-sex partnership between 1989 and 1997 and Danish women in general [13]. Lastly, Valanis and colleagues [3] found a lower self-reported prevalence of endometrial cancer among "lifetime" (pr=0.0 %) and adult (pr=1.5 %) lesbians relative to heterosexual women (pr=1.8 %) in a multisite study of predominately white U.S. women aged 50–79 years.

Sexual Orientation and Male Reproductive Cancers

Using pooled 2001, 2003, and 2005 CHIS data, Boehmer and colleagues [33] found statistically significant sexual orientation disparities in the self-reported prevalence of prostate cancer among U.S. men living in California, with a lower prevalence among self-identified gay men (pr = 5.28 %) compared to self-identified heterosexual (pr = 16.47 %) and bisexual (pr = 14.26 %) men ($p = 0.0009$). In Denmark, Frisch et al. [13] found no difference in the risk of developing prostate cancer between men in a registered same-sex partnership between 1989 and 1997 and men in general (SIR = 0.9; 95 % CI: 0.3, 2.4). In a population-based case-control study among predominately white men aged 40–64 years living in King County, Washington, Rosenblatt and colleagues [54] observed no statistically significant relationship between sexual orientation and prostate cancer; however, the numbers of gay and bisexual men and MSM participants were small. To my knowledge, no data are available on the prevalence or incidence of other male reproductive cancers—namely, penile and testicular cancer—by sexual orientation.

What Do we Know about the Epidemiology of Cancer by Gender Identity?

No population-based study has investigated the relationship between gender identity and cancer outcomes, and clinic-based studies on cancer prevalence, incidence, and mortality among transgender populations are scarce. However, a few researchers in Europe have examined whether transgender men and women receiving hormone therapy at a clinic are at higher risk than the general population of developing or dying of cancer. For example, Asscheman et al. [25] assessed whether, compared to the Dutch population in general, total cancer and cancer-specific mortality was elevated among 966 transgender women aged 16–76 years (mean age: 31.4 years) and 365 transgender men aged 16–75 years (mean age: 26.1 years) who received hormone therapy for one to 25 years (median: 18.5 years) at a gender clinic in the Netherlands between 1975 and 2007. The investigators found no evidence of a higher risk of death due to all cancers among transgender women or men relative to the general population [25]. However, they found statistically significant standardized mortality ratios for lung cancer (standardized mortality ratio [SMR] = 1.35; 95 % CI: 1.14, 1.58) and leukemia/lymphoma (SMR = 2.66; 95 % CI: 1.93, 3.60) for transgender women compared to the Dutch population in general, adjusting for age and gender [25]. The research team was not able to adequately assess the risk of dying of specific cancers among transgender men as a result of the population's relatively small size ($n = 365$) and young mean age (26.1 years) [25]. In Belgium, Wierckx et al. [55] conducted a clinic-based case-control study to determine the self-reported prevalence of all cancers among 214 transgender women (mean age: 43.7 years) and 138 transgender men (mean age: 37.5 years) who received hormone therapy at a gender clinic between 1986 and 2012 (mean follow-up: 7.4 years) relative to an age- and gender-matched control population. The researchers found a similar or lower prevalence of cancer among transgender women and men receiving estrogen or testosterone, respectively, compared to the control population [55]. However, they cautioned that these findings may be due to the relatively young age and short duration of hormone exposure among the transgender individuals in their study [55].

Scientists have hypothesized that transgender women receiving hormone therapy may be at elevated risk of developing estrogen-dependent tumors—namely, breast and prostate cancers—as a result of prolonged exposure to the hormone [25–27]. To date, two cases of breast cancer have been reported among transgender women [25–27, 56]. However, Asscheman and colleagues [25] could not assess the risk of developing or dying of breast cancer among transgender women receiving care at their clinic, where only one case had been diagnosed [25–27], because of participants' relatively young age (mean age: 31.4 years) and variable length of hormone therapy (1 to 25 years; median: 18.5 years). Additionally, four cases of prostate cancer have been identified among transgender women [26, 27, 57]; however, whether these tumors were caused by estrogen therapy has not been determined [26, 27]. Lastly, while scientists note that the risk of endometrial cancer is theoretically higher among transgender men receiving testosterone who have not obtained a hysterectomy relative to the population in general, no cases of the malignancy have been reported in this group [27].

Who and What is Missing in Research on the Epidemiology of Cancer by Sexual Orientation and Gender Identity?

Reviewing the literature on the epidemiology of cancer among LGBT populations shows that data on cancer disparities by sexual orientation and gender identity are not available for all types of cancer. Indeed, most studies have assessed how sexual orientation relates to breast cancer, the most common cancer among U.S. women [28], and anal cancer, which disproportionately affects MSM [19], especially those who are infected with HIV [18]. Although lung and colorectal cancer are the second and third most common cancers among U.S. men and women [58], respectively, only a few researchers have investigated sexual orientation disparities in these malignancies [3, 13, 48, 51]. Additionally, limited research exists on how sexual orientation relates to prostate cancer [13, 33, 54], the leading cause of new cancer cases among U.S. men in 2014 [58], and uterine cancer [13, 33], the most common reproductive cancer and fourth leading cause of new cancer cases among U.S. women in 2014 [58]. Further, research investigating the risk of developing specific cancers—including hormone-related breast, prostate, and uterine tumors—among transgender populations receiving hormone therapy is limited by small sample sizes, the relatively young age of transgender women and men using gender-related services, and the short duration of follow-up after hormone therapy in most studies [25–27].

Using the cancer disparities grid developed by Krieger [59], I found that research on the epidemiology of cancer among LGBT populations has not addressed sexual orientation and gender identity disparities along the full cancer continuum, across the lifecourse. While some population-based studies provided estimates of cancer risk behaviors, screening, prevalence, and incidence by sexual orientation, few studies focused on sexual orientation disparities in cancer mortality, and no epidemiologic study has assessed how sexual orientation relates to cancer detection, stage at diagnosis, treatment, or survival. Indeed, the majority of epidemiologic research on sexual orientation and cancer has relied on samples with wide age ranges and a relatively young mean or median age, which prevents investigators from studying outcomes that occur later in the lifecourse, when cancer is more likely to occur [58]. Additionally, given the absence of information on sexual orientation in cancer registries [1, 2], studies have used standardized incidence and mortality ratios to compare cancer incidence and mortality rates among LGBT populations to those among the population in general, which includes sexual and gender minorities and thus does not provide an appropriate comparison group for LGBT individuals. In order to estimate incidence and mortality rate ratios comparing sexual and gender minorities to their heterosexual and cisgender counterparts, researchers have predicted sexual orientation disparities in an individual's five-year and lifetime risk of developing certain cancers (namely, breast cancer) and estimated the relationship between the density of male and female same-sex partner households, which they used as a surrogate for gay and lesbian population density, and cancer incidence and mortality at the county level. Given the lack of sexual orientation and gender identity data in cancer registries [1, 2], no study has been able to assess disparities in observed cancer incidence and mortality rates among different sexual orientation and gender identity groups at the individual level. However, Boehmer and colleagues [60] suggested that, in the absence of relevant cancer surveillance information, researchers can use convenience sampling methods to recruit sexual minority cancer survivors, who were comparable to those captured in population-based cancer registries on several health and social characteristics, and estimate cancer outcomes, including survival and mortality, in these populations.

This review also shows that some LGBT populations are largely missing in existing research on sexual orientation and gender identity disparities in cancer [59]. In particular, all published studies have relied on samples of predominately white individuals [61], which precludes their generalizability to LGBT people of color, whose experiences along the cancer continuum may be influenced by not only heterosexism but also institutional and interpersonal racism [62–65]. Additionally, ecological studies that use the density of same-sex partner households as a surrogate for lesbian or gay population density fail to include LGBT individuals who are either single or partnered but living alone. However, these individuals may have social and economic resources and engage in cancer-related health behaviors that differ from those of LGBT persons living with a same-sex partner, such that existing estimates may not reflect their risk of developing or dying of certain cancers. Additionally, by using the density of same-sex partner households as a proxy for gay and lesbian population density, these studies conflate women living with a same-sex partner with lesbian and bisexual women and men living with a same-sex partner with gay and bisexual men. Thus, these research findings do not allow investigators to identify how sexual orientation identity and same-sex partner household status each independently relate to cancer outcomes or estimate the risk of developing or dying of certain cancers among bisexual women and men separately from lesbians and gay men, respectively. However, research shows that bisexual women in particular may experience a higher prevalence of adverse health outcomes, including cancer risk factors, relative to heterosexual women [66] and should be disaggregated from lesbians in studies of sexual orientation and cancer outcomes among women. Lastly, research on cancer incidence and mortality among transgender men and women is limited to a few investigations among individuals with access to university-based gender clinics [25–27, 55]. To date, no population-based study has assessed the burden of cancer among transgender populations, including individuals who do not use hormone therapy and persons who obtain hormones through means other than a health care provider (e.g., on the street), which may pose health concerns with implications for cancer. Moreover, no study has measured cancer outcomes among individuals whose identities do not conform to normative classifications of gender (e.g., genderqueer, masculine of center) and sexuality (e.g., queer, pansexual) and to whom estimates of cancer incidence and mortality among self-identified LGBT persons may not be applicable.

Moreover, limitations exist in the study of sexual orientation and gender identity disparities in cancer in relation to place and time [59]. In particular, all published studies pertaining to the population distribution of cancer by sexual orientation and gender identity were conducted in the United States, Europe, or Canada. Thus, no data exist on the epidemiology of cancer among LGBT populations in other areas of the world, including sub-Saharan Africa, Asia, Latin America, and the Caribbean. Similarly, with a few exceptions [67], there has been little attention to how, within the U.S., sexual orientation and gender identity may influence cancer outcomes differently across states based on varying laws and policies related to access to health care, public health prevention programs, and LGBT rights. Moreover, few studies have addressed how the lifecourse influences the existence and magnitude of cancer disparities by sexual orientation and gender identity. One notable exception is the study conducted by Austin et al. [17], in which the researchers used a modified version of the Rosner-Colditz prediction model to account for breast cancer risk factors that vary by age and reproductive history. Lastly, no study has investigated how historical period—in relation to changing norms pertaining to pregnancy and birth, the composition and use of oral contraceptives, the marketing of alcohol and tobacco to LGBT populations, and LGBT rights—affects sexual orientation and gender identity disparities in the risk of developing and dying of certain cancers over time.

Future Directions in Research on the Epidemiology of Cancer by Sexual Orientation and Gender Identity

The following recommendations provide guidance on future directions for population health research on the epidemiology of cancer among LGBT populations. First, for investigators to estimate the relationship between sexual orientation and observed cancer incidence and mortality rates among U.S. persons at the individual level, the SEER Program must collect and provide data on sexual orientation. Additionally, SEER data should include information on gender identity so that the risk of developing or dying of cancer among transgender persons relative to cisgender men and women can be ascertained and monitored. Second, given that the SEER Program does not currently collect data on sexual orientation at the individual level [1, 2], some researchers have assessed the relationship between the density of same-sex partner households, which they used as a surrogate for lesbian or gay population density, and cancer incidence and mortality at the county level. While this approach is a novel and resourceful one, findings gleaned using this methodology may be confounded by not only county level-factors—which the researchers have addressed by adjusting for race/ethnicity, federal poverty level, and, in some cases, education at the county level—but also neighborhood- and individual-level factors. Thus, data are needed at multiple levels of analysis to estimate the relationship between sexual orientation and cancer rates using multilevel models that account for potential confounding at the county, neighborhood, and individual levels.

Third, while some studies have assessed whether reproductive and other relevant factors (e.g., parity, breastfeeding, body mass index), hypothesized to be potential mediators, help explain sexual orientation disparities in breast cancer incidence [11], few investigators have identified the mechanisms that may underlie observed sexual orientation disparities in the incidence of other types of cancer. In order to determine the causal relationships between sexual orientation and gender identity, cancer outcomes, and potential mediators (e.g., cancer-related risk behaviors, reproductive history, health insurance status, access to and utilization of health services, institutional and interpersonal discrimination), longitudinal studies that provide data across the lifecourse among large numbers of individuals are needed [59]. Additionally, these studies should collect information on the potential mechanisms that may drive sexual orientation and gender identity disparities along the cancer continuum in multiple domains, including workplaces, neighborhoods, social relationships, laws, policies, and health care [59].

Fourth, studies should investigate inequalities *within* LGBT groups by gathering data on factors that may modify sexual orientation and gender identity disparities in cancer—including race/ethnicity, SEP, and immigrant status—and testing whether they interact with sexual orientation or gender identity [59]. In order to assess how sexual orientation and gender identity affect the population distribution of cancer singly and in conjunction with other forms of social inequality, studies should recruit large samples of LGBT persons and heterosexual cisgender men and women with sufficient numbers of people of color, poor and low-income individuals, and immigrant persons of diverse sexual orientation and gender identities. Additionally, studies that identify the societal determinants of cancer risk factors, screening, prevalence, incidence, diagnosis, treatment, survival, and/or mortality among LGBT people of color, poor and low-income LGBT individuals, and LGBT immigrants are needed to inform public health interventions tailored to the needs of these often ignored and marginalized populations.

Fifth, population theories of disease distribution can help guide the work of epidemiologists and other public health researchers investigating the population distribution of cancer by sexual orientation and gender identity [68–72]. Indeed, epidemiologic theories, such as ecosocial theory, can help inform the questions asked, measures considered, analyses conducted, and interpretations offered in the context of population health research [68–72]. Ecosocial theory, a multilevel theory of population disease distribution developed by Krieger, focuses on the central question of *"who and what drives social inequalities in health?"* The theory's core constructs include: (1) *embodiment*, which refers to how humans—as both social beings and biological organisms—literally incorporate and manifest lived experiences of social inequality throughout the lifecourse; (2) *pathways of embodiment*, or the multiple ways in which a range of exposures become incorporated as health and disease outcomes, as simultaneously structured by societal and biological constraints; (3) the *cumulative interplay between exposure, susceptibility, and resistance* at multiple levels, in multiple domains, and at multiple spatiotemporal scales; and (4) *accountability and agency*—not only in terms of who and what is responsible for the social patterning of disease and the (re)production of social inequalities in health, but also accountability and agency on the part of epidemiologists and other public health researchers for the theories they use, implicitly or explicitly, to describe and explain population distributions of disease, including health inequities [68–72].

In particular, ecosocial theory's core constructs of embodiment and pathways of embodiment can help investigators design epidemiologic studies that explicitly seek to identify the mechanisms through which sexual orientation and gender identity relate to cancer incidence and mortality. Additionally, the theory urges researchers to engage in nuanced population-level thinking about how and why the population distribution of cancer varies not only between but also *within* sexual orientation and gender identity groups—in relation to race/ethnicity, SEP, immigrant status, and other aspects of social inequality—across the lifecourse and in historical and ecological context [68–72]. Identifying how sexual orientation and gender identity intersect with other dimensions of social inequality to shape cancer outcomes is essential for designing interventions that meet the needs of all segments of the LGBT community—including sexual and gender minorities who are also marginalized and underserved as a result of other stigmatized social identities, such as LGBT people of color, poor and low-income LGBT individuals, and LGBT immigrants.

Policy Considerations for Decreasing Cancer among Lesbian, Gay, Bisexual, and Transgender Populations

In the United States, the burden of cancer among LGBT populations is compounded by pronounced sexual orientation disparities in health insurance and access to health care, especially among women [4, 6, 12, 73–75]. Using 1997 to 2003 National Health Interview Survey data on U.S. adults aged 18–64 years, Heck et al. [75] found that, adjusting for socio-demographic characteristics, women in same-sex relationships had significantly lower odds of health insurance (OR = 0.60; 95 % CI: 0.39, 0.92), having seen a health care provider in the last 12 months (OR = 0.66; 95 % CI: 0.46, 0.95), and having a usual source of care relative to women in different-sex relationships (OR = 0.50; 95 % CI: 0.35, 0.71). Additionally, the researchers' findings showed that, compared to women in different-sex relationships, women with same-sex partners had significantly higher odds of unmet medical needs as a result of cost issues (OR = 1.85; 95 % CI: 1.16, 2.96) [75]. Among U.S. men, Heck and colleagues [75] found some indication that those in same-sex relationships may have lower odds of health insurance compared to their counterparts in different-sex relationships (OR = 0.72; 95 % CI: 0.50, 1.06); however, this result was only marginally statistically significant. In contrast, men in same-sex relationships had significantly higher odds of having seen a health care provider in the last 12 months than men in opposite-sex relationships (OR = 1.63; 95 % CI: 1.19, 2.23) [75].

In an analysis of 2000 to 2007 Behavioral Risk Factor Surveillance System data, Buchmueller and Carpenter [74] showed that the lower adjusted odds of health insurance among U.S. women and men in same-sex relationships relative to those in different-sex relationships were largely due to differences in the prevalence of state-sanctioned marriage, through which individuals can obtain employer-sponsored health insurance for their spouse. Indeed, when the researchers distinguished married and unmarried individuals in different-sex relationships, they found that men and women in same-sex relationships had lower odds of being insured than married individuals in opposite-sex relationships but higher odds of having health insurance than unmarried individuals with different-sex partners [74]. Further using pooled data from the 2001, 2003, and 2005 CHIS, Ponce et al.'s [76] findings showed that differences in the prevalence of employer-sponsored dependent coverage, obtained through state-sanctioned marriage, between gays and lesbians and their heterosexual counterparts were at the root of observed sexual orientation disparities in health insurance. Specifically, the researchers found that, in California, partnered self-identified gay and lesbian individuals were 42 % and 28 % less likely than married self-identified heterosexual men and women, respectively, to report having employer-sponsored dependent coverage [76]. Similarly, using pooled 1996 to 2003 Current Population Survey data, Ash and Badgett [77] found that U.S. men and women with cohabitating same-sex and different-sex partners were less likely to have employment-based health insurance relative to married individuals with different-sex partners. Moreover, using 2008–2010 American Community Survey data, Gonzales and Blewett found that U.S. men and women aged 25–64 years in same-sex relationships were less likely to have employer-sponsored health insurance relative to their counterparts in married different-sex relationships, with the greatest disparities for men occurring in the South and for women occurring in the Midwest [78].

Because of discrimination in the employment [79, 80] and health insurance sectors [76, 77]—as well as restrictions in marriage, civil unions, and domestic partnerships for same-sex couples [78]—LGBT populations may lack the health coverage they need to access care related to the cancer continuum, including prevention, screening, detection, and treatment services. For example, studies have shown that lesbians are less likely to receive regular Pap tests, which detect changes in cells of the uterine cervix before cancer develops [58], compared to their heterosexual counterparts [6, 81–86]. Researchers have attributed sexual orientation disparities in Pap test use to a range of factors, including differences in health insurance and access to health care, heterosexism in the health care system, a lack of health care provider knowledge of and sensitivity toward same-sex sexuality, fear of disclosing one's sexual orientation to providers, and beliefs among women and providers that lesbians and women who have sex with women are not at risk of HPV [82–87]. Further, Cochran and colleagues [4] found that, adjusting for age, race/ethnicity, education level, and geographic region, lesbians aged 30–75 years had a significantly lower self-reported prevalence of mammographic screening, which was positively associated with health insurance status, relative to U.S. women in general (based on 1994 National Health Interview Survey, NHIS, data). In a cohort of predominately white (94%) U.S. women who participated in the Nurses' Health Study II from 1989 to 2005, Austin and colleagues [67] found small sexual orientation disparities in mammographic screening and none in colorectal screening. Additional research is needed to understand how health insurance and access to health care influence the use of cancer services among sexual and gender minorities of diverse racial/ethnic and socioeconomic backgrounds relative to their heterosexual counterparts.

Several recent policy decisions have the potential to improve LGBT individuals' access to health insurance [74, 76–78, 88, 89]. The Affordable Care Act (ACA), which was signed into law by President Obama in March 2010 and went into full effect in January 2014, provides expanded coverage for essential health benefits, including cancer screening and prevention services, through the expansion of Medicaid in some states (for individuals earning less than 138% of the federal poverty level, FPL) and the creation of federally-subsidized health insurance marketplaces (for individuals earning more than 138%, or 100% in states with no Medicaid expansion, but less than 400% of the FPL) [88]. Additionally, the ACA requires new private health plans to cover recommended preventive services—which include colorectal cancer screening, mammographic screening, cervical cancer screening, HPV DNA tests, and HPV vaccination—with no co-payments or deductibles [90, 91]. Moreover, as of January 1, 2014, individuals can no longer be denied health insurance due to a pre-existing condition—including HIV/AIDS, cancer, or "gender identity disorder," a psychiatric diagnosis necessary for transgender individuals to access gender-affirming care such as hormone therapy [88, 92]. Moreover, if a state requires coverage for hormone replacement therapy in all health plans, this procedure would have to be covered for all patients, regardless of gender identity [89]. However, transgender individuals will have to prove that hormone therapy is medically necessary to obtain coverage for the procedure, which may pose a barrier to care [89].

Lastly, the U.S. Department of Health and Human Services issued federal regulations that prohibit health insurance issues offering non-grandfathered health coverage, including health plans offered through the state Health Insurance Exchanges, from discriminating on the basis of sexual orientation in all states (i.e., a health insurance issuer that offers coverage of an opposite-sex spouse must also offer coverage, on the same terms and conditions, of a same-sex spouse) [88, 93, 94]. The ACA also calls for routine monitoring of health disparities, which could include sexual orientation and gender identity disparities in health outcomes, and measures of sexual orientation are being included in federal health surveys (e.g., 2013 NHIS), which will facilitate the assessment of sexual orientation disparities in health insurance, access to health care, and health behaviors and outcomes relevant to cancer prevention, detection, treatment, and survival [88, 89, 95, 96]. Similar efforts are ongoing to include measures of gender identity in federal surveys relevant to the assessment of health and health care disparities [96]. Given that national surveys include a small proportion of LGBT individuals, sub-national studies that focus on the health of sexual and gender minorities including those of diverse racial/ethnic, socioeconomic, and immigrant backgrounds, will continue to be essential for planning programs and interventions that meet the needs of diverse LGBT populations [97]. Additionally, the U.S. Supreme Court repealed Sect. 3 of the Defense of Marriage Act (DOMA) on June 26, 2013. As a result, married same-sex couples now have the same access to federal benefits as married different-sex couples, including health insurance for spouses of federal government employees, and military personnel living in states where same-sex marriage is legal, which will help improve access to health insurance for some LGBT people [88].

Recommendations for Clinical and Public Health Practice

The cancer prevention, screening, and treatment experiences of LGBT populations are further impacted by institutional and interpersonal discrimination related to sexual orientation [97–100] and gender identity [97, 101–103] within the health care system. Discrimination—including heterosexism and transphobia—can negatively impact cancer outcomes among sexual and gender minority groups by leading to delays in or avoidance of health care receipt or undermining patient-provider communication and trust [97–100]. Research shows that patient-provider communication, including heterosexist health care provider assumptions and health care provider responses to sexual orientation disclosure, influence the health care experiences of LGB persons [97, 104–106]. Some research suggests that sexual orientation disclosure can help improve care [97]—such as promoting lesbians' receipt of regular Pap smears [107]—by, for example, ensuring that clinicians have all of the information they need about individuals' sexual behavior to make appropriate health care recommendations [107, 108]. However, this will only occur if the disclosure of one's sexual orientation identity, gender identity, or sexual behavior is met with understanding and competent, well-informed care [97, 107]. Indeed, by being knowledgeable and non-judgmental about patients' sexual orientation and gender identity and taking sexual histories that ask open-ended questions that allow for non-heteronormative responses [108], clinicians can provide LGBT individuals with relevant, appropriate, and high-quality health information and care that meets their needs [98, 106].

Further, health care facilities can help ensure that their practice environment is welcoming to LGBT people by implementing a written policy that bans discrimination (including on the basis of sexual orientation and gender identity), training health care personnel in LGBT health issues, designing intake forms that are inclusive of persons in same-sex relationships and those who identify as transgender or gender non-conforming, displaying posters that represent diverse family structures, and offering brochures that are sensitive to the existence of LGBT populations and address their health concerns [97, 98, 101, 104, 106]. In order to meet the needs of LGBT cancer patients and survivors, hospitals can offer support groups for sexual and gender minority individuals and ensure that, if appropriate, partners of any sex or gender are welcome during family visiting hours, involved in healthcare decision-making, and valued as a source of support for patients [97, 100, 104, 106]. Lastly, health clinics, hospitals, and community-based organizations can offer tailored programs, for both LGBT individuals and health care providers, that promote awareness of and access to cancer prevention, screening, and treatment services among sexual and gender minority populations—who, studies suggest, experience a greater burden of cancer risk factors than heterosexual cisgender populations and may be at increased risk of developing or dying of certain cancers [97].

Conclusion

Epidemiologic research provides some evidence that sexual and gender minorities may be at higher risk than heterosexual and cisgender individuals of developing certain cancers—although several studies found no difference in cancer outcomes by sexual orientation or gender identity. In recent years, researchers have paid increased attention to the incidence of cancer among LGBT groups. However, given the lack of information on sexual orientation and gender identity in cancer registries [1, 2], investigators have not been able to assess sexual orientation and gender identity disparities in cancer incidence and mortality at the individual level. Instead, they have used a range of methods to help them estimate the risk of developing and dying of various malignancies among sexual and gender minorities relative to their heterosexual and cisgender counterparts—including ecological studies that make inferences at the county level, using same-sex partner households as a surrogate for sexual orientation identity, predicting individuals' risk of developing cancer based on their specific risk profile, and using the general population as a comparison group for LGBT populations. Until cancer registries such as the SEER Program in the United States include information on sexual orientation and gender identity, researchers will continue to lack the data they need to assess disparities in the observed risk of developing and dying of cancer among LGBT populations compared to their heterosexual and cisgender counterparts at the individual level. Identifying the epidemiology of cancer by sexual orientation and gender identity—including in relation to other dimensions of social inequality, such as race/ethnicity, SEP, and immigrant status, and over time and space—is essential for informing evidence-based policies and clinical and community based programs that promote the prevention, detection, and treatment of cancer among all segments of LGBT populations around the world and, ultimately, help advance health equity and social justice in our societies.

Acknowledgments I am grateful to Dr. Nancy Krieger, Professor of Social Epidemiology in the Department of Social and Behavioral Sciences at Harvard T.H. Chan School of Public Health, and Dr. S. Bryn Austin, Associate Professor in the Department of Social and Behavioral Sciences at Harvard T.H. Chan School of Public Health and Department of Pediatrics at Harvard Medical School, for their guidance and insights, which helped inform the content of this chapter.

References

1. Bowen DJ, Boehmer U. The lack of cancer surveillance data on sexual minorities and strategies for change. Cancer Cause Control. 2007;18(4):343–9.
2. Brown JP, Tracy JK. Lesbians and cancer: an overlooked health disparity. Cancer Cause Control. 2008;19(10):1009–20.
3. Valanis BG, Bowen DJ, Bassford T, Whitlock E, Charney P, Carter RA. Sexual orientation and health: comparisons in the Women's Health Initiative sample. Arch Fam Med. 2000;9:843–53.
4. Cochran SD, Mays VM, Bowen DJ, Gage S, Bybee D, Roberts S, Goldstein RS, Robison A, Rankow E, White J. Cancer-related risk indicators and preventive screening behaviors among lesbians and bisexual women. Am J Public Health. 2001;91:591–7.
5. Case P, Austin SB, Hunter DJ, Manson JE, Malspeis S, Willett WC, Spiegelman D. Sexual orientation, health risk factors, and physical functioning in the Nurses' Health Study II. J Womens Health. 2004;13(9):1033–47.
6. Diamant AL, Schuster MA, Lever J. Receipt of health care services by lesbians. Am J Prev Med. 2000;19(3):141–8.
7. Rosario M, Corliss HL, Everett BG, Reisner SL, Austin SB, Buchting FO, Birkett M. Sexual orientation disparities in cancer-related risk behaviors of tobacco, alcohol, sexual behaviors, and diet and physical activity: pooled Youth Risk Behavior Surveys. Am J Public Health. 2014;104(2):245–54.
8. Bowen DJ, Boehmer U, Russo M. Cancer and sexual minority women. In: Meyer IH, Northridge ME, editors. The health of sexual minorities: public health perspectives on lesbian, gay, bisexual, and transgender populations. New York: Springer; 2007. pp. 523–38.
9. Rankow EJ. Breast and cervical cancer among lesbians. Women's Health Issues. 1995;5: 123–9.
10. Zaritsky E, Dibble SL. Risk factors for reproductive and breast cancers among older lesbians. J Womens Health. 2010;19(1):125–31.
11. Kavanaugh-Lynch MHE, White E, Daling JR, Bowen DJ. Correlates of lesbian sexual orientation and the risk of breast cancer. J Gay Lesbian Med Assoc. 2002;6(3–4):91–5.
12. Committee on Lesbian, Gay, Bisexual, and Transgender Health Issues and Research Gaps and Opportunities, Board on the Health of Select Populations, Institute of Medicine. The health of lesbian, gay, bisexual, and transgender (LGBT) people: building a foundation for better understanding; 2011.
13. Frisch M, Smith E, Grulich A, Johansen C. Cancer in a population-based cohort of men and women in registered homosexual partnerships. Am J Epidemiol. 2003;157(11):966–72.
14. Boehmer U, Ozonoff A, Timm A. County-level association of sexual minority density with breast cancer incidence: results from an ecological study. Sex Res Soc Policy. 2011;8(2): 139–45.
15. Dibble SL, Roberts SA, Nussey B. Comparing breast cancer risk between lesbians and their heterosexual sisters. Women's Health Issues. 2004;14(2):60–8.
16. Brandenburg DL, Matthews AK, Johnson TP, Hughes TL. Breast cancer risk and screening: a comparison of lesbian and heterosexual women. Women Health. 2007;45(4):109–30.
17. Austin SB, Pazaris MJ, Rosner B, Bowen DJ, Rich-Edwards J, Spiegelman D. Application of the Rosner-Colditz risk prediction model to estimate sexual orientation group disparities in breast cancer risk in a U.S. cohort of premenopausal women. Cancer Epidemiol Biomark Prev. 2012;21(12):2201–08.
18. D'Souza G, Wiley DJ, Li X, Chmiel JS, Margolick JB, Cranston RD, Jacobson LP. Incidence and epidemiology of anal cancer in the Multicenter AIDS Cohort Study. J Aquitred Immune Defic Syndr. 2008;48(4):491–9.
19. Machalek DA, Poynten M, Jin F, Fairley CK, Farnsworth A, Garland SM, Hillman RJ, Petoumenos K, Roberts J, Tabrizi SN, Templeton DJ, Grulich AE. Anal human papillomavirus infection and associated neoplastic lesions in men who have sex with men: a systematic review and meta-analysis. Lancet Oncol. 2012;13(5):487–500.

20. Koblin BA, Hessol NA, Zauber AG, Taylor PE, Buchbinder SP, Katz MH, Stevens CE. Increased incidence of cancer among homosexual men, New York City and San Francisco, 1978–1990. Am J Epidemiol. 1996;144(10):916–23.
21. Chaturvedi AK, Madeleine MM, Biggar RJ, Engels EA. Risk of human papillomavirus–associated cancers among persons with AIDS. J Natl Cancer Inst. 2009;101(16):1120–30.
22. Dal Maso L, Polesel J, Serraino D, Lise M, Piselli P, Falcini F, Russo A, Intrieri T, Vercelli M, Zambon P, Tagliabue G, Zanetti R, Federico M, Limina RM, Mangone L, De Lisi V, Stracci F, Ferretti S, Piffer S, Budroni M, Donato A, Giacomin A, Bellù F, Fusco M, Madeddu A, Vitarelli S, Tessandori R, Tumino R, Suligoi B, Franceschi S; Cancer and AIDS Registries Linkage (CARL) Study. Pattern of cancer risk in persons with AIDS in Italy in the HAART era. Br J Cancer. 2009;100:840–7.
23. Piketty C, Darragh TM, Da Costa M, Bruneval P, Heard I, Kazatchkine MD, et al. High prevalence of anal human papillomavirus infection and anal cancer precursors among HIV-infected persons in the absence of anal intercourse. Ann Intern Med. 2003 138(6):453–60.
24. Daling JR, Madeleine MM, Johnson LG, Schwartz SM, Shera KA, Wurscher MA, Carter JJ, Porter PL, Galloway DA, McDougall JK. Human papillomavirus, smoking, and sexual practices in the etiology of anal cancer. Cancer. 2004;101(2):270–80.
25. Asscheman H, Giltay EJ, Megens JAJ, de Ronde W, van Trotsenburg MAA, Gooren LJG. A long-term follow-up study of mortality in transsexuals receiving treatment with cross-sex hormones. Eur J Endocrinol. 2011;164:635–42.
26. Gooren LJ, Giltay EJ, Bunck MC. Long-term treatment of transsexuals with cross-sex hormones: extensive personal experience. J Clin Endocrinol Metab. 2008;93(1):19–25.
27. Mueller A, Gooren LJ. Hormone-related tumors in transsexuals receiving treatment with cross-sex hormones. Eur J Endocrinol. 2008;159:197–202.
28. American Cancer Society. Breast cancer. 2014. http://www.cancer.org/cancer/breastcancer/detailedguide. Accessed 15 March 2014.
29. Surveillance, Epidemiology, and End Results Program. SEER Stat Fact Sheets: Breast Cancer. 2014. http://seer.cancer.gov/statfacts/html/breast.html. Accessed 15 March 2014.
30. American Cancer Society. Breast cancer facts and Figs. 2013–2014. 2013:1–37.
31. Bigby JA, Holmes MD. Disparities across the breast cancer continuum. Cancer Cause Control. 2005;16(1):35–44.
32. Meads C, Moore D. Breast cancer in lesbians and bisexual women: systematic review of incidence, prevalence and risk studies. BMC Public Health. 2013;13(1127).
33. Boehmer U, Miao X, Ozonoff A. Cancer survivorship and sexual orientation. Cancer. 2011;107(16):3796–804.
34. Aschengrau A, Seage GR. Essentials of epidemiology in public health. 2nd ed. Sudbury: Jones and Barlett; 2008.
35. Surveillance, Epidemiology, and End Results Program. About the SEER Program. 2014. http://seer.cancer.gov/about/. Accessed 15 March 2014.
36. McTiernan A, Kuniyuki A, Yasui Y, Bowen D, Burke W, Culver JB, Anderson R, Durfy S. Comparisons of two breast cancer risk estimates in women with a family history of breast cancer. Cancer Epidemiol Biomark Prev. 2001;10:333–8.
37. Costantino JP, Gail MH, Pee D, Anderson S, Redmond CK, Benichou J, Wieand HS. Validation studies for models projecting the risk of invasive and total breast cancer incidence. J Natl Cancer Inst. 1999;91(18):1541–8.
38. Roberts SA, Dibble SL, Scanlon JL, Paul SM, Davids H. Differences in risk factors for breast cancer: lesbian and heterosexual women. J Gay Lesbian Med Assoc. 1998;2(3):93–101.
39. Cochran SD, Mays VM. Risk of breast cancer mortality among women cohabiting with same sex partners: findings from the National Health Interview Survey, 1997–2003. J Womens Health. 2012;21(5):528–33.
40. American Cancer Society. Anal cancer. 2013. http://www.cancer.org/cancer/analcancer/detailedguide/index.htm. Accessed 15 March 2014.
41. Surveillance, Epidemiology, and End Results Program. SEER Stat Fact Sheets: Anal Cancer. 2014. http://seer.cancer.gov/statfacts/html/anus.html. Accessed 15 March 2014.

42. Silverberg MJ, Lau B, Justice AC, Engels E, Gill MJ, Goedert JJ, Kirk GD, D'Souza G, Bosch RJ, Brooks JT, Napravnik S, Hessol NA, Jacobson LP, Kitahata MM, Klein MB, Moore RD, Rodriguez B, Rourke SB, Saag MS, Sterling TR, Gebo KA, Press N, Martin JN, Dubrow R; North American AIDS Cohort Collaboration on Research and Design. Risk of anal cancer in HIV-infected and HIV-uninfected individuals in North America. Clin Infect Dis. 2012;54(7):1026–34.
43. National Cancer Institute. HPV and cancer. 2012. http://www.cancer.gov/cancertopics/factsheet/Risk/HPV. Accessed 15 May 2013.
44. American Cancer Society. Colorectal cancer. 2014. http://www.cancer.org/cancer/colonandrectumcancer/detailedguide/colon-rectum-cancer-detailed-guide-toc. Accessed 15 March 2014.
45. Surveillance, Epidemiology, and End Results Program. SEER Stat Fact Sheets: Colon and Rectum. 2014. http://seer.cancer.gov/statfacts/html/colorect.html. Accessed 17 March 2014.
46. U.S. Cancer Statistics Working Group. United States cancer statistics: 1999–2010 incidence and mortality web-based report. 2013.
47. Austin SB, Pazaris MJ, Wei EK, Rosner B, Kennedy GA, Bowen D, Spiegelman D. Application of the Rosner-Wei risk-prediction model to estimate sexual orientation patterns in colon cancer risk in a prospective cohort of U.S. women. Cancer Causes Control. 2014. doi:10.1007/s10552-014-0399-x.
48. Boehmer U, Ozonoff A, Miao X. An ecological analysis of colorectal cancer incidence and mortality: differences by sexual orientation. BMC Cancer. 2011;11(400):1–8.
49. Surveillance, Epidemiology, and End Results Program. SEER Stat Fact Sheets: Lung and Bronchus Cancer. 2014. http://seer.cancer.gov/statfacts/html/lungb.html. Accessed 15 March 2014.
50. American Cancer Society. Lung cancer (non-small cell). 2014. http://www.cancer.org/cancer/lungcancer-non-smallcell/detailedguide/index. Accessed 15 Month 2014.
51. Boehmer U, Ozonoff A, Miao X. An ecological approach to examine lung cancer disparities due to sexual orientation. Public Health. 2012;126(7):605–12.
52. Centers for Disease Control and Prevention. Basic information about lung cancer. 2014. http://www.cdc.gov/cancer/lung/basic_info/index.htm. Accessed 15 March 2014.
53. Lee JGL, Griffin GK, Melvin CL. Tobacco use among sexual minorities in the USA, 1987 to May 2007: a systematic review. Tob Control. 2009;18:275–82.
54. Rosenblatt KA, Wicklund KG, Stanford JL. Sexual factors and the risk of prostate cancer. Am J Epidemiol. 2001;153(12):1152–8.
55. Wierckx K, Elaut E, Declercq E, Heylens G, De Cuypere G, Taes Y, Kaufman JM, T'Sjoen G. Prevalence of cardiovascular disease and cancer during cross-sex hormone therapy in a large cohort of trans persons: a case–control study. Eur J Endocrinol. 2013;169:471–8.
56. Pritchard TJ, Pankowsky DA, Crowe JP, Abdul-Karim FW. Breast cancer in a male-to-female Transsexual: a case report. JAMA. 1988;259(15):2278–80.
57. Turo R, Jallad S, Prescott S, Cross WR. Metastatic prostate cancer in transsexual diagnosed after three decades of estrogen therapy. Can Urol Assoc J. 2013;7(7–8):E544–6.
58. American Cancer Society. Cancer facts and Figures 2014. 2014:1–68.
59. Krieger N. Defining and investigating social disparities in cancer: critical issues. Cancer Cause Control. 2005;16(1):5–14.
60. Boehmer U, Clark MA, Timm A, Glickman M, Sullivan M. Comparing sexual minority cancer survivors recruited through a cancer registry to convenience methods of recruitment. Womens Health Issues. 2011;21(5):345–52.
61. Boehmer U. Twenty years of public health research: inclusion of lesbian, gay, bisexual, and transgender populations. Am J Public Health. 2002;92(7):1125–30.
62. Wilson PA, Yoshikawa H. Improving access to health care among African-American, Asian and Pacific Islander, and Latino lesbian, gay, and bisexual populations. In: Meyer IH, Northridge ME, editors. The health of sexual minorities: public health perspectives on lesbian, gay, bisexual, and transgender populations. New York: Springer; 2007. pp. 607–37.

63. Stevens PE. The experiences of lesbians of color in health care encounters: narrative insights for improving access and quality. J Lesbian Stud. 1998;2(1):77–94.
64. Malebranche DJ, Peterson JL, Fullilove RE, Stackhouse RW. Race and sexual identity: perceptions about medical culture and healthcare among Black men who have sex with men. J Natl Med Assoc. 2004;96(1):97–107.
65. Mays VM, Yancey AK, Cochran SD, Weber M, Fielding J. Heterogeneity of health disparities among African American, Hispanic, and Asian American women: unrecognized influences of sexual orientation. Am J Public Health. 2002;92(4):632–9.
66. Fredriksen-Goldsen KI, Kim HJ, Barkan SE, Balsam KF, Mincer SL. Disparities in health-related quality of life: a comparison of lesbians and bisexual women. Am J Public Health. 2010;100(11):2255–61.
67. Austin SB, Pazaris MJ, Nichols LP, Bowen DJ, Wei EK, Spiegelman D. An examination of sexual orientation group patterns in mammographic and colorectal screening in a cohort of U.S. women. Cancer Cause Control. 2013;24(3):539–47.
68. Krieger N. Epidemiology and the web of causation: has anyone seen the spider? Soc Sci Med. 1994;39(7):887–903.
69. Krieger N. Epidemiology and the people's health: theory and context. New York: Oxford University Press, 2011.
70. Krieger N. Theories for social epidemiology in the 21st century: an ecosocial perspective. Int J Epidemiol. 2001;30(4):668–77.
71. Krieger N. A glossary for social epidemiology. J Epidemiol Commun Health. 2001;55: 693–700.
72. Krieger N. Got theory? On the 21st c CE rise of explicit use of epidemiologic theories of disease distribution: a review and ecosocial analysis. Curr Epidemiol Rep. 2014;1(1):45–56.
73. Solarz AL. Lesbian health: current assessment and directions for the future. 1999.
74. Buchmueller T, Carpenter CS. Disparities in health insurance coverage, access, and outcomes for individuals in same-sex versus different-sex relationships, 2000–2007. Am J Public Health. 2010;100(3):489–95.
75. Heck JE, Sell RL, Gorin SS. Health care access among individuals involved in same-sex relationships. Am J Public Health. 2006;96(6):1111–8.
76. Ponce NA, Cochran SD, Pizer JC, Mays VM. The effects of unequal access to health insurance for same-sex couples in California. Health Affairs. 2010;29(8):1539–48.
77. Ash MA, Badgett MVL. Separate and unequal: the effect of unequal access to employment-based health insurance on same-sex and unmarried different-sex couples. Contemp Econ Policy. 2006;24(4):582–99.
78. Gonzales G, Blewett LA. National and state-specific health insurance disparities for adults in same-sex relationships. Am J Public Health. 2014;104(2):e95–104.
79. Badgett MVL, Lau H, Sears B, Ho D. Bias in the workplace: consistent evidence of sexual orientation and gender identity discrimination. Williams Institute, UCLA School of Law. 2007.
80. Badgett MVL. Money, myths, and change: the economic lives of lesbians and gay men. Chicago: The University of Chicago Press; 2001.
81. Agénor M, Krieger N, Austin SB, Haneuse S, Gottlieb BR. Sexual orientation disparities in Papanicolaou test use among US women: the role of sexual and reproductive health services. Am J Public Health. 2014;104(2):e68–73.
82. Fish J. Cervical cancer screening in lesbian and bisexual women: a review of the worldwide literature using systematic methods. 2009. http://www.cancerscreening.nhs.uk/cervical/publications/screening-lesbians-bisexual-women.pdf.
83. Marrazzo JM, Koutsky LA, Kiviat NB, Kuypers JM, Stine KL. Papanicolaou test screening and prevalence of genital human papillomavirus among women who have sex with women. Am J Public Health. 2001;91(6):947–52.
84. Matthews AK, Brandenburg DL, Johnson TP, Hughes TL. Correlates of underutilization of gynecological cancer screening among lesbian and heterosexual women. Prev Med. 2004;38(1):105–13.

85. Hutchinson MK, Thompson AC, Cederbaum JA. Multisystem factors contributing to disparities in preventive health care among lesbian women. J Obstet Gynechol Neonatal Nurs. 2006;35(3):393–402.
86. Tracy JK, Lydecker AD, Ireland L. Barriers to cervical cancer screening among lesbians. J Womens Health. 2010;19(2):229–37.
87. Price JH, Easton AN, Telljohann SK, Wallace PB. Perceptions of cervical cancer and Pap smear screening behavior by women's sexual orientation. J Community Health. 1996;21(2):89–105.
88. Ranji U, Beamesderfer A, Kates J, Salganicoff A. Health and access to care and coverage for lesbian, gay, bisexual, and transgender individuals in the U.S. Kaiser Family Foundation. 2014.
89. Baker K, Krehely J. Changing the game: what health care reform means for gay, lesbian, bisexual, and transgender Americans. Center for American Progress, National Coalition for LGBT Health. 2011.
90. Kaiser Family Foundation. Preventive services covered by private health plans under the Affordable Care Act. 2011.
91. Department of Health and Human Services. Preventive services covered under the Affordable Care Act. 2012; http://www.hhs.gov/healthcare/facts/factsheets/2010/07/preventive-services-list.html#CoveredPreventiveServicesforChildren. Accessed 17 March 2014.
92. Davidson AJ. How Obamacare will affect trans folks and families. The Advocate 2013. http://www.advocate.com/politics/transgender/2013/11/01/how-obamacare-will-affect-trans-folks-and-families. Accessed 17 March 2014.
93. Cray A, Baker K. The Affordable Care Act: creating new health insurance marketplaces. Center for American Progress. 2013.
94. Keith K, Lucia K, Monahan C. Nondiscrimination under the Affordable Care Act. The Center on Health Insurance Reforms, Georgetown University Health Policy Institute. 2013.
95. Baker K, Cray A. FAQ: collecting sexual orientation and gender identity data. Center for American Progress. 2012.
96. National Coalition for LGBT Health. LGBT inclusion in federal health surveys. 2010.
97. Mayer KH, Bradford JB, Makadon HJ, Stall R, Goldhammer H, Landers S. Sexual and gender minority health: what we know and what needs to be done. Am J Public Health. 2008;98(6):989–95.
98. McNair RP. Lesbian health inequalities: a cultural minority issue for health professionals. Med J Aust. 2003;178(12):643–5.
99. Stevens PE. Lesbians and doctors: experiences of solidarity and domination in health care settings. Gend Soc. 1996;10(1):24–41.
100. Stevens PE. Structural and interpersonal impact of heterosexual assumptions on lesbian health care clients. Nurs Res. 1995;44(1):24–41.
101. Lombardi E. Enhancing transgender health care. Am J Public Health. 2001;91(6):869–72.
102. Lombardi E. Varieties of transgender/transsexual lives and their relationship with transphobia. J Homosex. 2009;56(8):977–92.
103. Bradford J, Reisner S, Honnold JA, Xavier J. Experiences of transgender-related discrimination and implications for health: results from the Virginia Transgender Health Initiative Study. Am J Public Health. 2013;103(10):1820–9.
104. Bonvicini KA, Perlin MJ. The same but different: clinician–patient communication with gay and lesbian patients. Patient Educ Couns. 2003;51(2):115–22.
105. Klitzman RB, Greenberg JD. Patterns of communication between gay and lesbian patients and their health care providers. J Homosex. 2002;42(4):65–75.
106. McNair R, Hegarty K. Guidelines for the primary care of lesbian, gay, and bisexual people: a systematic review. Ann Fam Med. 2010;8(6):533–41.
107. Diamant AL, Schuster MA, Lever J. Receipt of health care services by lesbians. Am J Prev Med. 2000;19(3):141–8.
108. Diamant AL, Schuster MA, McGuigan K, Lever J. Lesbians' sexual history with men: implications for taking a sexual history. Arch Intern Med. 1999;159(22):2730–6.

Chapter 9
Breast Cancer in Lesbian and Bisexual Women

Ulrike Boehmer

Abstract This chapter describes breast cancer survivorship of women who identify as lesbian or bisexual and of women who prefer or have a woman partner, all of which are captured under the term sexual minority women. Reviewed are what is known about sexual minority women with breast cancer, comparing sexual minority women to heterosexual women, when information is available, but also paying close attention to unique issues for sexual minority women with breast cancer. Throughout this chapter, shortcomings of the available information and gaps in knowledge are brought to the forefront. Finally, challenges for research are discussed, next steps for breast cancer research that focuses on sexual minority women are described, and a research trajectory for sexual minority women with breast cancer is outlined.

Within this chapter, the focus will be on breast cancer survivorship, that is, this chapter will begin with those who have been diagnosed with breast cancer. It will summarize the experiences of those living with breast cancer. While some transgender individuals or gay and bisexual men will develop breast cancer, given the dearth of research on these populations' experiences with breast cancer, they are omitted from this chapter with a call to conduct research on these populations' experiences. To date, lesbian or bisexual women and women who have a woman partner, defined as sexual minority women (SMW) with breast cancer, have almost exclusively occupied research on understanding cancer in sexual minority populations. Despite this focus, the current understanding of sexual minority women with breast cancer is nevertheless incomplete and patchy, which is why this chapter will present what is known but also describe areas of omission and point to questions that need to be answered in the future.

U. Boehmer (✉)
Department of Community Health Sciences, Boston University School of Public Health, Boston, MA, USA
e-mail: Boehmer@bu.edu

U. Boehmer, R. Elk (eds.), *Cancer and the LGBT Community*,
DOI 10.1007/978-3-319-15057-4_9

Demographic and Clinical Characteristics of Breast Cancer Survivors

Because cancer registries do not collect data on sexual orientation [1], it has hardly been assessed whether sexual orientation differences exist with respect to other demographic characteristics, stage at diagnosis, and receipt of life-saving treatments. So far, the best data on these characteristics stem from one population-based study, which recruited survivors of non-recurrent and non-metastatic breast cancer from a state cancer registry an average of 5 years after diagnosis [2]. When SMW, who participated in the study, were compared to the population of registry cases, SMW were significantly younger at diagnosis and less likely married, but similar with respect race or ethnicity [2]. In this study of ductal carcinoma in situ (DCIS) and stage I to III cancers, sexual minority women were more likely diagnosed with DCIS or stage I than the population of registry cases [2]. When the cancer treatments of the heterosexual and sexual minority women who participated in the survey study were compared, breast-conserving lumpectomy was more common among sexual minority than heterosexual women, and among women who underwent mastectomy, comparatively fewer sexual minority than heterosexual women opted for breast reconstruction [3]. Receipt of adjuvant therapies, that is radiation, chemotherapy, and/or anti-estrogen treatments, however, was similar for heterosexual and sexual minority women. Convenience samples confirm this pattern [4] of SMW having earlier diagnoses of breast cancer and receiving more breast-conserving surgical treatment. Nevertheless, caution is required when interpreting these results because the inclusion and exclusion criteria limited this study to women who were alive approximately 5 years after their diagnosis, all treatment data were self-reported, stage IV breast cancers and recurrences were excluded, and the study's geographic scope was limited to one US state in the Northeast with a pre-dominantly white population. These inclusion and exclusion criteria may have biased the results towards an equal or possibly even favorable diagnosis stage and treatment pattern for sexual minority compared to heterosexual breast cancer survivors.

Treatment Decision-Making

The role of sexual minority women in treatment decision-making, their preferences for treatments when presented with a choice, and issues of adherence to treatments have rarely been the focus of studies. So far, there is an absence of knowledge about sexual minority women's preferred role in decision-making, a lack of information about their process of decision-making, including to what extent they obtain second opinions on treatment regimens, their uptake of referrals to specialists, and whether clinical trial participation is weighed as an option. Further, it is unclear if SMW of reproductive age who receive a diagnosis of breast cancer receive information about fertility options, and whether retaining their ability to have children later is taken into account when determining treatment options, as suggested for young, heterosexual women with breast cancer. Information about SMW's decision-making stems from four studies. Two studies focused on LGB's participation in clinical trials, yet neither study focused on breast cancer specifically, both included sexual minority men, and the two studies report contradictory results [5, 6]. Egleston et al. conducted a review of the ClinicalTrials.gov database, which includes detailed information on more than 80,000 clinical trials sponsored by the National Institutes of Health, other governmental agencies, and private industry. They concluded that lesbian and gay men are frequently excluded from clinical trials and that their exclusion is particularly likely when studies focus on sexual function [6]. The second study analyzed self-reported data on clinical trial participation, comparing gay, bisexual, and lesbian individuals to heterosexual individuals, concluding that gay, bisexual, and lesbian individuals have a greater likelihood of participating in clinical trials, again referring to clinical trials in general, not breast cancer specifically [5]. Because both studies included sexual minority men, it is unclear to what extent these findings are impacted by HIV/AIDS-related clinical trials. From two qualitative studies with SMW surgically treated with mastectomy, insights can be gained about SMW's decision-making regarding breast reconstruction [7, 8]. According to Boehmer et al. when deciding for or against breast reconstruction, SMW prioritize a sense of well-being, which includes body strength, survival, and physical function, over outward appearance and normative standards of beauty [7]. SMW who decide against reconstruction perceived breast reconstruction not contributing to their well-being, in that it did not provide them with an improved physical function. SMW who chose reconstruction hoped it would enhance their well-being, preventing depression triggered by their breast loss, but some reported regrets when they did not achieve an enhanced well-being from reconstructive surgery [7]. Rubin and Tannenbaum's findings are generally consistent with the earlier study. Their findings expand the earlier study by stating SMW's decision-making about reconstruction is influenced by sexual, gender, and political identities, as well as by experiences with physicians. Further, Rubin and Tannenbaum state that SMW deciding about breast reconstruction weigh reasons and concerns similar to those reported in the literature as reasons that heterosexual women consider when deciding about reconstruction [8].

Breast cancer treatments have known side effects and long-term effects, including arm morbidity, lymphedema due to surgical treatments and radiation, but also cardiovascular disease, chest pain, myocardial infarction, cardiac toxicity due to radiation and other adjuvant systemic therapy. The prevalence of symptoms and side effects varies greatly among breast cancer survivors in general. While disease-related factors explain much of breast cancer survivors' perceptions, survivor characteristics, including demographics, make an additional contribution towards explaining symptoms. So far, two studies focused on sexual minority status, assessing the subjective impact of breast cancer treatments approximately 5 years after diagnosis, using breast cancer survivors' self-reports of their side effects. When lesbians were compared to heterosexual women, lesbians reported more chemotherapy-induced side effects [9]. The second study reported greater physical impairments in sexual minority women following surgery, radiation, and hormone therapy compared to heterosexual survivors, indicating sexual minority women's poorer perception of these treatments [10]. The paucity of information about SMW's treatment decision-making, their perceptions of breast cancer treatments, including SMW's responses to mastectomy, hair loss, pain, discomfort, and ovarian failure, speak to the need for future studies on these topics.

Such future studies should assess SMW's perceptions and decision-making, to ensure SMW achieve their desired role in decision-making, are fully informed about treatments and their side effects, receive appropriate attention to alleviate the side effects, and are supported in coping with the side effects of treatments.

Interactions with Health Care Providers and the Health Care System

From the moment, a breast cancer diagnosis is made, women are engaged with health care providers and navigate the health care system to address their life threatening disease. Little is known about SMW's perceptions of this process, such as their access through health insurance coverage, their ability to find providers that specialize in breast cancer, and their navigation of the oncology world while they are undergoing life-saving treatments for many weeks or months. To date, much of the research of the general (that is non-cancer population) reports on sexual minority women's greater prevalence of being uninsured compared to heterosexual women [11, 12]. Positive changes are expected in the future due to the Affordable Care Act and the legalization of same-sex marriage in more states, which contributes to SMW's access to health insurance through their spouses. To date, the effects of being uninsured on SMW's use of health care and their breast cancer survival have not been assessed. Research that assessed breast cancer survivors who were alive 5 years after their diagnosis, concluded that there were no differences in insurance status by sexual orientation [3], suggesting that SMW who survive breast cancer have gained access to health insurance, possibly relying on Medicaid or Medicare if they meet eligibility criteria.

Qualitative studies inform about SMW's perceptions of their interactions with health care providers. SMW actively disclosed their sexual minority status to physicians, whereas none of the physicians actively inquired about sexual orientation [13]. The majority of SMW with breast cancer disclosed their sexual orientation to their breast cancer providers, nevertheless SMW perceived their relationship with their providers as difficult [13]. Women who took it upon themselves to tell their breast cancer providers about their sexual minority status were more open about their sexual orientation to others in their social network than women who decided against disclosing their sexual minority status to their provider. Both groups of SMW perceived themselves to be in a life-threatening emergency situation and evaluated their personal safety when deciding whether to disclose their sexual minority status. The disclosers had more personal resources available, which reassured them that disclosure was safe. Nondisclosers had fewer resources available, feared homophobia, and perceived disclosure as unsafe [13]. SMW with breast cancer reported a preference for female providers [14]. Nevertheless, the study ultimately concluded that physicians of either gender can achieve satisfying sexual minority patient-provider relationships. Learned provider traits, consisting of positive interpersonal behaviors, e.g., expressions of respect, seeking a connection with and showing an interest in the patient, perceiving the patient as an equal, and having good communication skills, as well as providers' medical expertise are linked to SMW's satisfaction with their physician relationship [14]. Qualitative as well as quantitative studies that compare lesbian to heterosexual women with breast cancer reported that lesbians were less satisfied with the care they received, and were less satisfied with their health care providers [15, 16]. Yet sexual minority women did not differ from heterosexual women in their rating of their communication with providers [16]. A study of breast cancer survivors, 5 years post diagnosis, found that sexual minority and heterosexual women reported similar levels of trust in their physicians, [17]. Interestingly, when lesbian women were compared to bisexual women with breast cancer, bisexual women reported significantly less trust in their providers [18]. A qualitative study of lesbians diagnosed with breast or gynecological cancers reported on their experiences with providers [19]. In this study, most lesbians described negative experiences with providers, yet reported not feeling discriminated against. Few described being targeted, denied standard care, or that aspects of their identity and social context relevant to cancer care were dismissed [19]. Another study of SMW assessed discrimination experiences in the health care system, concluding SMW's discrimination experiences are low [20]. When discrimination experiences captured everyday life experiences and not discrimination in the health care setting specifically, sexual minority women with breast cancer reported more experiences of discrimination than heterosexual women [17]. Overall, the research to date describes a complex relationship between SMW and their providers and the health care system, pointing to opportunities to improve the quality of care for SMW. Recently, the Institute of Medicine placed much emphasis on improving the quality of care cancer survivors receive [21], recommending the use of survivorship care plans to facilitate coordination of care and adherence to the recommended follow up care. While there is variation in the implementation of such plans and their use is still infrequent [22], it is unclear if SMW with breast cancer are considered equally in this quality improvement and whether SMW's survivorship plans are tailored to address their unique needs.

Secondary Survivors and Social Support of Breast Cancer Survivors

In this chapter, the term 'secondary survivor' refers to spouses, partners, friends, or family members of the breast cancer survivor. Some may be more familiar with the term informal caregiver, to describe loved ones or friends to a person living with cancer. NCI defines loved ones as secondary providers to signify that they are a part of cancer survivorship. Because of the stress associated with a cancer diagnosis and the impact of the cancer treatments, sexual minority survivors who are diagnosed with breast cancer are likely utilizing their social support network for a variety of tasks, which may range from providing transportation, assisting with treatment decision-making, and providing care as well as emotional or spiritual support.

So far, one study provides information about the sources of social support for SMW with breast cancer, in that survivors were asked to identify "their trusted other" or most important support person for their cancer experience [23], without forcing a particular choice of type of support provider. This approach resulted in 10 % of SMW with breast cancer reporting not having such a person. Another 10 % reported having such a person, but did not allow the researchers to contact their support person because they currently had a strained relationship or felt it be too upsetting for their support person. Of the contacted support providers, all but one agreed to participate in the study [23]. All support providers were female, 79 % were relationship partners, 13 % were friends, and 9 % relatives. Further, having a support provider was independent of the size of the survivors' social network, yet partnered sexual minority women were more likely to have a support person. Finally, those who had a support provider available to them reported greater social support than SMW who did not have a designated person, from which one can infer that single SMW are at risk of not being supported when dealing with breast cancer [23]. Some hypothesized that sexual minority survivors of breast cancer will be at risk for low support, in that they may not be able to rely on support from their families of origin. Therefore, a number of studies have evaluated the available social support of SMW with breast cancer [16]. Two studies, using different measures of social support and assessing breast cancer survivors at different time points in their survivorship, concluded that sexual minority women with breast cancer have the same level of support as heterosexual survivors [17, 24]. However, when studies assessed the sources of social support, differences between heterosexual and sexual minority women became apparent. Lesbians relied less on relatives and more on friends for support compared to heterosexual women, who relied more on relatives and less on friends [16, 24]. Some studies focused on the spouses or partners of breast cancer survivors. So far, the results are less than conclusive, in that one study found that heterosexual and lesbian women with breast cancer reported similar relationship satisfaction and relationship fighting or friction [24]. Further, the two survivor groups were similar on their perceptions of their partners being bothered by their surgical scars, on the amount of affection their partners expressed, and their partners' reaction to breast cancer as a threat to their lives [24]. Fobair and colleagues, however, found differences in that lesbians were more likely to report feeling loved and supported by their partners, while heterosexual women more likely reported their partners made too many demands on them [16]. The latter findings were echoed by a qualitative study that found female partners are the most valuable source of support for SMW and that female partners provide support by fulfilling complex social support functions, which may range from discussing the survivor's distress to managing the home [25]. An important aspect put forth by this qualitative study is SMW's perception of their partners being stressed and greatly burdened by their breast cancer diagnosis and by providing support to them [25].

An important gap in the literature is that with the exception of one study, the experiences of secondary breast cancer survivors have not been assessed. Comparing breast cancer survivors and their support providers who were mostly relationship partners, some friends, and some family members, showed that support providers had less support available and a trend towards a smaller social network than the breast cancer survivor. Survivors and their support providers reported similar levels of mood disturbance and sexual orientation disclosure [23]. So far the experiences of secondary survivors is a particularly underdeveloped aspect of cancer survivorship, indicating that more research is needed to understand these secondary survivors' experiences, allowing for a wide range of secondary survivors, including relationship partners and children of SMW with breast cancer. Despite an absence of studies that inform in much detail about the social support needs of sexual minority survivors of breast cancer and their secondary survivors, it is of note that throughout the country, in urban areas and online, cancer support services are available that focus specifically on SMW and in some cases their partners. One study that compared heterosexual and sexual minority survivors of breast cancer concluded that sexual minority survivors more likely attend cancer support groups and are also more likely seek out mental health counseling to deal with their breast cancer compared to heterosexual survivors [26]. However, this study did not assess whether sexual minority survivors' use of cancer support groups referred to lesbian or sexual minority specific groups. Three qualitative studies reported on sexual minority women's experiences with cancer support groups made up of predominantly heterosexual group members [15, 27, 28]. These studies reported on SMW's "otherness" and alienation from the heterosexual women in the group, reporting that heterosexual group members lacked awareness and openness for sexual minority women's lives, which caused sexual minority women to conceal their sexual orientation, leave the group, or perceive diminished benefit from the group meetings [15, 27, 28]. Therefore, it is necessary for future studies to carefully measure that SMW's rates of support group use refers to continued social support group attendance and having support needs met, rather than a reflection of short-term utilization followed by dropping out of groups due to a lack of benefit. Secondary support providers' use and interest in support groups and mental health counseling due to the stress of the survivors' breast cancer is unknown to date. However, finding appropriate and positive support groups for partners that match their needs is likely magnified and an unmet need to date [28].

Quality of Life and Psychological Adjustment

Much of the research to date focused on assessing SMW's coping with a breast cancer diagnosis, their quality of life, and psychological adjustment after breast cancer. Several studies report that sexual minority women's coping styles differ from heterosexual women's coping, revealing mostly areas of strengths in sexual minority women's coping. Compared to heterosexual women, lesbians use less cognitive avoidance, less denial, less anxious preoccupation, and less hopelessness coping, which are strengths. Other strengths are SMW's greater expression of anger, increased venting, and more positive reframing [16, 24, 26]. Compared to heterosexual survivors, sexual minority survivors show vulnerabilities too, in that one study found lesbians have less fighting spirit [16]. However, a later study concluded that sexual minority women were similar to heterosexual women with respect to fatalism and fighting spirit coping [26]. According to one qualitative study, at the time of diagnosis lesbian women experience significantly more stress than heterosexual women [15]. Most other studies that assessed stress, anxiety and depression, reported on sexual minority survivors at later time points, frequently years after their diagnosis.

Breast cancer studies consistently concluded heterosexual and sexual minority survivors have similar quality of life, anxiety, depression, and mood disturbance [3, 15, 16, 20, 29]. This is contrary to expectations, given findings in the general population of sexual minority women having more mental health problems than heterosexual women [30, 31]. Benefit finding is a reflection of a person's changed beliefs and life lessons learned from a traumatic event such as breast cancer, and sexual minority and heterosexual survivors shared similar levels of benefit finding [26]. In addition, with respect to physical health, contrary to expectations, overweight and obesity rates and sexual well-being were similar in sexual minority and heterosexual survivors of breast cancer [16, 17, 24, 32]. When considering breast cancer survivors' body image, sexual function, and sexual enjoyment, sexual minority and heterosexual women were similar [17]. Because of differences in sexual expressions and sexual activities, one can call into question whether heterosexual women are an appropriate comparison group for sexual minority women. Therefore, one study compared age- and partner-status matched samples of SMW with breast cancer to SMW without cancer and found overall risk of sexual dysfunction did not differ between these two groups [33]. However, the SMW who had a history of breast cancer reported lower sexual frequency, lower desire, lower ability to reach orgasm, and more pain related to sexual activity compared to SMW without cancer [33]. Moreover, the same study also compared these two groups of women on quality of life, anxiety and depression, concluding breast cancer survivors' quality of life, anxiety and depression was similar [34]. As one would expect, given the cancer treatments the survivors had been exposed to, sexual minority women who are breast cancer survivors were more likely menopausal compared to age-matched controls without cancer [34].

Understanding Quality of Life and Mechanisms to Affect Psychological Adjustment

Much attention focused on understanding why SMW might have better than expected quality of life and psychological adjustment. Arena and colleagues hypothesized that lesbians who are already living in a hostile environment due to their sexual minority status, might perceive breast cancer as one more stressor, while among heterosexual women the diagnosis of breast cancer and its treatments might constitute the first major adversity in their lives [24]. The finding that lesbian's obesity after breast cancer is similar to heterosexual women's rate, despite much evidence in the non-cancer population of lesbians having higher obesity rates, has been interpreted as an indication that lesbians might more likely improve their weight-related behaviors after cancer than heterosexual women [32]. Only longitudinal studies with data prior to and post-diagnosis of breast cancer can positively confirm these speculations. It is important to note that findings of similar quality of life and psychological adjustment after breast cancer in sexual minority and heterosexual women is not an indication of an absence of anguish and suffering in sexual minority women after breast cancer. Rather, these findings suggest sexual minority women's psychological responses and reactions to breast cancer are at comparable levels to heterosexual women's, despite much evidence of sexual minority women being underserved and at a disadvantage due to their sexual minority status.

Much effort focused on explaining SMW's quality of life and psychological adjustment. Ultimately, this type of inquiry, which focuses on understanding the factors that contribute to sexual minority women's quality of life and psychological adjustments, is formative for the selection of suitable interventions to improve sexual minority women's quality of life and reduce their mood disturbance, anxiety, and depression. With interventions in mind, it is of particular importance to highlight mutable factors, which are suitable intervention targets. Among such mutable factors are SMW's coping responses to the breast cancer diagnosis. Positive attitudes, cognitive avoidance, and hopelessness coping are linked to finding benefit in the breast cancer experience [26]. Coping responses in general and in some instances, sexual minority women's different coping styles are linked to quality of life, anxiety, and depression [17]. Specifically, sexual minority women's fighting spirit coping is linked to sexual minority women's reduced anxiety compared to heterosexual survivors' anxiety [17]. Fatalism coping was identified as another strength of sexual minority women, which then linked to sexual minority women's better mental health and less depression, while coping via anxious preoccupation correlated to quality of life, anxiety and depression for both groups of survivors [17]. Other aspects associated with better quality of life, less anxiety and depression, were body image and perceptions about one's future health [17]. Body image was associated with mental health, anxiety and depression in both sexual minority and heterosexual survivors, suggesting changing women's perceptions of their bodies through targeted interventions may improve their well-being [17]. Moreover, heterosexual women with breast cancer generally have a better perception of their future than sexual minority women. However, when sexual minority women perceived their future positively, they had fewer depression symptoms than heterosexual women, indicating one may be able to affect sexual minority women's depression through an improved perception of their future health [17].

So far, only one intervention study sought to intervene on lesbians' psychological responses, using supportive-expressive group therapy intervention [35]. This small study reported positive results in that after the 12-week intervention, lesbians reported less emotional distress, intrusiveness, avoidance, and better coping with their breast cancer [35]. However, lesbians' body image, sexuality, and attitudes towards health care providers remained unaffected by the intervention. To date no other intervention studies have been conducted with SMW who are living with breast cancer, pointing to an area of dire need. A study of SMW's sexual function after breast cancer linked women's perceived sexual attractiveness and urogenital symptoms to their sexual function. When focusing on partnered women only, relationship cohesion and their menopausal status had an additional impact on their sexual function after breast cancer [34]. The study concluded education about the need for greater intensity and duration of genital stimulation and use of mechanical devices might be useful to address sexual minority survivors' urogenital symptoms, while psychosocial interventions might be helpful to address sexual minority women's perceived sexual attractiveness and relationship concerns [34].

Other potential intervention targets for this population of breast cancer survivors could be these women's unique self-perceptions stemming from their sexual minority identity. One of the early studies linked internalized homophobia, a negative self-perception of one's sexual minority status, to greater distress in lesbians with breast cancer [36], while showing disclosure of sexual orientation was unrelated to distress. Later studies are somewhat confirmative of sexual minority-specific issues relating to psychological outcomes in sexual minority survivors. One study of lesbian and bisexual survivors of breast cancer linked the perception that one's sexual minority identity has been difficult to greater depression [18]. In addition, lesbian and bisexual survivors' openness, that is, disclosure of one's sexual minority identity to coworkers and heterosexual friends, linked to lower anxiety, with the caveat that lesbians showed more openness about disclosing their sexual orientation to others, including health care providers, and displayed more trust in their health care providers than bisexual survivors [18]. However, having trust in health care providers did not significantly contribute to explaining lesbian and bisexual breast cancer survivors' quality of life, anxiety, and depression [18]. Similarly, a study of SMW confirmed that disclosure of a lesbian identity to providers does not result in lower distress [37]. A study with dyadic data, from SMW with breast cancer and their support providers sheds further light on the issue of disclosure or openness about one's sexual minority identity [23]. This study found that when focusing on breast cancer survivors and support providers' mood disturbance, being open about one's identity is associated with less distress in the women with breast cancer and the support provider. However, when assessing the dyad of breast cancer survivor and support provider, discordance in openness, consisting of the support provider being more open about her sexual minority identity than the sexual minority woman with breast cancer, negatively affects the survivor, in that she shows more emotional distress [23]. Furthermore, this study's dyadic data point to the need for assistance and possibly interventions that address survivors' support providers. For example, these supporters of SMW with breast cancer were primarily these women's partners, had less support than survivors, and had generally a smaller social network than women with breast cancer [23]. Finally, the well-being of support providers and SMW with breast cancer was interrelated, in that their level of distress was about equal, meaning a distressed survivor matched a distressed support provider. This may create opportunities to affect breast cancer survivors' well-being through alleviating their support providers' distress, possibly improving both parties' well-being [23]. Consistent with this are findings that show sexual minority women who live with their partners report more anxiety than heterosexual women [17], a possible indication that sexual minority women's partners are more distressed than heterosexual women's partners. This again opens up the possibility of affecting the well-being of sexual minority survivors of breast cancer via services, programs, and support for these women's partners.

Despite an absence of evidence-based interventions and programs for SMW with breast cancer, findings indicate that SMW on their own find means to improve their well-being. Specifically, sexual minority women's greater use of cancer support groups and mental health counseling for breast cancer-related issues compared to heterosexual women correlated with better mental health in sexual minority than heterosexual women [17], indicating that sexual minority women were more likely to meet their needs for psychosocial services than heterosexual women. However, future studies will need to distinguish between sexual minority- or non-specific support groups to identify the benefits that sexual minority survivors obtain from either one of the respective social support groups. The evidence for the benefits of psychopharmacological interventions on the other hand is mixed. SMW had a positive response to anti-anxiety medications but those on mood stabilizers did not have a positive response to the medication. Those on mood stabilizers reported an increase in symptoms of depression [17].

Consistent with expectations, social support greatly benefits SMW with breast cancer, improving their quality of life [20] and depression [18]. In addition, social support has been shown to be of equal importance for sexual minority and heterosexual survivors' anxiety, while sexual minority women with social support have lower levels of depression than comparable heterosexual women [17]. However, the few studies that paid close attention to the sources of social support suggest that having one specific designated support provider available does not in itself improve sexual minority women's adjustment or coping responses [23], indicating the breadth of the social support network and level of support received contributes to positive well-being for sexual minority women. This is a particularly informative finding, suggesting single SMW are not necessarily at a disadvantage, assuming they can find the support from others in their social support network, and underscores the opportunity of assisting SMW of any partner status through social support services. As previously discussed, having a partner can also increase distress in sexual minority women under certain conditions. A study of lesbian and bisexual women who were with a female partner, a male partner, or were without a partner, found sexual minority women with a female partner had significantly better mental health than those who were with a male partner [18], supporting sexual minority women's positive perceptions of their female partners [25]. Partner status itself has been linked to physical health, with partnered sexual minority women showing significantly better physical health than partnered heterosexual women [17].

From some findings, one can infer opportunities exist for interventions or programs in the health care setting, by changing care delivery. For example, sexual minority women who were on anti-estrogen therapy, a treatment typically lasting about 5 years, showed better mental health than heterosexual survivors on this therapy. This possibly indicates that sexual minority women derive benefits from actively addressing their cancers and having a prolonged interaction with the health care system [17]. Further, because of the strong effects of systemic side effects and arm morbidities on survivors' well-being, rehabilitation services and better control of long-term and late effects of breast cancer will likely improve sexual minority women's physical and emotional well-being [17, 38]. Taken together these findings may indicate that SMW are an opportune target group for survivorship care plans and increased monitoring through health care providers. Other findings point to additional opportunities to intervene in the health care system through educational trainings for health care providers and staff to increase their level of competency when dealing with sexual minority women. For example, the previously noted strained interactions between SMW and their health care providers, point to opportunities for improvement. Specifically, studies indicating that health care providers do not ask about their patients' sexual orientation, leaving it up to SMW to bring this aspect of their lives to their providers' attention [13]. The fact that lesbian-identified women's greater rate of disclosure, compared to bisexual women's, does not improve their well-being as one would expect [36, 37], raises questions about health care providers' ability to respond to these disclosures and about their ability to make these women comfortable and support them appropriately. However, more research needs to be done on specifically understanding SMW's needs with respect to sexual minority status disclosure and their experiences of discrimination in the health care setting to more fully inform provider and staff training and increase their cultural competency. So far, qualitative studies show sexual minority survivors' negative experiences with providers, while insisting that they did not feel discriminated against [39]. Similarly, sexual minority women framed breast cancer as a "women's issue, not a lesbian issue," highlighting their ability to manage their sexual minority identity in the context of breast cancer and not perceiving themselves as disadvantaged [40]. Another study concluded discrimination experiences in the health care setting are low [20]. However, the study failed to assess sexual minority women's disclosure to health care providers, and given that many sexual minority women in their sample endorsed "being perceived by doctors and nurses as heterosexually-identified" it appears many sexual minority women concealed their sexual minority identity, which this study related to better quality of life [20]. A study that measured sexual minority and heterosexual survivors' discrimination experiences in everyday life integrated discrimination due to sexual orientation as one response choice along with other choices such as feeling discriminated due to one's gender, age, income, race/ethnicity, appearance and having cancer [3]. As one would expect, SMW reported more experiences of discrimination than heterosexual survivors. However, upon further examination it became clear that less than half of SMW reported discrimination due to their sexual orientation. Rather sexual minority women reported more gender, cancer, and race/ethnicity discrimination than heterosexual women, despite sharing with heterosexual women being female, having cancer, and their race/ethnicity. Furthermore, sexual minority breast cancer survivors were younger and had higher income than heterosexual survivors; nevertheless, they reported more discrimination due to age and income, suggesting that that sexual minority women appraise discrimination differently, frequently attributing it to factors other than their sexual orientation [3]. The diversity and inconsistency of findings of discrimination in the context of receiving breast cancer care highlight the complexity of attribution of discrimination. It may be that quantitative measures of discrimination are not yet sufficiently refined to collect data on sexual minority women's discrimination. For example, sexual minority women may perceive the care they receive as better than they expected or may perceive providers and the health care system as heteronormative, consistent with the heteronormative society they live in, which may explain reports of no or low experiences of discrimination. Similarly, as has been shown for other minority groups, sexual minority women may maximize their perception of control, while minimizing discrimination because the consequences of minimizing discrimination are psychologically beneficial [41, 42]. Therefore, future research is needed to fully understand how appraisal of discrimination experiences affect sexual minority women's experiences with the health care setting and providers specifically. So far, studies have been able to link discrimination to anxiety and depression, even when other factors were controlled [17, 29].

While the previously-mentioned studies provide information about mechanisms that can be targeted by interventions, inferences can also be made about subgroups among SMW who are at risk for worse outcomes after breast cancer diagnosis and its treatments. Sexual minority breast cancer survivors with health insurance had worse physical health than heterosexual survivors with insurance, which has been interpreted as an indication that SMW with poor physical health may be able to obtain insurance through Medicaid and Medicare [17]. Not surprisingly, having a later stage of breast cancer linked to worse mental health and depression [17], suggesting these sexual minority women have more needs for support and assistance to alleviate their suffering. Findings of lesser depression in survivors with more education and those who are employed likely speaks to greater resources available to these women [17]. On the other hand, it is also possible that this finding indicates a return to work is less likely for women who suffer from depression due to their breast cancer. This is a hypothesis to be explored by later studies that have pre- and post-diagnosis information on breast cancer survivors, along with an assessment of breast cancer's economic impact on sexual minority women, which is so far unknown. Residing in more impoverished neighborhoods has been linked to worse mental health and to greater anxiety specifically [17], pointing to a vulnerability in cancer survivors who live in resource-poor neighborhoods, which needs to be further explored to fully understand which aspect of the neighborhood impacts breast cancer survivors' mental health. Given the increasing legal opportunities for sexual minority women to enter into same-sex marriages, it is also of note that sexual minority women's marital status has been linked to their adjustment after breast cancer. Being married has been shown to be related to less depression and anxiety in breast cancer survivors [17], suggesting benefits of marriage to which sexual minority women finally have access to as more states make same-sex marriage an option. A particular oversight of breast cancer studies to date is information about breast cancer survivors who are sexual minorities, but also report as racial or ethnic minorities. While studies included racial and ethnic minority women, the numbers of sexual minority women who are also racial and ethnic minorities are too small to assess whether these women have additional disadvantages, a possible double jeopardy due to their dual minority status.

Conclusions and Next Steps

While breast cancer is the most thoroughly evaluated cancer type in SMW, many questions and needs for future studies remain. As indicated previously, we still lack information about SMW with stage IV breast cancer, breast cancer recurrences, and second cancers. So far, breast cancer studies focused mostly on women who are many years past their diagnosis, meaning early survivorship, including responses to their diagnosis, their decision-making, and their experiences while undergoing treatments are still areas in need of exploration. Further, studies must give attention to SMW in different life circumstances. For example, lacking are breast cancer studies of SMW who are racial or ethnic minorities, different age cohorts, sexual minorities who live in poverty, with children, and those who live in rural areas, areas where few sexual minority women live, or areas without a strong presence of a lesbian, gay, bisexual community. The economic burden of breast cancer on sexual minority women's lives, families, and relationships is also unexplored. Therefore issues such as whether SMW return to their same workplace or need to switch jobs, whether sexual minorities' partners or spouses have dedicated time or the ability to go on medical leave to take care of their spouse or partner who is undergoing cancer treatment is unknown. Little is known about the partners, nothing about children of SMW with breast cancer, and next to nothing about changes to these relationships due to breast cancer. So far, almost all information about SMW with breast cancer has been derived from cross-sectional studies, which means we have no information about changes over time, including about the long-term and late effects of breast cancer and its treatments. Pre-diagnosis data on SMW with breast cancer are needed to more fully understand the changes brought on by breast cancer. Along those lines, changes to the health behaviors of breast cancer survivors have to be explored, which include not smoking, moderate alcohol use, having a healthy diet, regular physical activity, surveillance to detect recurrences, second cancers, and late effects and long-term effects of breast cancer treatments.

A few studies characterized SMW's perceptions of their healthcare providers, from which one can at least cursorily infer that this is an important area for improvement. However, no research to date focused on the health care providers who interact with and care for SMW with breast cancer, which means their perceptions, attitudes, knowledge, and skill caring for these patients is still unknown. Future research with health care professionals may help answer the question whether health care professionals are open to changing their approach or whether they feel their knowledge of breast cancer is sufficient because the disease does not present differently in sexual minority versus heterosexual women.

A widely acknowledged challenge for researchers is the identification of SMW with breast cancer and gaining their participation in breast cancer studies. One of the earliest studies recruited 29 lesbians with breast cancer in the San Francisco Bay area [16]. They reported relaxing their eligibility criteria, spending more time recruiting the lesbian sample, and that despite their extensive outreach, the number of lesbian study participants fell short of the estimated number of lesbians with the disease in the San Francisco Bay area [16]. Most studies used similar recruitment strategies, that is, advertising the study through flyers, the internet, and other means of reaching the sexual minority community. However, one study used a statewide cancer registry to find sexual minority women and a heterosexual comparison sample of breast cancer survivors [2]. Their detailed evaluation of their recruitment strategy noted that their process was not only labor intensive, but they also reported reasons why in their experience sexual minority women were not eager to participate in the study, which ranged from a perceived invasion of privacy to likely leading busier and more stressful lives than heterosexual women [2]. Researchers will need to plan on dedicating considerable resources, e.g., spending more time and money on the recruitment of sexual minority women compared to heterosexual women with breast cancer. The difficulties of recruitment and SMW's hesitancy to participate are likely major obstacles for intervention studies with SMW with breast cancer, especially if the intervention depends on repeated face-to-face contacts and participants' willingness to commit to an extended timeframe. To stimulate more intervention studies with breast cancer survivors who are sexual minorities, researchers may need to consider other means of delivering interventions, e.g., via the telephone and the internet.

As noted, to date there exists only one intervention study with lesbians with breast cancer [35]. Much of what has been reported in this chapter about sexual minority women with breast cancer shows that in many respects, they mirror the quality of life, coping, and psychological adjustments of heterosexual women with breast cancer. While these findings are unexpected in that sexual minority women with breast cancer apparently do better than expected, this absence of a disparity must not be interpreted as lack of need for programs for and interventions with SMW who live with breast cancer. To the contrary, the goal of fully understanding the needs of SMW with breast cancer and then intervening with programs and services for the purpose of alleviating suffering and improving these women's well-being remains.

References

1. Bowen DJ, Boehmer U. The lack of cancer surveillance data on sexual minorities and strategies for change. Cancer Causes Control. 2007;18(4):343–9.
2. Boehmer U, Clark M, Glickman M, Timm A, Sullivan M, Bradford J, et al. Using cancer registry data for recruitment of sexual minority women: successes and limitations. J Women's Health. 2010;19(7):1289–97.

3. Boehmer U, Glickman M, Milton J, Winter M. Health-related quality of life in breast cancer survivors of different sexual orientations. Qual Life Res. 2012;21(2):225–36.
4. Dibble SL, Roberts SA. A comparison of breast cancer diagnosis and treatment between lesbian and heterosexual women. J Gay Lesbian Med Assoc. 2002;6(1):9–17.
5. Jabson JM, Blosnich JR. Representation of lesbian, gay, and bisexual people in clinical cancer trials. Ann Epidemiol. 2012 Nov;22(11):821–3.
6. Egleston BL, Dunbrack RL, Jr., Hall MJ. Clinical trials that explicitly exclude gay and lesbian patients. N Engl J Med. 2010;362(11):1054–5.
7. Boehmer U, Linde R, Freund KM. Breast reconstruction following mastectomy for breast cancer: the decisions of sexual minority women. Plast Reconstr Surg. 2007;119(2):464–72.
8. Rubin LR, Tanenbaum M. "Does that make me a woman?": breast cancer, mastectomy, and breast reconstruction decisions among sexual minority women. Psychol Women Q. 2011;35(3):401–14.
9. Dibble SL, Roberts SA. A comparison of breast cancer diagnosis and treatment between lesbian and heterosexual women. J Gay Lesbian Med Assn. 2002;6(1):9–17.
10. Boehmer U, Glickman M, Winter M, Clark MA. Long-term breast cancer survivors' symptoms and morbidity: differences by sexual orientation? J Cancer Surviv. 2013;7(2):203–10 (Comparative Study Research Support, Non-U.S. Gov't).
11. Heck JE, Sell RL, Sheinfeld Gorin S. Health care access among individuals involved in same-sex relationships. Am J Public Health. 2006;96(6):1111–8.
12. Ponce NA, Cochran SD, Pizer JC, Mays VM. The effects of unequal access to health insurance for same-sex couples in California. Health Aff (Millwood). 2010;29(8):1539–48.
13. Boehmer U, Case P. Physicians don't ask, sometimes patients tell: disclosure of sexual orientation among women with breast carcinoma. Cancer. 2004;101(8):1882–9 (Research Support, Non-U.S. Gov't).
14. Boehmer U, Case P. Sexual minority women's interactions with breast cancer providers. Women Health. 2006;44(2):41–58.
15. Matthews AK, Peterman A, Delaney P, Menard L, Brandenburg D. A qualitative exploration of the experiences of lesbian and heterosexual patients with breast cancer. Oncol Nurs Forum. 2002;29(10):1455–62.
16. Fobair P, O'Hanlan K, Koopman C, Classen C, Dimiceli S, Drooker N, et al. Comparison of lesbian and heterosexual women's response to newly diagnosed breast cancer. Psychooncology. 2001;10(1):40–51.
17. Boehmer U, Glickman M, Winter M, Clark MA. Breast cancer survivors of different sexual orientations: which factors explain survivors' quality of life and adjustment? Ann Oncol. 2013;24(6):1622–30.
18. Boehmer U, Glickman M, Winter M, Clark MA. Lesbian and bisexual women's adjustment after a breast cancer diagnosis. J Am Psych Nurs Ass. 2013;19(5):280–92.
19. Sinding C, Barnoff L, Grassau P. Homophobia and heterosexism in cancer care: the experiences of lesbians. Can J Nurs Res. 2004;36(4):170–88.
20. Jabson JM, Donatelle RJ, Bowen D. Breast cancer survivorship: the role of perceived discrimination and sexual orientation. J Cancer Surviv: Res Pract. 2011;5(1):92–101 (Research Support, N.I.H., Extramural Research Support, Non-U.S. Gov't).
21. Institute of Medicine. Editor. From cancer patient to cancer survivor: lost in transition. Washington, DC: The National Academies Press; 2005.
22. Salz T, Oeffinger KC, McCabe MS, Layne TM, Bach PB. Survivorship care plans in research and practice. CA Cancer J Clin. 2012;62(2):101–17.
23. Boehmer U, Freund KM, Linde R. Support providers of sexual minority women with breast cancer: who they are and how they impact the breast cancer experience. J Psychosom Res. 2005;59(5):307–14.
24. Arena PL, Carver CS, Antoni MH, Weiss S, Ironson G, Durán RE. Psychosocial responses to treatment for breast cancer among lesbian and heterosexual women Women Health. 2006;44(2):81–102.

25. White JL, Boehmer U. Long-term breast cancer survivors' perceptions of support from woman partners: an exploratory study with sexual minority women. Oncol Nurs Forum. 2012;39(2):210–7.
26. Boehmer U, Glickman M, Winter M, Clark MA. Coping and benefit finding among long-term breast cancer survivors of different sexual orientations. Women & Therapy. 2014;37(3–4):222–41.
27. Fish J. Coming out about breast cancer in lesbian and bisexual women. Leicester: health policy research unit; De Montfort University Funded by the NHS National Cancer Action Team; 2010. http://hdl.handle.net/2086/4744. Accessed 21 June 2014.
28. Paul LB, Pitagora D, Brown B, Tworecke A, Rubin L. Support needs and resources of sexual minority women with breast cancer. Psychooncology. 2014;23(5):578–84.
29. Boehmer U, Glickman M, Winter M. Anxiety and depression in breast cancer survivors of different sexual orientations. J Consult Clin Psychol. 2012;80(3):382–95.
30. King M, Semlyen J, Tai SS, Killaspy H, Osborn D, Popelyuk D, et al. A systematic review of mental disorder, suicide, and deliberate self harm in lesbian, gay and bisexual people. BMC Psychiatry. 2008;8:70.
31. Bostwick WB, Boyd CJ, Hughes TL, McCabe SE. Dimensions of sexual orientation and the prevalence of mood and anxiety disorders in the United States. Am J Pub Health. 2010;100(3):468–75.
32. Boehmer U, Mertz M, Timm A, Glickman M, Sullivan M, Potter J. Overweight and obesity in long-term breast cancer survivors: how does sexual orientation impact BMI?. Cancer Invest. 2011;29(3):220–8.
33. Boehmer U, Ozonoff A, Timm A, Winter M, Potter J. After breast cancer: sexual functioning of sexual minority survivors. J Sex Res. 2014;51(6):681–9.
34. Boehmer U, Timm A, Ozonoff A, Potter J. Explanatory factors of sexual function in sexual minority women breast cancer survivors. Ann Oncol. 2012;23(11):2873–8.
35. Fobair P, Koopman C, Dimiceli S, O'Hanlan K, Butler L, Classen C, et al. Psychosocial intervention for lesbians with primary breast cancer. Psychooncology. 2002;11(5):427–38.
36. McGregor BA, Carver CS, Antoni MH, Weiss S, Yount SE, Ironson G. Distress and internalized homophobia among lesbian women treated for early stage breast cancer. Psychol Women Q. 2001;25(1):1–9.
37. Boehmer U, Linde R, Freund KM. Sexual minority women's coping and psychological adjustment after a diagnosis of breast cancer. J Women's Health. 2005;14(3):214–24.
38. Boehmer U, Glickman M, Winter M, Clark MA. Long-term breast cancer survivors' symptoms and morbidity: Differences by sexual orientation? Journal of Cancer Survivorship. 2013;7(2):203–10.
39. Sinding C, Barnoff L, Grassau P. Homophobia and heterosexism in cancer care: the experiences of lesbians. CJNR: Can J Nurs Res. 2004;36(4):170–88.
40. Boehmer U, White JL. Sexual minority status and long-term breast cancer survivorship. Women Health. 2012;52(1):71–87.
41. Ruggiero KM, Taylor DM. Why minority group members perceive or do not perceive the discrimination that confronts them: the role of self-esteem and perceived control. J person soc psychol. 1997;72(2):373–89.
42. Contrada RJ, Ashmore RD, Gary ML, Coups E, Egeth JD, Sewell A, et al. Ethnicity-related sources of stress and their effects on well-being. Curr dir Psychol Sci. 2000;9(4):136–9.

Chapter 10
Gay Men and Prostate Cancer: Opportunities to Improve HRQOL and Access to Care

Gilad E. Amiel, Heather H. Goltz, Evan P. Wenker, Michael R. Kauth, Tae L. Hart and David M. Latini

Abstract Little previous research has focused on gay and bisexual men who develop prostate cancer. However, a few small studies have recently been published that begin to tell the story of the specific problems gay and bisexual men with prostate cancer face. In this chapter, we summarize this recent literature and offer specific suggestions for changes to made by urologists and other cancer treatment providers to address the unique needs of gay and bisexual men for survivorship services. In addition, we discuss techniques that providers can use to make their practice more welcoming for gay and bisexual men facing prostate cancer.

D. M. Latini (✉) · G. E. Amiel · E. P. Wenker
Scott Department of Urology, Baylor College of Medicine, Houston, TX, USA
e-mail: Latini@bcm.edu

H. H. Goltz
Social Work Program, University of Houston—Downtown, Houston, TX, USA

Section of Infectious Diseases, Department of Medicine, Baylor College of Medicine, Houston, TX, USA

M. R. Kauth
VA South Central Mental Illness Research, Education and Clinical Center, Houston, TX, USA

D. M. Latini · M. R. Kauth
Mental Health Care Line, Michael E. DeBakey VA Medical Center, Houston, TX, USA

M. R. Kauth
Center for Innovations in Quality, Effectiveness and Safety, Michael E. DeBakey VA Medical Center, Houston, TX, USA

Department of Psychiatry & Behavioral Sciences, Baylor College of Medicine, Houston, TX, USA

T. L. Hart
Department of Psychology, Ryerson University, Toronto, ON, Canada

U. Boehmer, R. Elk (eds.), *Cancer and the LGBT Community*,
DOI 10.1007/978-3-319-15057-4_10

Overview

Prostate cancer (PCa) is the most common male malignancy. There were an estimated 240,000 new cases and over 2.6 million survivors in the United States in 2013 [1]. While there has been no large-scale, population-based study examining the prevalence of prostate cancer by sexual orientation, some work has suggested that gay and bisexual (G/B) men may be diagnosed less frequently than heterosexual men [2]. However, using a conservative estimate of the prevalence of G/B men in the general population of 2–3 %, at least 5000 G/B men are diagnosed with prostate cancer each year; over 50,000 are still living following treatment [3].

Compared to their heterosexual counterparts, G/B men face several unique challenges in healthcare settings. A long-standing concern is that G/B men are likely to have prostate cancer diagnosed at a later stage relative to heterosexual men. Many in the gay community believe that gay men are likely to receive inadequate prostate care, citing discomfort coming out to physicians [4], lack of adequate social support [5], and the possibility of excessively rough or violent rectal exams by homophobic practitioners [6]. Stigma around homosexuality may be related to negative experiences in the health care system, such as providers failing to ask about sexual orientation and assuming heterosexuality [7]. Race and ethnicity may compound stigma further, as data from large study of California men suggests that G/B African-American men receive prostate specific antigen testing less frequently than heterosexual African-American men or G/B Caucasian men [8]. Taken together, negative experiences with the healthcare system are likely related to the poorer health outcomes experienced by lesbian, gay and bisexual persons [9].

Like many heterosexual men, gay men have limited understanding of their prostate or the range of sexual challenges associated with prostate cancer and its treatment [4]. With hundreds of thousands of G/B men facing the prospect of future prostate disease, it is essential for this population to be knowledgeable about their risk, options for treatment, ways to improve health-related quality of life (HRQOL) after treatment, and what to expect from their health care providers. By the same token, providers need to understand the challenges faced by G/B with PCa, some of which are unique to this population. In this chapter, we briefly outline the treatments for PCa and typical changes in HRQOL post-treatment. We then describe the unique concerns that G/B men with PCa may have, summarize the limited existing literature on HRQOL for G/B men with prostate cancer, and suggest ways in which health care professionals may provide more patient-centered, affirming care for G/B men with PCa.

Prostate Cancer Treatment and Health-Related Quality of Life

The currently available treatments for localized prostate cancer carry the risk of a number of possible iatrogenic symptoms, primarily urinary and bowel incontinence and erectile dysfunction (ED) [10]. The issue of iatrogenic symptoms is particularly important to men with prostate cancer because their prognosis, relative to other cancers is very good and the potential treatment-related symptoms can have such important implications for HRQOL. Because of early prostate cancer's long natural history, men who develop iatrogenic symptoms will experience those symptoms for years [11].

Treatment-related symptoms vary by the treatment received. Men who receive a radical prostatectomy (RP) are more likely to have problems with urinary and sexual functioning. Radiotherapy patients are more likely to experience bowel problems [10, 11]. However, this symptom picture may change over time. Surgery patients frequently report substantial improvements in their urinary and sexual functioning 12 months after treatment [12]. A recently published study shows that overall quality of life, sexual desire and function, bladder function, and fatigue are the symptoms that persist at 30 months post-treatment for surgery patients [13]. Patients receiving radiotherapy have a different prognosis. While their urinary functioning remains fairly stable, sexual functioning for radiotherapy patients declines steadily over time [12, 14]. Radiotherapy patients also report substantial declines in bowel function [15]. Hormone therapy patients report both localized problems (e.g., ED) and systemic concerns, such as fatigue, depression, hot flashes [16].

The Concerns of Gay and Bisexual Men

Various treatment modalities have different implications for G/B men when compared with heterosexual men. Researchers have hypothesized that the effects of external pelvic beam radiation may more severely affect G/B men because of the nature of the side effects on G/B men's sexual practices. Despite advances in radiation therapy, significant percentages of patients who undergo pelvic radiotherapy for prostate cancer are affected by fecal urgency, involuntary flatulence, and incontinence. Furthermore, many men will suffer from significantly decreased sphincter pressure and rectal capacity [17]. These iatrogenic changes are likely to significantly impact the sexual function of G/B men, particularly those who are primarily anal-receptive in their sexual behavior, as severe anal damage may be a contraindication to anal intercourse.

There has also been concern that the ED patients experience following surgery may be more difficult to treat effectively in G/B men [3]. First-line oral ED treatments are designed to enable vaginal intercourse and may not be capable of enabling erections sufficient for anal penetration given the increased pressure of the anal sphincter [18, 19]. After anal penetration, the insertive partner also may have difficulty maintaining their erections, if penetration forces blood from the penis [18].

Ejaculatory dysfunction after PCa treatment causes distress for many men but may be particularly problematic for G/B men. Research with G/B men has documented the cultural significance among gay men around the eroticization of ejaculate and semen [4, 20]. Ejaculation has been described as crucial to satisfying sex and maintaining relationships with partners [4]. Thus, the loss of ejaculation after PCa treatment is a side-effect that will impact HRQOL among many G/B men and that providers should warn G/B men about this side-effect before treatment.

Health-Related Quality of Life in Gay and Bisexual men—What Do We Know?

Until recently, little was known about HRQOL in G/B men with PCa or how it might differ from their heterosexual counterparts. Several small-to-medium size studies have begun to appear in the literature. Like heterosexual men, G/B men experience PCa as having a substantial impact on HRQOL though some report transforming the experience into a positive effect on their life [21]. A qualitative study by Thomas and colleagues eloquently described the struggles with post-treatment symptoms of incontinence and sexual dysfunction. Participants also noted that urologists need to understand that gay men's experience of PCa may be substantively different than heterosexual men [21]. In particular, participants noted the dismissive attitude that many perceived from their urologists, prompting some to seek out another provider.

Another small study examined differences in sexual functioning before and after the introduction of hormonal therapy in a sample of heterosexual and gay men [22]. Gay men ($N=12$) were more adversely affected in the areas of sexual arousal, orgasm function, sexual desire, and overall sexual satisfaction after treatment with bicalutamide when compared with heterosexual men. This difference may arise from an increased importance of androgen, especially for ejaculation, in G/B sexuality [22]. A pilot study of 15 gay men treated with radiation or surgery examined disease-specific HRQOL using the Expanded Prostate Cancer Index (EPIC) [23], a widely-used, validated measure, and the ejaculatory function and bother scores from the Men's Sexual Health Questionnaire (MSHQ) [24]. While the small sample size precluded formal statistical testing, radiation patients were better able to maintain insertive and receptive anal intercourse [25]. Most participants reported difficulties with urinary, bowel, and ejaculatory functioning and reported being "bothered" by their ejaculatory difficulties [25].

Three larger cross-sectional studies have examined difference in HRQOL between G/B and heterosexual men. Men in the US, Australia, Canada, United Kingdom, and other countries completed an anonymous, online survey using the EPIC [23]. The authors compared heterosexual ($N=460$) and G/B ($N=96$) men on a range of diagnostic and HRQOL outcomes [26]. G/B men were diagnosed with PCa at significantly younger ages in this study. There were no differences between the two groups in the type of PCa treatment selected. On the EPIC, the two groups did not differ on sexual functioning or urinary incontinence. In both groups, 60% of the respondents reported "never or almost never" being able to achieve an erection during sex. Among the respondents who could achieve an erection sufficient to attempt penetration, more than one-third of each group reported "never or almost never" achieving satisfaction with orgasm. G/B men in the study reported significantly greater "bother" with their sexual functioning. G/B men also reported worse ejaculatory functioning than heterosexual men and greater "bother" because of their diminished ejaculation [26].

In the second large cross-sectional study, 341 heterosexual men and 111 gay men were interviewed about their post-treatment HRQOL [27]. Gay men reported significantly worse urinary and bowel functioning than heterosexual men. Among gay men, younger men reported lower HRQOL than older men. Gay men reported significantly lower masculine self-esteem, less affection from their partners, and more treatment regret than heterosexual men. Unlike the previous studies, no differences in sexual functioning were found between heterosexual and gay men. It should be noted that a different HRQOL instrument was used in this study, meaning direct comparisons with other studies that used the EPIC difficult. Differences in question wording may have affected the investigators' ability to detect differences in sexual functioning.

The third large cross-sectional study also compared HRQOL among G/B men and heterosexual men after treatment [28]. Ninety-two men completed an internet-based survey using the EPIC and MSHQ to measure disease-specific HRQOL and validated measures of fear of recurrence [29], illness intrusiveness [30], and general HRQOL [31]. Data were compared to published means from heterosexual samples of PCa survivors. Gay men reported better sexual functioning, with no differences between groups on sexual "bother." Gay men reported significantly more "bother" in the urinary, bowel, and hormonal domains of the EPIC. Gay men reported greater psychosocial impairment than heterosexual men, including greater fear of cancer recurrence and worse scores on the Short Form-36 mental composite score. Even though sexual functioning was higher among gay men, they reported a number of concerns related to ejaculatory difficulties, climacturia, and changes in their primary relationship because of changes in sexual functioning. When asked to compare pre- and post-treatment functioning, 40 % of the gay men reported their frequency of sexual activity decreased "a lot." For many men, their erectile difficulties prevented them from resuming insertive sexual activity after treatment.

To summarize the changes in HRQOL published in the literature, several patterns emerge. In studies where comparisons were made with heterosexual men, G/B men generally reported significantly worse urinary and bowel function. Sexual functioning and bother varied across studies. These variable results in sexual functioning may be related to the use of different instruments or to differences in sampling strategies. It is clear that changes in ejaculatory functioning after treatment are perceived as greater by gay men and result in higher ejaculatory "bother" scores.

Gay and Bisexual Specific Needs

G/B men treated for PCa report significant decrements in several areas of physical symptoms after treatment, compared with their heterosexual counterparts. Thus, G/B men may be in even greater need of self-management programs that help manage post-treatment symptoms [32–35]. In particular, sexual rehabilitation may be especially problematic. The number of men who retain the ability to ejaculate after PCa treatment is limited. For G/B men, the loss of ejaculate is especially difficult, given the premium placed on ejaculation as a visible sign of sexual completion in the G/B community [4, 20].

Health care providers working with G/B PCa survivors on sexual rehabilitation may find that first-line oral therapies for ED are less effective for men who wish to resume their role as the insertive partner during sex. Thus, urologists may need to consider other options. One promising treatment approach may be a combination of oral therapy and vacuum erection devices [36]. Interest in vacuum erection devices is resurging because they are cost-effective, less invasive treatment option that increases blood flow to the penile structures [37–39]. Our clinical experience also suggests that some gay men have incorporated vacuum devices into their sexual repertoire independent of use after PCa. Thus, the device may be especially appropriate for G/B men.

If oral therapies and vacuum devices are unsuccessful, urologists may need to move more quickly to more invasive approaches such as intracavernosal injections or uretheral suppositories. Health care providers also need to be mindful of possible rectal difficulties after PCa treatment that may affect G/B men's ability to function as the receptive partner for anal sex. Assessment and treatment so that men can resume receptive anal sex may be an important part of sexual rehabilitation for many G/B men.

Sex therapists and other mental health providers can assist G/B men struggling with sexual rehabilitation concerns. For some men, resuming their previous role in sexual activity may not be possible because of ED or rectal damage. In one study, men who were unable to go back to pre-treatment roles reported a negative impact on their primary relationship [28]. Another study noted that although some men may be willing to adapt their sexual repertoire after treatment, many would find doing so problematic [4]. Sex therapists may also be important resources to help men grieve for their loss of their sexual identity and spontaneity because of their PCa treatment [40]. Sex therapists can help men who are open to changing their sexual repertoire to include new sexual activities and improve communication with sexual partners. Mental health providers may also be able to address the other psychosocial decrements such as fear of cancer recurrence or perceived stigma reported in some studies [27, 28].

The unique characteristics and challenges of the G/B community require that physicians modify their practice to ensure they are providing high-quality care. Gay men may experience difficulty interacting with a medical community comprised mainly of heterosexual providers. Indeed, some surveys have indicated that G/B men are wary of real or perceived homophobia and physicians' heteronormative focus [6]. In a survey that included lesbian, gay, bisexual, transgender, and queer partners and caregivers, the participants expressed similar concerns about their disenfranchisement within the medical system, compared to heterosexual partners and caregivers [41]. Partners of G/B men also need to be considered in pre-treatment decision-making, treatment preparation, and in survivorship services in the same way that heterosexual partners are. Furthermore, a recent study has shown a general disquiet among G/B men concerning the professional attributes of their urologists. Specifically, patients have reported that communication with urologists is extremely problematic because practitioners often fail to explain potential treatment-related side effects or appreciate the psychological impact of therapy [21].

G/B men are less likely to be in long-term monogamous relationships at the time of prostate cancer diagnosis, and are less likely to have established social support systems in place compared to heterosexual men [21]. While health care providers cannot replace these social institutions, they can work with G/B patients to enable men facing prostate cancer to establish and use their own support systems effectively. Face-to-face support groups (e.g., Us TOO, American Cancer Society) and specialized LGBT resources (e.g., Male Care, Inc., Metropolitan Community Church) exist in many communities or online, and efforts should be made to mobilize existing resources in meeting the diverse needs of patients, including gay and bisexual men [3]. For those who are uncomfortable with in-person groups, online support groups have been found to be valuable for many men [42].

Creating a More Welcoming Practice

Creating a welcoming clinical environment for G/B men begins with how a clinic/department advertises their services and progresses down to the clinic encounter. G/B men may seek out providers who list their association with G/B health organizations (e.g., Gay/Lesbian Medical Association) or who publicize G/B health as a specialty. From the moment that G/B men walk into the waiting room, they are gathering an impression about how welcoming toward and knowledgeable about G/B men the practice is. If the waiting room has photos of families, magazines on a coffee table, or information about community resources, a welcoming environment would include same-sex couples in the photos, gay community magazines, and local G/B resource information. Another approach to creating a positive clinical atmosphere is to have an internal or institutional non-discrimination policy that includes sexual orientation and post the policy where it is visible [43]. Further, staff training on dealing with diversity in sexuality and other areas is available for free from the Gay/Lesbian Medical Association (GLMA) and Fenway Health Institute websites.

Intake forms that ask about marital status project a heterosexist bias and fail to recognize that G/B men may be partnered, but not legally married, and perhaps cannot be married depending on the state of residence [44]. Additionally, lifetime relationship and marital status histories may be complex. For example, how would a G/B male patient respond to the standard intake question about marital status if he was previously married to a woman, but has lived with his male partner for the past 10 years? A more informed and welcoming strategy is to ask about "Current relationship status" with the following options: single, married, domestic partnership/civil union, partnered, involved with multiple partners, separated from spouse/

partner, divorced/permanently separated from spouse/partner, other (please specify). In addition, it is useful to ask about "Current living situation" (live alone, live with a spouse/partner, live with roommate(s), live with parents or family members, other) since many G/B men have families of choice and may not live with their romantic partner. Further, a provider who is conscious of the health disparities experienced by G/B men might include a question about "Sexual orientation" (gay, lesbian, heterosexual/straight, bisexual, not sure, prefer not to answer, other) on the intake form [6, 45]. The provider can then follow up during the visit with appropriate questions about sexual activity, sexual functioning, health risks, etc. [46]. The goal is for G/B male patients to perceive that this is a medical practice that expects to see G/B people and feels comfortable with this population.

During the clinic visit, providers demonstrate a welcoming environment by being respectful and not asking questions to satisfy curiosity [43]. The presence of someone with a non-heterosexual sexuality is not a training opportunity. Welcoming providers are aware of their attitudes and biases and strive to respond to patients in a positive, helpful manner. Providers demonstrate sensitivity by asking about sexuality and sexual health, using inclusive, non-heterosexist language, and modeling their language after the patients' [44]. That is, providers avoid gender role terms like "wife," avoid highly technical language, and refer to the patient and the patient's relationships with the same terms the patient uses. Lastly, welcoming, sensitive providers have G/B community resources (e.g., support groups) at their fingertips or can direct patients to Internet resources [6]. Again, the goal is for G/B male patients to feel that the practice is comfortable treating G/B men.

The challenges in providing appropriate care to G/B men with prostate cancer are numerous, but there is ample opportunity for improvement. By treating each individual patient with respect and sensitivity, providers can build trust and relationships that enable effective care. And as with any other group of patients, the G/B men have needs specific to their circumstances. Being knowledgeable about what these needs are and how to most effectively respect the unique context will enable improved care.

Conclusions

Ultimately, the provider's office can serve as a mechanism for helping PCa patients and survivors access and utilize support systems to enable emotional and psychological recovery and a return to pre-treatment quality of life. Providers and researchers should continue to investigate the particular effects of PCa diagnosis and therapy on G/B men. Further study will continue to provide insights valuable in improving health and decreasing morbidity in this community.

Acknowledgements The views expressed reflect those of the authors and not necessarily the views of the Department of Veterans Affairs or Baylor College of Medicine.

References

1. Surveillance Epidemiology and End-Results Program SEER Stat Fact Sheets: Prostate Cancer. 2013. http://seer.cancer.gov/statfacts/html/prost.html.
2. Boehmer U, Miao X, Ozonoff A. Cancer survivorship and sexual orientation. Cancer. 2011;117(16):3796–804.
3. Blank TO. Gay men and prostate cancer: invisible diversity. J Clin Oncol. 2005;23(12):2593–6.
4. Asencio M, et al. The prospect of prostate cancer: a challenge for gay men's sexualities as they age. Sex Res Soc Policy. 2009;6:28–51.
5. Berger, RM. Gay and gray: the older homosexual man. Urbana: The University of Illinois Press; 1982.
6. Gay and Lesbian Medical Association and LGBT health experts. Healthy people 2010: lesbian, gay, bisexual, and transgender health. San Francisco: Gay and Lesbian Medical Association; 2001.
7. Mitteldorf D. Psychotherapy with gay prostate cancer patients. In: Perlman G, Drescher J, Editors. A gay man's guide to prostate cancer. Binghamton: The Haworth Medical Press; 2005. p. 57–67.
8. Heslin KC, et al. Sexual orientation and testing for prostate and colorectal cancers among men in California. Med Care. 2008;46(12):1240–8.
9. Institute of Medicine. The health of lesbian, gay, bisexual, and transgender people: building a foundation for better understanding. Washington: National Academies Press; 2011.
10. Litwin MS, et al. Quality-of-life outcomes in men treated for localized prostate cancer. JAMA. 1995;273(2):129–35.
11. Talcott JA. Quality of life in early prostate cancer: do we know enough to treat? Hematol Oncol Clin North Am. 1996;10:691–701.
12. Lubeck DP, et al. Changes in health-related quality of life in the first year after treatment for prostate cancer: results from CaPSURE. Urology. 1999;53(1):180–6.
13. Matthew AG, et al. Health-related quality of life following radical prostatectomy: long-term outcomes. Qual Life Res. 2014;23(8):2309–17.
14. Talcott JA, et al. Patient-reported symptoms after primary therapy for early prostate cancer: results of a prospective cohort study. J Clin Oncol. 1998;16:275–83.
15. Potosky AL, et al. Health outcomes after prostatectomy or radiotherapy for prostate cancer: results from the Prostate Cancer outcomes study. J Natl Cancer Inst. 2000;92(19):1582–92.
16. Holzbeierlein JM, McLaughlin MD, Thrasher JB. Complications of androgen deprivation therapy for prostate cancer. Curr Opin Urol. 2004;14(3):177–83.
17. Berndtsson I, Lennernas B, Hulten L. Anorectal function after modern conformal radiation therapy for prostate cancer: a pilot study. Tech Coloproctol. 2002;6(2):101–4.
18. Goldstone SE. The ups and downs of gay sex after prostate cancer treatment. In: Perlman G, Drescher J, Editors. A gay man's guide to prostate cancer. Binghamton: The Haworth Medical Press; 2005. p. 43–55.
19. Kleinmann N, et al. The effect of ethnicity and sexual preference on prostate-cancer-related quality of life. Nat Rev Urology. 2012;9(5):258–65.
20. Schilder AJ, et al. It's like the treasure: beliefs associated with semen among young HIV-positive and HIV-negative gay men. Cult Health Sex. 2008;10(7):667–79.
21. Thomas C, Wootten A, Robinson P. The experiences of gay and bisexual men diagnosed with prostate cancer: results from an online focus group. Eur J Cancer Care. 2013;22(4):522–9.
22. Motofei IG, et al. Preliminary study with bicalutamide in heterosexual and homosexual patients with prostate cancer: a possible implication of androgens in male homosexual arousal. BJU Int. 2011;108(1):110–5.
23. Wei JT, et al. Development and validation of the expanded prostate cancer index composite (EPIC) for comprehensive assessment of health-related quality of life in men with prostate cancer. Urology. 2000;56(6):899–905.

24. Rosen RC, et al. Development and validation of four-item version of male sexual health questionnaire to assess ejaculatory dysfunction. Urology. 2007;69(5):805–9.
25. Lee TK, Breau RH, Eapen L. Pilot study on quality of life and sexual function in men-who-have-sex-with-men treated for prostate cancer. J Sex Med. 2013;10(8):2094–100.
26. Wassersug RJ, et al. Diagnostic and outcome differences between heterosexual and nonheterosexual men treated for prostate cancer. Urology. 2013;82(3):565–71.
27. Allensworth-Davies D. Assessing localized prostate cancer post-treatment quality of life outcomes among gay men. In School of Public Health. Boston: Boston University; 2012.
28. Hart T, et al. Changes in sexual roles and quality of life for gay men after prostate cancer: challenges for sexual health providers. J Sex Med. 2014;11(9):230817.
29. Mehta SS, et al. Fear of cancer recurrence in patients undergoing definitive treatment for prostate cancer: results from CaPSURE. J Urol. 2003;170(5):1931–3.
30. Devins GM. Using the illness intrusiveness ratings scale to understand health-related quality of life in chronic disease. J Psychosom Res. 2010;68(6):591–602.
31. Ware JE, Snow KK, Kosinski M. SF-36 health survey: manual and interpretation guide. Lincoln: QualityMetric, Inc.; 2000.
32. Latini DM, et al. Prostate Cancer Patient Education Project (PCPEP)—prostate cancer symptom management in low-literacy men. In: Elk R, Landrine H, Editors. Cancer health disparities: causes and evidence based solutions. New York: Springer; 2011. p. 393–414.
33. Maliski SL, Clerkin B, Letwin MS. Describing a nurse case manager intervention to empower low-income men with prostate cancer. Oncol Nurs Forum. 2004;31(1):57–64.
34. Giesler RB, et al. Improving the quality of life of patients with prostate carcinoma: a randomized trial testing the efficacy of a nurse-driven intervention. Cancer. 2005;104(4):752–62.
35. Lepore SJ, et al. Improving quality of life in men with prostate cancer: a randomized controlled trial of group education interventions. Health Psychol. 2003;22(5):443–52.
36. Canguven O, et al. Combination of vacuum erection device and PDE5 inhibitors as salvage therapy in PDE5 inhibitor nonresponders with erectile dysfunction. J Sex Med. 2009;6(9):2561–7.
37. Brison D, Seftel A, Sadeghi-Nejad H. The resurgence of the vacuum erection device (VED) for treatment of erectile dysfunction. J Sex Med. 2013;10(4):1124–35.
38. Pahlajani G, et al. Vacuum erection devices revisited: its emerging role in the treatment of erectile dysfunction and early penile rehabilitation following prostate cancer therapy. J Sex Med. 2012;9(4):1182–9.
39. Hoyland K, Vasdev N, Adshead J. The use of vacuum erection devices in erectile dysfunction after radical prostatectomy. Rev Urol. 2013;15(2):67–71.
40. Wittmann D, Foley S, Balon R. A biopsychosocial approach to sexual recovery after prostate cancer surgery: the role of grief and mourning. J Sex Marital Ther. 2011;37(2):130–44.
41. Valenti K, Katz A. Needs and perceptions of LGBTQ caregivers: the challenges of services and support. J Gay Lesbian Soc Serv. 2014;26:70–90.
42. Klemm P, et al. Online cancer support groups: a review of the research literature. Comput Inform Nurs. 2003;21(3):136–42.
43. The Joint Commission. Advancing effective communication, cultural competence, and patient- and family-centered care for the lesbian, gay, bisexual, and transgender (LGBT) community: a field guide. Oak Brook: Joint Commission; 2001.
44. Makadon HJ, et al. (Editors). Fenway guide to lesbian, gay, bisexual, and transgender health. Philadelphia: American College of Physicians; 2008.
45. Bradford JB, et al. How to gather data on sexual orientation and gender identity in clinical settings. The Fenway Institute, 2012.
46. Kauth MR, Meier C, Latini DM. A review of sexual health among lesbian, gay, and bisexual veterans. Current Sexual Health Reports, 2014.

Chapter 11
HIV-Associated Cancers

Missak Haigentz, Jr.

Abstract The HIV/AIDS epidemic, now in its 4th decade, has seen major shifts in epidemiology, with survival of infected persons increasingly approximating that of the general population and resulting in an aging population increasingly susceptible to cancer. Furthermore, cancer, a historically important manifestation of HIV/AIDS, has also changed epidemiology over time, where the prevalence of the "non-AIDS-defining" cancers (including cancers of the lungs, liver, head and neck, and anus—all seen in excess among HIV-infected populations) now exceeds that of the AIDS-defining cancers (Kaposi sarcoma, non-Hodgkin lymphoma and cervical carcinoma). As approximately 9% of LGBT persons aged 50 or older have HIV infection, cancer is an important heath concern and cause of mortality in this demographic. This chapter will review the current epidemiology and clinical considerations and treatment for HIV-associated malignancies as it pertains to LGBT populations.

Introduction

The HIV/AIDS epidemic, now in its 4th decade, has seen major shifts in epidemiology leading to an aging population increasingly susceptible to cancer. The advent of effective combination antiretroviral therapies (cART) associated with immune system reconstitution and improved HIV care has dramatically improved the life expectancy of infected persons. By the end of 2012, an estimated 35.3 million people worldwide were living with HIV infection [1].

In developed nations, HIV infection, once considered a death sentence, is now a chronic and treatable comorbidity in many persons living otherwise normal and healthy lives, even decades after infection. The improved survival of infected persons with a declining incidence of new infections [1] has resulted in an aging HIV population. In high-income countries, nearly a third of adults living with HIV are over age

M. Haigentz, Jr. (✉)
Departments of Medicine (Oncology) and Otorhinolaryngology-Head and Neck Surgery, Albert Einstein College of Medicine, Montefiore Medical Center, Bronx, NY, USA
e-mail: mhaigent@montefiore.org

U. Boehmer, R. Elk (eds.), *Cancer and the LGBT Community*,
DOI 10.1007/978-3-319-15057-4_11

50 [2]. As a result of the changing demographics, cancer diagnoses are frequent, diagnosed in up to 40% of persons with HIV infection [3]. Furthermore, malignancy has become an important cause of death of persons with HIV infection, noted as a cause of 28% of deaths in one French study [4]. And as cancer is a disease of aging, it should not be a surprise that cancer will continue to be a major concern in this population. This chapter will review the current epidemiology and clinical considerations and treatment for HIV-associated malignancies as it pertains to LGBT populations.

Demographics of HIV in LGBT Populations

In addition to the aging of HIV infected persons, major shifts in the demographics of HIV infection have also been observed since HIV emerged in the 1980s. HIV infection, initially seen almost exclusively in gay men and intravenous drug users (IDU), is no longer considered a gay men's disease, as high-risk heterosexual transmission has increased and women now make up over 50% of the worldwide HIV population. In the United States, women comprise over 25% of the nearly 900,000 people living with diagnosed HIV infection [5].

The primary behavioral routes of HIV acquisition remain IDU and sexual intercourse. Although IDU accounted for only 8% of estimated incident HIV infections in 2011 [5], it is one of the higher risks of HIV acquisition, estimated at 63 in 10,000 exposures. Regarding sexual transmission of HIV, receptive anal intercourse is associated with much higher risk (138/10,000) than receptive vaginal intercourse (8/10,000). The risk of HIV acquisition with insertive anal or vaginal intercourse is also lower, at 11 and 4 in 10,000 exposures, respectively [6]. In 2012, the FDA approved Truvada® (tenofovir/emtricitabine) for pre-exposure prophylaxis (PrEP) of HIV-negative adults with ongoing sexual activity with a partner who is HIV infected or who engages in high-risk behaviors [7].

Although great efforts in the prevention of sexual transmitted diseases have historically focused on gay men, the need to address this important health issue in the broader LGBT community has become increasingly important. An estimated 64% of all newly diagnosed HIV infections in the United States in 2009 were in men who have sex with men (MSM) [8], a term which includes not only gay- and bisexual-identified men but also MSM who identify as heterosexual, and which does not adequately describe specific sexual practices and even less accurately accounts for transgender persons. Aging with HIV infection is a particular concern in the LGBT older adult community. Approximately 9% of LGBT persons aged 50 or older have HIV infection, with most occurring in gay or bisexual men [9]. Other LGBT populations, including lesbian and transgender persons, have had considerably less research focus.

HIV infection has continued to disproportionately affect minority populations. The Centers for Disease Control and Prevention (CDC) has estimated that among newly infected MSM in 2006, 46% were white, 35% were black and 19% were Hispanic. Among women, high-risk sexual contact accounted for 80% of new HIV transmissions [10], and also disproportionately affects racial minorities.

AIDS-Defining and Non-AIDS Defining Cancers

Cancers in HIV infection are generally classified in the literature as being AIDS defining or non-AIDS-defining. Since 1993, the CDC definition of AIDS has included three specific malignancies associated with immunosuppression: non-Hodgkin lymphoma (NHL), Kaposi sarcoma (KS) and invasive cervical cancer [11]. Under this definition, persons with HIV infection diagnosed with one of these malignancies had AIDS, regardless of other measures of immunosuppression, including low CD4+ T-cell subset or prior opportunistic infection. These malignancies (particularly NHL and KS) are generally associated with advanced immunosuppression and are termed AIDS-defining cancers (ADCs). In contrast, other malignancies are termed non-AIDS defining cancers (NADCs).

Early in the course of the HIV epidemic where antiretroviral therapy was either not available or of limited efficacy, the vast majority of malignancies in the setting of HIV infection were ADCs. These malignancies were often the presenting symptom of patients with advanced HIV infection and were associated with dismal prognoses.

The widespread availability of combination antiretroviral therapy (cART) regimens, generally considered post-1996 with the protease inhibitors, has led to effective, at least partial reconstitution of patient immune systems resulting in marked declines in ADC incidence [12], particularly for NHL and KS. Although persons with HIV infection remain at marked risk for ADCs, cART improves immunologic, virologic and clinical outcomes [13]. The Swiss HIV Cohort Study included 9429 patients with 54,715 person-years of follow-up and evaluated cancers in the pre- (1985–1996), early- (1997–2001) and late- (2002–2006) cART periods; as compared to the non-HIV infected population, the incidence of ADCs in the HIV-infected population progressively declined over these periods (Standardized Incidence Ratios [SIRs] of 136, 27.7, and 14.7, respectively) [14]. Data from United States AIDS and cancer registries have also noted declines in incidence of KS and NHL in the cART era [15].

Conversely, the improved survival among persons with HIV infection in the cART era has led to an aging HIV population, resulting in increased prevalence of NADCs to the extent that the number of NADCs diagnosed each year in the US now exceeds those of ADCs [16]. Some studies, including the Swiss HIV Cohort Study, have noted increased incidence of NADCs, which have been stable over the study intervals (SIRs of 2.3, 2.7, and 2.2, respectively) [14]. Although NHL remains the most common malignancy in persons with HIV infection, cancers of the lung, liver, and head and neck, anus as well as Hodgkin lymphoma, all NADCs, are being seen more frequently in this aging population. Moreover, these NADCs are seen in excess in HIV populations in several cohort studies, suggesting increased risk. Furthermore, many of these malignancies are diagnosed at an early age, on average a decade and a half earlier than the general population. As a result of the shifting cancer epidemiology, the distinction/classification of ADCs and NADCs has become blurred and in several ways outdated, though the terms remain in widespread use [17].

AIDS-Defining Cancers (ADCs)

Non-Hodgkin Lymphomas

Non-Hodgkin Lymphomas (NHLs) are a heterogeneous group of malignancies of the lymphatic system with wide variation of tumor biology and disease aggressiveness. Some NHL types are indolent, associated with prolonged survival, and others are far more aggressive. Most NHL types are sensitive to chemotherapy but differ in curability, often with more aggressive diseases associated with higher curative potential.

NHLs are the most common malignancy types in persons with HIV infection and are generally associated with advanced immunosuppression and low CD4+ cell counts, with cohort studies demonstrating risk of HIV infected persons 23- to 353-fold that of non-immunocompromized persons [18]. The most common NHL types seen in HIV-infected persons are of B-cell lineage and are associated with aggressive course, including Burkitt lymphoma, diffuse large B-cell lymphoma and plasmablastic lymphoma, which can be associated with Epstein-Barr virus infection. Other NHLs associated with severe immunosuppression include primary central nervous system (PCNS) lymphoma and primary effusion lymphoma (PEL, also known as body cavity lymphoma).

The overall incidence of NHL in HIV infection has declined with the widespread use of cART [19]. However, the incidence of lymphoma remains highest in the first 6 months of cART initiation, possibly associated with immunosuppression that led to cART or to unmasking due to immune reconstitution inflammatory syndrome (IRIS) [20].

Despite the association of NHL with immunosuppression, patients with AIDS-associated NHL have been able to tolerate and benefit from aggressive lymphoma type and stage-specific chemotherapy regimens [21]. Generally, antiretroviral therapy should be initiated or modified (if already begun) at the time of diagnosis to control HIV infection and should be continued during the chemotherapy regimen.

Kaposi Sarcoma

Kaposi Sarcoma (KS) is a low-grade vascular tumor associated with human herpesvirus—8 infection (HHV-8) [also known as Kaposi Sarcoma Herpesvirus, KSHV]. KS, a common presentation of HIV infection in the early years of the AIDS epidemic often with an aggressive course, has fortunately markedly dropped in incidence in the cART era and in many patients has been a chronic disease. Although KS has been reported in all risk groups for HIV infection it has been seen most commonly in MSM. The incidence of KS in HIV infected men appears most strongly associated with current CD4+ cell count, and survival of KS patients has improved in the cART era [22]. Similar to NHL, however, the incidence seems highest immediately (within the first 6 months) following cART initiation, possibly related to IRIS [20].

Although KS can affect any site of the body, cutaneous disease is most common. The skin lesions of KS and resulting edema and inflammation can be debilitating and remains an important chronic health issue with patients associated with psychosocial distress. Combination antiretroviral therapy is recommended for all patients with AIDS-associated KS and may be the only therapy required for disease control and symptom palliation. KS is also responsive to systemic chemotherapy (generally liposomal doxorubicin and paclitaxel). However, the toxicities of chronic therapy (myelosuppression with doxorubicin, neuropathy with paclitaxel) may be limiting.

Cervical Cancer

The incidence of invasive cervical cancer and its precursor, cervical intraepithelial neoplasia (CIN) is significantly higher in HIV-infected compared to uninfected women [23, 24]. Of note, high-grade squamous intraepithelial lesions of the cervix were 4–5 times higher in HIV-infected adolescents as compared to HIV-uninfected adolescent girls with high-risk sexual behaviors [25].

Cervical cancer, though markedly declining in incidence in the developed world, remains a deadly disease that can be prevented by early detection with routine Papanicolaou (Pap) screening. The cause of nearly all cervical cancer is oncogenic HPV infection, commonly involving several high-risk genotypes (HPV types 16, 18, 31, 33). Prophylactic administration of HPV vaccines Gardasil® (Merck, quadravalent vaccine against HPV types 6, 11, 16 and 18) and Cervarix® (GlaxoSmithKline, a vaccine against HPV types 16 and 18) has been demonstrated to prevent cervical cancer in the general population. These vaccines can be administered safely to HIV infected persons and have been advocated in the guidelines for primary care of the HIV-infected patient younger than age 26.

Select Non-AIDS-Defining Cancers (NADCs)

Lung Cancer

Lung cancer, the most common NADC in the cART era, is also the most common cause of cancer death in persons with HIV infection [26], similar to that in populations without HIV infection, and yet is seen in 3–5 fold excess in cohort studies of cancer in HIV infection [19]. This increased lung cancer risk has been attributed to increased smoking among HIV-infected populations, but the risk remains despite accounting for smoking [27, 28].

Case series of lung cancer in HIV infection have demonstrated similar histology distributions, with adenocarcinoma and squamous cell carcinoma being most common, though all disease histologies, including small cell histology, have been represented [29, 30]. Of note, lung cancer has been diagnosed at young age, often diagnosed in the fourth decade of life and has been associated with advanced stage at diagnosis and poor prognoses [31]. However, more recent data support detection of potentially surgically resectable (and therefore curable) early stage (stage I and II) disease [30]. Some reports have suggested that HIV-infected patients with lung cancer have had lower rates of stage-appropriate cancer treatment [32], suggesting some of the historically poor survival rates are related to treatment disparities. A clinical trial mounted by the AIDS Malignancy Consortium (AMC) is currently investigating the safety and tolerability of erlotinib, an FDA-approved lung cancer therapy in persons with advanced lung cancer and HIV infection (AMC-090, NCT02134886).

Most recently, the National Lung Screening Trial (NLST), enrolling 53,454 participants with heavy smoking histories, has demonstrated a 20 % reduction in lung cancer mortality with annual low dose computed tomography (CT) scan [33]. The study also demonstrated a 7 % improvement in all-cause mortality, and as a result several health organizations are developing guidelines for screening the general population. The eligibility criteria for this study included persons aged 55–74 years with at least a 30 pack-year smoking history and who had quit within 15 years prior to screening. Although the NLST did not exclude persons with HIV infection, additional evaluation in the setting of HIV infection is warranted to evaluate its utility and efficacy in this high-risk population.

Liver Cancer

Hepatocellular carcinoma is remains one of the most common NADCs. Etiologies include alcoholic and viral hepatitis, including Hepatitis B (HBV) and Hepatitis C (HCV) infections. HBV infections are endemic worldwide and coinfection with HCV and HIV is common due to similar routes of transmission. HBV prophylactic vaccination is preventive, and although vaccination against HCV is not currently available, HCV treatment can cure the infection in high rates, including in persons with HIV infection. Surgical procedures including orthotopic liver transplantation can be curative and safely performed in HIV infected patients with liver cancer [34]. Unresectable disease, however, is generally incurable; systemic treatment with sorafenib, a targeted palliative therapy approved for advanced hepatocellular carcinoma, may be considered for these patients [35].

Head and Neck Cancer

Head and neck squamous cell carcinoma is the 5th most common malignancy worldwide and appears to be at 3-fold increased risk efforts in HIV infected populations. Although tobacco carcinogen exposure remains a significant risk factor for this malignancy, oncogenic HPV infection (specifically HPV 16) has been implicated in the pathogenesis of oropharyngeal cancers (including the tonsils, base of tongue, soft palate and posterior pharyngeal wall) and has been associated with favorable prognosis. Although head and neck cancers regardless of etiologies generally affect males, HPV-associated head and neck cancers share similar sexual risk associations with cervical cancers, namely multiple sexual partners (specifically high number of lifetime vaginal and oral sex partners) [36]. Although the viral etiology of a subset of these cancers has made viral co-infection a tempting explanation for the increased risk observed in HIV-infection, preliminary investigations have not shown excess HPV infection in HIV-associated tumors [37, 38].

Patients with head and neck cancer often present with locoregionally advanced disease and are treated with curative-intent multimodality therapy (combinations of surgery, radiotherapy, and chemotherapy). Despite prolonged disease-free survival, frequent survivorship issues of patients include chronic toxicities of therapy (e.g., xerostomia, swallowing dysfunction, hypothyroidism) and high rates of second primary malignancies related to field effects of tobacco carcinogen exposure.

Anal Cancer

Although anal cancer is a NADC, it is seen in over 30-fold excess in HIV infection, and is similar to cervical cancer in that most cases are associated with high-risk HPV types.

In the United States, anal squamous cell cancer incidence rates are increasing in both men and women, [39] and there is markedly higher incidence of high-grade anal intraepithelial neoplasia (AIN) in HIV-infected men, particularly affecting MSM [40]. For HIV-infected MSM, a recent meta-analysis of 53 studies reporting on anal HPV detection, AIN and anal cancer in MSM demonstrated 35.4 (95 % CI: 32.9–37.9) pooled prevalence of HPV-16, 29.1 % (22.8–35.1) prevalence of high-grade AIN, and anal cancer incidence of 45.9 per 100,000 (31.2–60.3) [41].

The quadravalent HPV vaccination is safe and highly immunogenic in HIV-infected MSM and may prevent anal cancer [42]. Baseline anal cancer screening with cytology may be considered for HIV-infected MSM and women with history of receptive anal intercourse or abnormal cervical Papanicolaou (Pap) results, and those with genital warts [43]. Persons with abnormal cytology and all HIV-infected patients with anorectal symptoms should have high resolution anoscopy (HRA) and biopsy. Patients with anal cancer often present with locoregional disease and can be treated with curative-intent. Preliminary results of a prospective study of chemoradiotherapy for anal cancer in HIV infection demonstrate that patients can tolerate a therapy [44].

Hodgkin Lymphoma

Hodgkin lymphoma, a disease arising from germinal center or post-germinal center B-cells, though considered a NADC, is seen at 15 to 30-fold excess in HIV infection [45]. It has a unique cellular composition (presence of Reed-Sternberg neoplastic cells in an inflammatory background) and clinicopathological features with several described histological types. Among patients with HIV infection, almost all cases of Hodgkin lymphoma are Epstein-Barr virus (EBV)-positive and have unfavorable histology and advanced stage disease at presentation. In contrast with aggressive AIDS-defining NHL, antiretroviral therapy has not reduced the incidence of this lymphoma. However, with use of cART and chemotherapy, 5-year survival rates have been reported in excess of 60 % [46].

Cancers of the Breast, Prostate, and Colon

These cancers are not known to be associated with excess risk in persons with HIV infection. Although these malignancies are far more prevalent in the general population, the aging of the HIV infected population will likely result in growing prevalence of these malignancies as well. Current age and risk-based cancer screening guidelines should apply for HIV infected populations.

Cancer Etiologies

Immunosuppression

The development of cancer in HIV infection is quite similar to that of persons with solid tumor organ transplantation receiving chronic immunosuppressive therapies and persons with impaired cell-mediated immunity. As noted above, KS and NHL incidence has closely followed immunologic outcomes of persons with HIV infection.

Direct effects of HIV infection may have effects on varied cellular processes that contribute to carcinogenesis (including activation of oncogenes, inhibition of tumor suppressors, and alterations in cell-cycle regulation).

Viral Co-infections

Epstein Barr Virus (EBV) is associated with nasopharyngeal cancer, and among persons with HIV infection, both AIDS defining NHL (including plasmablastic, large cell and PCNS lymphomas) and Hodgkin lymphoma.

Human herpesvirus-8 (HHV-8) [also known as Kaposi Sarcoma Herpesvirus (KSHV)] infections are associated with KS tumors. HHV-8 is also found in the multicentric form of Castleman's disease and primary effusion lymphoma (PEL), both of which have been associated with HIV-infection.

Human Papillomavirus (HPV) infections cause cervical cancer, anogenital (anal, penile and vulvar) cancers and a subset of head and neck cancers (specifically in the oropharynx). As a result of T-cell deficiency, HIV infected persons may have had decreased clearance and persistence of oncogenic HPV infections associated with carcinogenesis. HPV vaccination can protect against select high-risk genotypes and is recommended for HIV-positive men and women age 26 and younger who have not been adequately immunized [47].

Chronic Hepatitis B Virus (HBV) and Hepatitis C Virus (HCV) infections are associated with cirrhosis and inflammation resulting in hepatocellular carcinoma. In persons with HIV Infection, routine hepatitis B vaccination and treatment of chronic hepatitis infections may prevent the development of this malignancy.

Merkel Cell Polyomavirus is associated with Merkel Cell Carcinoma, a rare and aggressive skin malignancy associated with HIV infection and other forms of severe immunosuppression.

Tobacco Carcinogen Exposure

Tobacco carcinogen exposure is by far the most preventable cause of cancer, and HIV infected populations generally have higher smoking rates [48, 49]. In several case series, nearly all patients with HIV-associated lung cancers were smokers [31].

Other Mechanisms

Chronic inflammation has been suggested as one mechanism of carcinogenesis in persons with HIV infection, possibly accounting for early onset of malignancy in this population.

The concomitant decreased incidence of ADCs coupled with the increased prevalence of NADCs during the cART era has led to speculation on the carcinogenic potential of antiretroviral agents. Though limited in number, current evidence does not suggest a strong and consistent link of antiretrovirals to specific NADCs.

Obesity has become an increasingly understood cancer risk for breast and uterine malignancies and possibly others. The role of hormone exposure in transgender persons and cancer risk is an area needing additional cancer research, addressed in other chapters.

Issues Pertaining to LGBT Cancer Patients with HIV Infection

Research in HIV associated cancers is limited, and even more limited is evidence-based recommendations in LGBT populations. Sexual histories are often inadequately obtained in routine medical care, contributing to the limited data. Even in

Western and developed nations where LGBT populations are openly accepted, underrepresented demographic characteristics (HIV infection, LGBT identity, racial minorities) can contribute to health care disparities, discrimination and marginalization of this vulnerable population [50].

Cancer Treatment Disparities

In a recent study of HIV and cancer registry data from Connecticut, Michigan and Texas, HIV infected persons with several types of common cancers (diffuse-large B-cell lymphoma, Hodgkin lymphoma, lung cancer, prostate cancer and colorectal cancer) were approximately 2-fold less frequently treated for their cancer than their HIV-uninfected counterparts [51]. Of particular concern was that the results applied also to early stage cancers with curative potential. Proposed explanations for treatment disparities in this population include increased comorbid burden or worse functional status of patients limiting treatment, or worse perceived prognosis by clinicians. HIV infected patients may also elect to forgo treatment due to inadequate knowledge of the benefits of cancer treatment or a fear of its toxicity. The results, though not specific to sexual orientation or gender identity (approximately half of HIV-infected persons in the registry were MSM), underscore the need educate both clinicians and the HIV-infected community on cancer screening and early and appropriate cancer treatment.

HIV Testing

In 2006, the CDC recommended routine HIV testing as a component of routine health care for all persons, regardless of sexual orientation or gender identity [52]. Despite these recommendations and increased risk of several malignancies in HIV infection (including the ADCs and several NADCs), oncologists have not adequately performed HIV testing in their cancer patients [53]. Routine testing for HIV will improve the health of all persons, including those with cancer, and should contribute to reduced transmission rates.

Cancer Prevention

Although there is no consistent evidence linking antiretroviral therapy with increased NADC risk, its use has been associated with marked declines in ADCs and therefore is an important cancer prevention measure in persons with HIV infection.

Tobacco cessation remains critical to cancer prevention in all populations. Prophylactic HPV vaccination (protective against anogenital and head and neck malignancies) can be administered safely to HIV infected persons and has been advocated in the guidelines for primary care of the HIV-infected patient younger than age 26. Hepatitis B vaccination and treatment of known chronic active hepatitis (Hepatitis B and C) infections may be protective against hepatic carcinogenesis.

Cancer Screening Recommendations

Although several major health organizations have developed guidelines for screening of average and at risk patient populations for several malignancies (including breast, prostate, colorectal and cervical cancers), guidelines for HIV infected populations have been lagging. As noted above, lung cancer screening with low-dose CT imaging has been supported by a prospective study demonstrating reduction in lung cancer and all cause mortality in heavy smokers. Although additional research is warranted, there is no reason to exclude otherwise fit HIV-infected persons from age-specific cancer screening.

Cancer screening guidelines are extremely limited for the HIV infected LGBT population. That said, the New York State Department of Health has had guidelines for the primary care of persons with HIV infection incorporating cancer screening recommendations [54] and has recently developed specific guidelines for care of HIV-infected transgender persons [55]. Generally, screening guidelines for the general population should be employed for screening of breast and prostate cancers. Of note, appropriate screening of "birth-gender" cancers should be continued in transgender persons, though additional consideration for breast cancer screening should be given to female to male (FtM) patients with remaining breast tissue or male to female (MtF) transgender patients with breast tissue who have received hormone therapy for at least 5 years [55]. In addition to known cancer risks associated with viral infections and exposure to tobacco carcinogens, the role of exogenous hormone use in transgender individuals, associated with increased cancer risk for several malignancies (breast, uterine and ovarian), and its effects during cancer therapy deserves additional study.

Cervical Papanicolaou (Pap) screening should be performed in all persons with a cervix (including lesbian and FtM transgender patients), and anal cytology may be considered for all HIV infected individuals. Current guidelines from the American College of Obstetricians and Gynecologists (ACOG) recommend cervical cancer screening twice in the first year of HIV infection and then annually [56]. Ablative treatment of precancerous, high-grade squamous intraepithelial anal lesions in persons with HIV infection is the subject of a recently activated prospective national trial (ANCHOR study, NCT02135419).

Cancer Treatment Recommendations

Cancer treatment recommendations for HIV infected patients have similar challenges of limited evidence-based data. HIV-specific prospective clinical trial data is most robust for patients with NHL and KS, with studies supporting aggressive cancer treatment in all but the most immunosuppressed patients. In contrast, evidence-based treatment recommendations for NADCs are very limited due to frequent and often arbitrary exclusion of persons with HIV infection in cancer clinical trials [57, 58]. In the absence of data to suggest otherwise, HIV-infected persons with cancer should receive the same therapy as their HIV-uninfected counterparts; this position has recently been supported by the British HIV Association [59].

Continuation of antiretrovirals is generally considered safe during cancer therapy and is required for effective treatment of cancers associated with advanced immunosuppression such as Kaposi sarcoma and AIDS-associated lymphoma. Caution is warranted to prevent worsening immunosuppression as well as potentiation of adverse effects of cancer therapy on other HIV-associated comorbidities (e.g., myelosuppression, neuropathy or renal dysfunction) or on toxicities of antiretrovirals (e.g., nausea). Additionally, an awareness of potential drug-drug interactions of systemic cancer therapies with antiretroviral therapies is necessary. These interactions may affect the metabolism of systemic cancer therapies or antiretrovirals and may affect the therapeutic ratio, resulting in increased drug exposure (increasing toxicity) or decreased exposure (decreasing therapeutic efficacy). For transgender persons treated with hormones, additional concerns include potential for drug-interactions with antiretrovirals as well as impact of continued hormone therapy on cancer treatment outcomes. The AIDS Malignancy Clinical Trials Consortium (AMC) is actively evaluating the tolerability and efficacy of standard and novel systemic therapies for HIV-infected patients with cancer. Whenever possible, patients should be encouraged to participate in these trials.

Psychosocial Concerns of HIV-Infected LGBT Cancer Patients

Psychosocial and survivorship concerns of cancer patients have only recently received research attention, and research data specifically in the HIV-infected LGBT population is sparse. However, LGBT cancer patients with HIV infection are a particularly vulnerable population due to the burden of managing both cancer and HIV infection, as well as being stigmatized by their sexual orientation or gender identity. There is therefore a need for evaluating the impact of physical and psychosocial concerns and the sexuality of patients on cancer treatment choices and on survivorship. Given the variability in cancer diagnoses and treatments and their expected toxicities, as well as inadequate sexual histories obtained in routine clinical practice, this field should be ideally evaluated with prospective studies for specific cancers.

Of note, a recent single institution case-control study reported prostate cancer treatment involving 43 HIV infected patients and 86 HIV negative controls [60]. Although prostate cancer was largely appropriately treated in the HIV-infected patients, HIV-infected men received more radiotherapy and less radical prostatectomies. Although this would have been a great opportunity to identify differences in treatment as well as toxicities by sexual orientation, the study was unable to ascertain HIV risk factors, though the MSM frequency of HIV infected persons in the study region (Chicago, IL) was estimated at 70 %. Whether the choice for nonsurgical therapy for HIV-infected patients was patient or physician-directed is not known.

Summary

Despite remarkable improvements in treatment of HIV infection resulting in long-term survival from reduction of opportunistic infections and cancers traditionally associated with immunodeficiency, cancer continues to be a major cause of death of persons with HIV infection and a growing health concern for the older adult HIV-infected LGBT community.

Although aging will continue to account for the increased prevalence of NADCs, the apparent higher risk for and early onset of several malignancies in HIV-positive populations suggest other responsible associations. Currently understood cancer etiologies in this population include chronic inflammation, exposure to carcinogens (particularly those from tobacco), as well as chronic immunosuppression and viral co-infections. A growing number of malignancies (NHL, KS, cervical cancer, head and neck cancer, anal cancer and liver cancer) have been attributed to oncogenic viruses, and future research may possibly identify other associations.

The cancer epidemiology may need us to refocus cancer prevention efforts in HIV infected populations. Although the incidence of ADCs has markedly declined in the cART era, NHL remains the most frequent cancer in HIV infected persons. In contrast, lung cancer has become second in frequency but has now become the most common cause of cancer death in this population. Although great research attention has appropriately been focused on NHL over the decades of the HIV epidemic, lung cancer biology and management in this population will require increased study. Continued consistent antiretroviral use should be recommended. Tobacco cessation efforts cannot be overemphasized in this high-risk population where cancer often strikes in the 4th decade of life, and current cancer screening efforts for the general population should be applied to HIV-infection while research tests the utility of these interventions.

The LGBT population is at particular risk for marginalization and health disparities. In addition to prevention education, prophylactic vaccination of HBV and HPV and when appropriate, drug prophylaxis (PrEP) of HIV infection, HIV testing and HIV treatment are necessary, as are targeted smoking cessation, age-specific cancer screening and treatment of HBV and HCV infection in primary care practice. Cultural competency programs for healthcare professionals should be developed to improve provider knowledge and competency in clinical care and address the treatment disparities and survivorship issues specific to this population. Only focused clinical research in this specific population will provide evidence-based recommendations.

Acknowledgements The author gratefully acknowledges the critical review of this chapter by Dr. Jack E. Burkhalter. This work was funded by the Clinical Core of the Center for AIDS Research at the Albert Einstein College of Medicine and Montefiore Medical Center (NIH AI-51519) and the AIDS Malignancy Consortium grant (U01CA121947).

References

1. http://www.unaids.org/en/media/unaids/contentassets/documents/epidemiology/2013/gr2013/UNAIDS_Global_Report_2013_en.pdf. Accessed 30 July 2014.
2. http://www.unaids.org/en/media/unaids/contentassets/documents/unaidspublication/2013/20131101_JC2563_hiv-and-aging_en.pdf. Accessed 30 July 2014.
3. Akanmu AS. AIDS-associated malignancies. Afr J Med Med Sci. 2006;(35 Suppl):57–70.
4. Bonnet F, Lewden C, May T, Heripret L, Jougla E, Bevilacqua S, Costagliola D, Salmon D, Chêne G, Morlat P. Malignancy-related causes of death in human immunodeficiency virus-infected patients in the era of highly active antiretroviral therapy. Cancer. 2004;101(2):317–24.
5. CDC HIV Surveillance Report. 2011. http://www.cdc.gov/hiv/pdf/statistics_2011_HIV_Surveillance_Report_vol_23.pdf. Accessed 30 July 2014.
6. Patel P, Borkowf CB, Patel P, Borkowf CB, Brooks JT, Lasry A, Lansky A, Mermin J. Estimating per-act HIV transmission risk: a systematic review. AIDS. 2014;28(10):1509–19.
7. http://www.cdc.gov/hiv/pdf/guidelines/PrEPguidelines2014.pdf. Accessed 8 Aug 2014.
8. Centers for Disease Control and Prevention (CDC). HIV infections attributed to male-to-male sexual contact—metropolitan statistical areas, United States and Puerto Rico, 2010. MMWR Morb Mortal Wkly Rep. 2012;61(47):962–6.
9. Emlet CA, Fredriksen-Goldsen KI, Kim HJ. Risk and protective factors associated with health-related quality of life among older gay and bisexual men living with HIV disease. Gerontologist. 2013;53(6):963–72.
10. Centers for Disease Control and Prevention (CDC). Subpopulation estimates from the HIV incidence surveillance system—United States, 2006. MMWR Morb Mortal Wkly Rep. 2008;57(36):985–9.
11. Centers for Disease Control and Prevention. 1993 revised classification system for HIV infection and expanded surveillance case definition for AIDS among adolescents and adults. MMWR Recomm Rep. 1992;41(RR-17):1–19.
12. Bonnet F, Balestre E, Thiébaut R, Morlat P, Pellegrin JL, Neau D, Dabis F, Groupe d'Epidemiologie Clinique du SIDA en Aquitaine. Factors associated with the occurrence of AIDS-related non-Hodgkin lymphoma in the era of highly active antiretroviral therapy: Aquitaine Cohort, France. Clin Infect Dis. 2006;42(3):411–7.
13. Grabar S, Le Moing V, Goujard C, Leport C, Kazatchkine MD, Costagliola D, Weiss L. Clinical outcome of patients with HIV-1 infection according to immunologic and virologic response after 6 months of highly active antiretroviral therapy. Ann Intern Med. 2000;133(6):401–10.
14. Franceschi S, Lise M, Clifford GM, Rickenbach M, Levi F, Maspoli M, Bouchardy C, Dehler S, Jundt G, Ess S, Bordoni A, Konzelmann I, Frick H, Dal Maso L, Elzi L, Furrer H, Calmy A, Cavassini M, Ledergerber B, Keiser O, Swiss HIV Cohort Study. Changing patterns of cancer incidence in the early- and late-HAART periods: the Swiss HIV cohort study. Br J Cancer. 2010;103(3):416–22.
15. Biggar RJ, Chaturvedi AK, Goedert JJ, Engels EA, HIV/AIDS Cancer Match Study. AIDS-related cancer and severity of immunosuppression in persons with AIDS. J Natl Cancer Inst. 2007;99(12):962–72.
16. Shiels MS, Pfeiffer RM, Gail MH, Hall HI, Li J, Chaturvedi AK, Bhatia K, Uldrick TS, Yarchoan R, Goedert JJ, Engels EA. Cancer burden in the HIV-infected population in the United States. J Natl Cancer Inst. 2011;103(9):753–62.
17. Gopal S, Achenbach CJ, Yanik EL, Dittmer DP, Eron JJ, Engels EA. Moving forward in HIV-associated cancer. J Clin Oncol. 2014;32(9):876–80.

18. Grulich AE, van Leeuwen MT, Falster MO, Vajdic CM. Incidence of cancers in people with HIV/AIDS compared with immunosuppressed transplant recipients: a meta-analysis. Lancet. 2007;370(9581):59–67.
19. Engels EA, Pfeiffer RM, Goedert JJ, Virgo P, McNeel TS, Scoppa SM, Biggar RJ, HIV/AIDS Cancer Match Study. Trends in cancer risk among people with AIDS in the United States 1980–2002. AIDS. 2006;20(12):1645–54.
20. Yanik EL, Napravnik S, Cole SR, Achenbach CJ, Gopal S, Olshan A, Dittmer DP, Kitahata MM, Mugavero MJ, Saag M, Moore RD, Mayer K, Mathews WC, Hunt PW, Rodriguez B, Eron JJ. Incidence and timing of cancer in HIV-infected individuals following initiation of combination antiretroviral therapy. Clin Infect Dis. 2013;57(5):756–64.
21. Carbone A, Vaccher E, Gloghini A, Pantanowitz L, Abayomi A, de Paoli P, Franceschi S. Diagnosis and management of lymphomas and other cancers in HIV-infected patients. Nat Rev Clin Oncol. 2014;11(4):223–38.
22. Lodi S, Guiguet M, Costagliola D, Fisher M, de Luca A, Porter K, CASCADE Collaboration. Kaposi sarcoma incidence and survival among HIV-infected homosexual men after HIV seroconversion. J Natl Cancer Inst. 2010;102(11):784–92.
23. Frisch M, Biggar RJ, Goedert JJ. Human papillomavirus-associated cancers in patients with human immunodeficiency virus infection and acquired immunodeficiency syndrome. J Natl Cancer Inst. 2000;92(18):1500–10.
24. Ellerbrock TV, Chiasson MA, Bush TJ, Sun XW, Sawo D, Brudney K, Wright TC Jr. Incidence of cervical squamous intraepithelial lesions in HIV-infected women. JAMA. 2000;283(8):1031–7.
25. Moscicki AB, Ellenberg JH, Crowley-Nowick P, Darragh TM, Xu J, Fahrat S. Risk of high-grade squamous intraepithelial lesion in HIV-infected adolescents. J Infect Dis. 2004;190(8):1413–21.
26. Simard EP, Pfeiffer RM, Engles EA. Cumulative incidence of cancer among individuals with acquired immunodeficiency syndrome in the United States. Cancer. 2011;117(5):1089–96.
27. Kirk GD, Merlo C, O'Driscoll P, Mehta SH, Galai N, Vlahov D, Samet J, Engels EA. HIV infection is associated with an increased risk for lung cancer, independent of smoking. Clin Infect Dis. 2007;45(1):103–10.
28. Engels EA, Brock MV, Chen J, Hooker CM, Gillison M, Moore RD. Elevated incidence of lung cancer among HIV-infected individuals. J Clin Oncol. 2006;24(9):1383–8.
29. Pakkala S, Chen Z, Rimland D, Owonikoko TK, Gunthel C, Brandes JR, Saba NR, Shin DM, Curran WJ Jr, Khuri FR, Ramalingam SS. Human immunodeficiency virus-associated lung cancer in the era of highly active antiretroviral therapy. Cancer. 2012; 118(1):164–72.
30. Shcherba M, Hosgood HD, Lin J, Hanna D, Felsen UR, Ginsberg M, Fisher L, Wilson K, Chung J, Xue X, Anastos K, Piperdi B, Spivack S, Keller SM, Strickler HD, Haigentz M. Characteristics of HIV+ lung cancer cases in a large clinical population: implications for lung cancer screening. J Clin Oncol. 2014;32:5s (suppl; abstr 1569).
31. Mani D, Haigentz M Jr, Aboulafia DM. Lung cancer in HIV infection. Clin Lung Cancer. 2012;13(1):6–13.
32. Suneja G, Shiels MS, Melville SK, Williams MA, Rengan R, Engels EA. Disparities in the treatment and outcomes of lung cancer among HIV-infected individuals. AIDS. 2013;27(3):459–68.
33. National Lung Screening Trial Research Team, Aberle DR, Adams AM, Berg CD, Black WC, Clapp JD, Fagerstrom RM, Gareen IF, Gatsonis C, Marcus PM, Sicks JD. Reduced lung-cancer mortality with low-dose computed tomographic screening. N Engl J Med. 2011;365(5):395–409.
34. Di Benedetto F, Tarantino G, Ercolani G, Baccarani U, Montalti R, De Ruvo N, Berretta M, Adani GL, Zanello M, Tavio M, Cautero N, Tirelli U, Pinna AD, Gerunda GE, Guaraldi G. Multicenter italian experience in liver transplantation for hepatocellular carcinoma in HIV-infected patients. Oncologist. 2013;18(5):592–9.
35. Berretta M, Di Benedetto F, Dal Maso L, Cacopardo B, Nasti G, Facchini G, Bearz A, Spina M, Garlassi E, De Re V, Fiorica F, Lleshi A, Tirelli U. Sorafenib for the treatment of unresectable hepatocellular carcinoma in HIV-positive patients. Anticancer Drugs. 2013;24(2):212–8.

36. D'Souza G, Kreimer AR, Viscidi R, Pawlita M, Fakhry C, Koch WM, Westra WH, Gillison ML. Case-control study of human papillomavirus and oropharyngeal cancer. N Engl J Med. 2007;356(19):1944–56.
37. McLemore MS, Haigentz M Jr, Smith RV, Nuovo GJ, Alos L, Cardesa A, Brandwein-Gensler M. Head and neck squamous cell carcinomas in HIV-positive patients: a preliminary investigation of viral associations. Head Neck Pathol. 2010;4(2):97–105.
38. D'Souza G, Carey TE, William WN Jr, Nguyen ML, Ko EC, Riddell J 4th, Pai SI, Gupta V, Walline HM, Lee JJ, Wolf GT, Shin DM, Grandis JR, Ferris RL. Epidemiology of head and neck squamous cell cancer among HIV-infected patients. J Acquir Immune Defic Syndr. 2014;65(5):603–10.
39. Nelson RA, Levine AM, Bernstein L, Smith DD, Lai LL. Changing patterns of anal canal carcinoma in the United States. J Clin Oncol. 2013;31(12):1569–75.
40. Palefsky JM, Holly EA, Ralston ML, Jay N, Berry JM, Darragh TM. High incidence of anal high-grade squamous intra-epithelial lesions among HIV-positive and HIV-negative homosexual and bisexual men. AIDS. 1998;12(5):495–503.
41. Machalek DA, Poynten M, Jin F, Fairley CK, Farnsworth A, Garland SM, Hillman RJ, Petoumenos K, Roberts J, Tabrizi SN, Templeton DJ, Grulich AE. Anal human papillomavirus infection and associated neoplastic lesions in men who have sex with men: a systematic review and meta-analysis. Lancet Oncol. 2012;13(5):487–500.
42. Wilkin T, Lee JY, Lensing SY, Stier EA, Goldstone SE, Berry JM, Jay N, Aboulafia D, Cohn DL, Einstein MH, Saah A, Mitsuyasu RT, Palefsky JM. Safety and immunogenicity of the quadrivalent human papillomavirus vaccine in HIV-1-infected men. J Infect Dis. 2010;202(8):1246–53.
43. Aberg JA, Gallant JE, Ghanem KG, Emmanuel P, Zingman BS, Horberg MA, Infectious Diseases Society of America. Primary care guidelines for the management of persons infected with HIV: 2013 update by the HIV Medicine Association of the Infectious Diseases Society of America. Clin Infect Dis. 2014;58(1):e1–34.
44. Garg M, Lee JY, Kachnic LA, Catalano PJ, Henry DH, Cooley TP, Ratner L, Wachsman W, Aboulafia DM, Benson AB, Palefsky J, Whittington R, Mitsuyasu RT, Sparano JA, Eastern Cooperative Oncology Group (ECOG), AIDS Malignancy Consortium (AMC). Phase II trials of cetuximab (CX) plus cisplatin (CDDP), 5-fluorouracil (5-FU) and radiation (RT) in immunocompetent (ECOG 3205) and HIV-positive (AMC045) patients with squamous cell carcinoma of the anal canal (SCAC): safety and preliminary efficacy results. J Clin Oncol. 2012;30 (suppl; abstr 4030).
45. Deeken JF, Tjen-A-Looi A, Rudek MA, Okuliar C, Young M, Little RF, Dezube BJ. The rising challenge of non-AIDS-defining cancers in HIV-infected patients. Clin Infect Dis. 2012;55(9):1228–35.
46. Gopal S, Patel MR, Yanik EL, Cole SR, Achenbach CJ, Napravnik S, Burkholder GA, Reid EG, Rodriguez B, Deeks SG, Mayer KH, Moore RD, Kitahata MM, Eron JJ, Richards KL. Temporal trends in presentation and survival for HIV-associated lymphoma in the antiretroviral therapy era. J Natl Cancer Inst. 2013;105(16):1221–29.
47. ACIP Adult Immunization Work Group, Bridges CB, Woods L, Coyne-Beasley T, Centers for Disease Control and Prevention (CDC). Advisory Committee on Immunization Practices (ACIP) recommended immunization schedule for adults aged 19 years and older—United States, 2013. MMWR Surveill Summ. 2013;62(Suppl 1):9–19.
48. Burkhalter JE, Springer CM, Chhabra R, Ostroff JS, Rapkin BD. Tobacco use and readiness to quit smoking in low-income HIV-infected persons. Nicotine Tob Res. 2005;7(4):511–22.
49. Centers for Disease Control and Prevention. Vital signs: current cigarette smoking among adults aged > or = 18 years—United States, 2009. MMWR Morb Mortal Wkly Rep. 2010;59(35):1135–40.
50. Emlet CA, Fredriksen-Goldsen KI, Kim HJ. Risk and protective factors associated with health-related quality of life among older gay and bisexual men living with HIV disease. Gerontologist. 2013;53(6):963–72.
51. Suneja G, Shiels MS, Angulo R, Copeland GE, Gonsalves L, Hakenewerth AM, Macomber KE, Melville SK, Engels EA. Cancer treatment disparities in HIV-infected individuals in the United States. J Clin Oncol. 2014;32(22):2344–50.

52. Branson BM, Handsfield HH, Lampe MA, Janssen RS, Taylor AW, Lyss SB, Clark JE, Centers for Disease Control and Prevention (CDC). Revised recommendations for HIV testing of adults, adolescents, and pregnant women in health-care settings. MMWR Recomm Rep. 2006;55(RR-14):1–17.
53. Chiao EY, Dezube BJ, Krown SE, Wachsman W, Brock MV, Giordano TP, Mitsuyasu R, Pantanowitz L. Time for oncologists to opt in for routine opt-out HIV testing? JAMA. 2010;304(3):334–9.
54. New York State Department of Health. Primary care approach to the HIV-infected patient. New York (NY): New York State Department of Health. (2011 April). http://www.guideline.gov/content.aspx?id=34268&search=hiv+cancer. Accessed 1 Nov 2014.
55. New York State Department of Health. Care of the HIV-infected transgender patient. New York (NY): New York State Department of Health. (2012 January). http://www.guideline.gov/content.aspx?id=37877&search=hiv+cancer. Accessed 1 Nov 2014.
56. ACOG Committee on Practice Bulletins Gynecology. ACOG practice bulletin No. 117: gynecologic care for women with human immunodeficiency virus. Obstet Gynecol. 2010;116(6):1492–509.
57. Persad GC, Little RF, Grady C. Including persons with HIV infection in cancer clinical trials. J Clin Oncol. 2008;26(7):1027–32.
58. Weiss SA, Gajavelli S, Negassa A, Sparano JA, Haigentz M. Evaluation of cancer trial eligibility criteria (with focus on non-AIDS—defining cancers) for inclusion of persons with HIV infection. Poster Presentation. J Clin Oncol. 2011;29(suppl; abstr 6092).
59. Bower M, Palfreeman A, Alfa-Wali M, Bunker C, Burns F, Churchill D, Collins S, Cwynarski K, Edwards S, Fields P, Fife K, Gallop-Evans E, Kassam S, Kulasegaram R, Lacey C, Marcus R, Montoto S, Nelson M, Newsom-Davis T, Orkin C, Shaw K, Tenant-Flowers M, Webb A, Westwell S, Williams M, British HIV Association. British HIV Association guidelines for HIV-associated malignancies 2014. HIV Med. 2014;15(Suppl 2):1–92.
60. Murphy AB, Bhatia R, Martin IK, Klein DA, Hollowell CM, Nyame Y, Dielubanza E, Achenbach C, Kittles RA. Are HIV-infected men vulnerable to prostate cancer treatment disparities? Cancer Epidemiol Biomarkers Prev. 2014;23(10):2009–18.

Chapter 12
Provider-Patient Issues for the LGBT Cancer Patient

Michele J. Eliason and Suzanne L. Dibble

Abstract In this chapter we describe some of the issues LGBT cancer patients experience when they must engage with healthcare systems including providers who are uninformed about the terminology, partner/family issues, or health care concerns of LGBT individuals. We review the sparse literature about healthcare professionals' education about LGBT issues and LGBT patients' experiences with healthcare. Then we recommend a framework of healthcare microaggressions to describe the climate in which cancer care often occurs. Finally, we offer suggestions for healthcare providers working with LGBT patients to alter their individual behavior and to improve the healthcare system experience for their patients.

> Jason is a 47 year old African American bisexual man in a relationship with Tomas, a Latino gay man. They have been together for 16 years and arrive at an appointment with the gastroenterologist to discuss Jason's colonoscopy results. At the reception desk, Jason explains that Tomas is his partner and the receptionist gets flustered when she cannot find a field on the computer registration form to record this relationship. She announces "I have to list you as single." Other patients in the waiting area are staring at Jason and Tomas after this exchange. When the nurse comes to the door and announces Jason's name, they stand up together and the nurse says, "You can wait for your friend here, sir" to Tomas. Tomas insists that he is coming in with Jason, and the nurse just shrugs and leads them to an exam room. When the physician comes in, she introduces herself to Jason and starts talking before Jason can introduce Tomas. Dr. Anders never makes eye contact with Tomas as she delivers the news that Jason has colon cancer and starts to outline the treatment options. When she leaves the room, Tomas starts to cry. The nurse returns to give Jason some paperwork and says, "Well, you don't have to get all emotional about it. Your friend will be fine." Jason and Tomas leave the appointment in a great deal of stress about the upcoming treatment, and feeling demoralized by their "care" in the clinic.

A cancer diagnosis is one of the most frightening and stressful experiences anyone can have in a healthcare setting. For LGBT patients, this terrifying diagnosis means that one will have to spend precious energy surviving through intensive and ongoing contact in a potentially insensitive and culturally inappropriate setting. The

S. L. Dibble (✉)
Institute of Health and Aging, School of Nursing, University of California, San Francisco, CA, USA
e-mail: sue.dibble@gmail.com

M. J. Eliason
Department of Health Education, San Francisco State University, San Francisco, CA, USA

U. Boehmer, R. Elk (eds.), *Cancer and the LGBT Community*,
DOI 10.1007/978-3-319-15057-4_12

past ten years have brought almost unbelievable progress in legal protections for LGBT people and in positive societal attitudes toward LGBT individuals. However, disclosing personal information about gender, sexuality, and family structures to healthcare providers can still be fraught with stress for LGBT patients and their partners/families. As the opening case study of Jason and Tomas reveals, most LGBT people no longer face refusals of care or overtly negative treatment, but instead, are challenged by more subtle discrimination and invalidations. In this chapter, we review the sparse literature about healthcare provider attitudes and knowledge, healthcare training/education about LGBT issues, and LGBT patients' experiences in healthcare. Then we recommend a framework of "healthcare microaggressions" to explore how LGBT cancer patients may experience their ongoing care within the U.S. healthcare system. We end with recommendations for individual healthcare providers and healthcare delivery systems to improve the quality of care to LGBT patients and their families.

Knowledge and Attitudes of Health Care Providers

Unfortunately, healthcare professional training typically has not included much information about LGBT health issues. Research about medical and nursing curricula show that this content has not been a priority [1, 2] and there has even been some resistance in the past about the relevance of this content. The "we treat everyone the same" argument has often been used to justify this lack in the education of healthcare professionals, who are assumed to be impartial, all-knowing authorities [3].

Physicians

Medical school and residency education rarely contain much information about LGBT issues beyond HIV/AIDS. Even LGBT physicians report a lack of education about LGBT issues. In a recent survey of LGBT physicians [4], most had not received education about LGBT issues in medical school (61 % had no education about lesbian health; 49 % had no content about gay men's health; 78 % were not informed about bisexual health, and 76 % had received no training on transgender health). These LGBT physicians often encountered examples of discrimination and harassment on the workplace: 15 % had been harassed by a colleague and 22 % had experienced social ostracizing. They had also witnessed disparaging remarks about LGBT patients (65 %), discriminatory care of an LGBT patient (34 %), or disrespect of an LGBT patient's partner (36 %). One study reported that students in healthcare professional training (medicine, physical therapy, physician assistant) heard disparaging remarks about LGBT people from residents or other students (25 %) or faculty (7 %) [5]. Among medical students in New York City with some exposure to LGBT patient care, 28 % were uncomfortable addressing the patient's healthcare needs and fewer than half reported screening for same-sex activity when taking a sexual history; consequently, more than half never or rarely discovered a patient's sexual orientation [6].

Nurses

Until recently, nursing education had a nearly total silence about LGBT issues [7]. In the past few years, more guidance is available about infusing the nursing curriculum with LGBT content (e.g. [1, 8–11]). Older studies reported high levels of negativity about LGBT people among nurse educators [12] and nursing students [13–15] but more recent studies find lower rates of overt negativity among nursing students [16] and practicing nurses [17]. In a recent study, nurse educators [18] agreed that teaching nursing students about LGBT issues is very important (79% of a sample of over 1000 nurse educators in the U.S.), but 72% reported that they were not at all prepared to teach about LGBT issues. Unfortunately, a minority of nurses continue to hold negative beliefs about LGBT people [19, 20], and LGBT nurses report being treated differently from heterosexual nurses [21].

LGBT Patient's Experiences in Healthcare Settings

In a qualitative study of LGBT patients in the Pacific Northwest, Rounds and colleagues [22] reported that participants described two qualities to be desirable in their primary care providers: basic knowledge of LGBT issues and good communication and interpersonal skills. These basic skills were lacking in some health care providers, resulting in a poorer quality of care. Patient care experiences reported by LGBT individuals included issues related to disclosure of sexuality and/or gender, actual care given by providers, heterosexism noted on the forms and policies/procedures, lack of recognition of partners and family, and differences related to the specificity of one's identities. In addition, the importance of LGBT community support was often ignored. These issues are discussed below.

Disclosure

> [It was important] to not be dancing around with who I am as a person and who my support people are. [23, p. 204]

The first issue that LGBT patients have is deciding whether, and how, to disclose their sexual or gender identity to a healthcare provider. There are a number of factors that predict whether someone might or might not disclose. For LGB men and women in one study [24], being bisexual, having a higher degree of internalized oppression, and having less connection to LGB communities were predictive of *not* disclosing. Gender differences were also noted. Among women, additional predictors were having a racial/ethnic minority identification, lower educational attainment, and having children. Among men, further predictors were being younger, being born outside of the U.S., and being older when they first recognized their sexuality. Patients may decide to disclose or not depending on: the nature of the presenting problem (if acute and ongoing care involving a partner might be needed), if sexuality or gender are relevant to the health problem (a one-time ER visit for a sprained ankle is less critical for disclosure than ongoing monitoring of cancer treatment), behaviors of the healthcare provider and the reputation of the agency/institution or characteristics of the healthcare provider [8].

Disclosure is not an all or none event, but an ongoing and sometimes unclear process. Eliason and Schope [25] reported that a convenience sample of lesbians and gay men from the Midwest used four different disclosure strategies. In active disclosure, the person directly told a provider of their sexual identity. In passive disclosure, the patient assumed that the provider knew because the patient had a same-sex partner in the room or wore a t-shirt or button that declared their sexual orientation. In active non-disclosure, the patient deliberately lied to the provider about their sexuality or relationships. A common scenario was passive non-disclosure, or the classic "'don't ask, don't tell" situation. When healthcare providers and written forms do not provide any openings for the patient to disclose, patients often do not volunteer this information. Disclosure is important to get appropriate care, and one study reported that lesbians who disclosed to their healthcare providers were more likely to get regular care and when their physicians asked about sexual orientation, 100% of the respondents disclosed [26].

Clinical Care Issues

Very little research has focused on LGBT people's experiences with cancer care. Dibble and Roberts [27] reported that among the 80 women in their study, the lesbians delayed seeing a physician after being suspicious that something was wrong when compared to the heterosexual women. The researchers postulated that there may have been a failure in the relationship between the lesbian and her health care provider. Boehmer and Case [28] interviewed 39 sexual minority women with breast cancer about their experiences with healthcare providers. They reported that women desired providers who were competent caregivers and who had warm communication styles and a patient-centered approach that included their families and partners. One older study [29] reported that compared to heterosexual women, lesbians with breast cancer got more support from their partner and friends, but felt less satisfied with their medical care. Harding and colleagues [30] reviewed the literature about end of life and palliative care for LGBT patients and reported only 12 articles, mostly focused on the experiences of gay and lesbian individuals, with few bisexual and no transgender individuals included. The evidence from these studies is clear and repetitive of the need for health care providers to have training in order to: (1) facilitate disclosure of sexual orientation; (2) determine ways to minimize heterosexual assumptions; (3) identify and diminish bias; and (4) promote com-

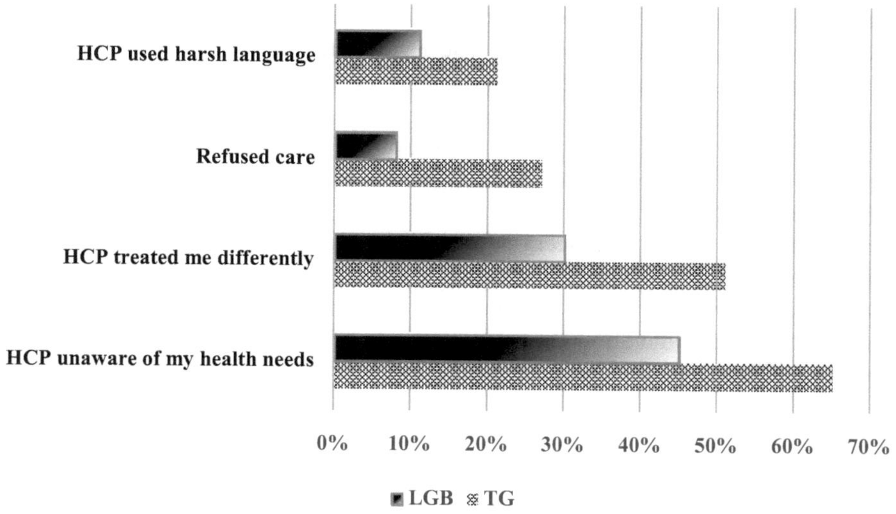

Fig. 12.1. Healthcare experiences by LGB and TG (transgender) people ($n=4916$) [Adapted from Lambda Legal, 2010]

fort and acceptance. They also reported that providers must respect the patient's wishes, include the partner in decision making, and educate themselves about the legal implications for same sex couples in their area when a partner is terminally ill. Harding et al. also noted the importance of asking about spirituality rather than religion. Also, many participants in these studies reported that their healthcare provider never asked them who should make medical decisions for them if they were unable to do so.

There is ample evidence that discrimination and poor treatment are still problems in healthcare settings. A portion of the results for the Lambda Legal Health Care Fairness Survey [31] are summarized in Fig. 12.1 below, showing experiences in healthcare settings of nearly 5000 LGBT individuals. In every case, transgender or gender non-conforming patients experienced more discrimination and harassment than LGB patients. For example, 50 % of transgender and 30 % of LGB people felt that a healthcare provider had treated them differently than other patients. The most common problem was encountering a healthcare provider who knew nothing about LGBT patient care needs.

Heterosexist and Gender Normative Language and Policies

Heterosexism refers to deeply ingrained beliefs that everyone is, or should be, heterosexual. Gender normativity refers to beliefs that there are only two sexes, male and female, and that our gender derives from our sex at birth. These two belief systems are embedded in U.S. culture and also in healthcare institutional practices, from the written forms to the history-taking interviews to informal interactions with patients and their families. LGBT patients encounter these beliefs throughout their navigation of the healthcare system. The forms often do not allow for recording one's personal sexual or gender identities, nor do they allow for identification of one's partner or families. Patients have to make a decision whether to disclose at this point (many would prefer to wait and see how open-minded the provider seems to be) or to lie. Later on, a provider may discuss their health history and progress since the last visit, often in a rushed manner. Rarely does this process allow LGBT patients to raise issues of concern or allow healthcare providers to signal their acceptance of LGBT patients. If the patient does experience discrimination or mild harassment, does the agency have a policy that includes sexual orientation and gender identity that would allow their complaints to be taken seriously? Is the healthcare provider aware of the policy?

Partners and Families

Laura is a 58 year-old single lesbian with advanced breast cancer. She is about to enter a hospice wing of a hospital, and requests that her social network, a circle of 5 women, including two ex-lovers, all be equally included in her care and able to visit at any time of the day or night. One of her social support system overheard a nursing assistant at the nurses' station say to a colleague, "It's not natural to have such a close relationship with an ex. Do you think they all sleep with each other?" One of the members of the circle was told by the daughter of another patient to stay away from her mother, who was "deeply religious" and should not have to look at gay people when she was dying.

LGBT patients may have strained relationships or even been rejected by their families of origin, so "families of choice" become the main support for their care. Many LGBT patients have had experiences of partners being ignored, excluded, or treated badly by healthcare providers [28].

LGBT Community Support

McGregor and colleagues [32] reported that lesbians with breast cancer had greater distress if they had higher internalized homophobia scores. Internalized oppression is the result of believing negative stereotypes about one's own group, and consists of shame, guilt, and fear related to one's sexuality or gender. These negative emotions are an additional source of stress that impacts wellbeing and the capacity to cope with challenging physical illnesses. Boehmer and coauthors [33] reported that women who self-identified as lesbian or bisexual had better coping strategies for cancer than women with same-sex partners who did not self-identify. Presumably, this is related to having a more supportive community if one is out and identified with the LGBT community. Durso and Meyer [24] also reported that those with stronger ties to LGB community were more likely to disclose to healthcare providers. Having the support of a community may be a significant predictor of adjustment and well-being for LGBT individuals (and for reducing internalized homophobia/biphobia/transphobia).

Sinding et al. [34] studied community support of lesbians with breast and gynecologic cancers, and reported that some of their participants had the perception that lesbians get better support from their partners and communities than heterosexual women. Some, though, noted that they felt isolated and had difficulty talking openly about their cancer. “Cancer scares the shit out of people and they don’t know what to do with you” (p. 69), said one participant. Some respondents felt that lesbians’ involvement in the HIV/AIDS community support/care movements in the 1980s made them more prepared to deal with other illnesses in the community.

Many LGBT survivors do not feel welcome or understood in mainstream support groups, and transgender survivors have been especially challenged. Most of the few LGBT-specific cancer support groups across the country are in major metropolitan areas. Access to 24/7 online support is an important small step toward providing encouragement and assistance for those living with a cancer diagnosis. Recently the National LGBT Cancer Network received funding to set up free online support groups for lesbian, bisexual and transgender breast cancer survivors (See http://cancer-network.org/support_groups_for_survivors). Another online support service for LGBT folks comes from The National LGBT Cancer Project (See http://lgbt-cancer.com).

Diversity Within LGBT Communities

There is a dearth of information about LGBT people’s healthcare experiences in general, but particularly about experiences with cancer care. There seems to be more research about lesbians than any other group, but it is difficult to know if lesbians’ experiences are the same as gay, bisexual, or transgender people. It is also highly likely that there are differences among LGBT people’s experiences with cancer care based on age, race, ethnicity, level of education, income, geographic location, and many other factors as well. Differences such as these are found among heterosexuals and it is likely that a similar diversity exists within LGBT communities. This section offers some suggestions about the diversity of experiences that LGBT cancer survivors might have.

Lesbian/Bisexual Women Some authors speculate that lesbian and bisexual women have very different experiences, partly depending on whether they are currently partnered with men, women, or both. Research needs to consistently separate out individuals by their sexuality and gender to study the nuances of experience [35, 36]. To study the possible differences among breast cancer survivors by lesbian or bisexual orientation, Boehmer and colleagues [37] used Massachusetts Cancer Registry data to find sexual minority women with breast cancer histories, and then supplemented the sample by convenience sampling from across the U.S., resulting in 180 participants: 161 lesbian and 19 bisexual women. This study identified few differences by sexual identity. The bisexual women had a higher level of education, but the groups were similar on other demographic, cancer-clinical presentation and treatment variables, body image, sexual functioning, and side effects of treatment. There were no differences in physical or mental health outcomes. However, lesbians were more likely to trust their physicians, be partnered (and have a female partner), live with a partner, and be open about their sexuality. Having a partner was associated with better physical health, and having a female partner was associated with better mental health. In another report from the same sample of cancer survivors [38], fewer of the lesbian women treated with mastectomy chose to have breast reconstruction (3 % of lesbians, 15 % of heterosexual and 17 % of bisexual women), but more were on mood stabilizers and anti-depressant medications (40 % sexual minority and 21 % heterosexual). On the other hand, there was no difference in current anxiety or depression by sexual orientation. Arena and colleagues [39] reported that lesbians had fewer concerns about sexuality after a breast cancer diagnosis than did heterosexual women, and were also less concerned about physical appearance changes, experienced less disruption of their sexual relationships, had less denial, and demonstrated more positive coping strategies. Other studies report that quality of life is not different for sexual minority women with cancer compared with heterosexual women [40, 41].

Gay/Bisexual Men Thomas and colleagues [42] interviewed 9 gay and one bisexual man with prostate cancer and reported that their sexual identities were often wrapped up in sexual practices, so that altered sexual functioning after prostate cancer affected self-worth and increased performance anxiety. Most thought of themselves as "damaged goods," although one participant thought that cancer was an opportunity to redefine his sexuality from a genital focus to a greater focus on intimacy. The men were generally unhappy with the communication with their urologists, who they perceived as lacking in empathy and poor at caring for emotional needs, but described their relationship with their primary healthcare providers as more satisfactory. Because of sample size limitations more research is needed to explore these findings. Some gay/bisexual men appear to fragment their healthcare by seeking sexual health care separately from primary care to avoid embarrassment, shame, or lack of respect from their primary care doctors [43].

Transgender Patients Healthcare providers appear to be the least prepared to deal with healthcare issues of transgender patients, and transgender patients may be the most likely to experience overt discrimination in healthcare settings [44, 45], although we could not find any studies particularly about cancer treatment. The following case study highlights some of the issues that trans women might face.

> Emily is a 66 year old woman, who was born male and transitioned to a female role and body 25 years earlier. She has throat cancer and was hospitalized for symptom management during radiation therapy. She became a source of deep curiosity and gossip among the hospital staff. Every day a different caregiver helped her with her bath, and there was a constant stream of housekeepers, residents, medical students, and dieticians gawking at her as they passed by in the hallway. No one was blatantly discriminatory or harassing to her, but she often heard giggles from the nurses' station when she was escorted to therapy in a wheelchair. One day, she was handed her chart to hold while she was transported to the clinic, and she found that all the formal documents referred to her as "he" and "male." Her birth name was used on many of the recent progress reports rather than her legally changed new name. When she pointed this out to her physician, he said "our system has no option for transgender." She gently replied that she was now a woman, but the doctor said, "You cannot change your DNA. That is still male."

In conclusion, research on LGBT people's experiences with cancer care are very limited, but it appears that LGBT patients and their families encounter some of the same types of discrimination, harassment, and even violence that they may experience in the outside world.

Healthcare Microaggressions and Cancer Care

It is no longer socially acceptable to engage in overtly discriminatory and rejecting ways in healthcare settings, like hospitals and clinics [46], however, a minority of the population, including some healthcare providers, still harbor overtly negative attitudes. Hate crimes based on sexual orientation and gender identity increased in the late 2000s whereas racial, ethnic, and religious-based hate crimes remained steady [47]. Some LGBT patients will continue to encounter blatant differential treatment such as refusals of care and inappropriate care. However, the majority will experience a more subtle form of discrimination. Sue and colleagues [48] called the subtle daily assaults on minority peoples "micro-aggressions." They happen daily, briefly, and are covert, and people with minority identifications must learn to cope with these ongoing assaults to their well-being, creating a condition of daily stress (called minority stress). Homophobia, biphobia, transphobia, heterosexism, and gender normativity are so deeply imbedded in the culture that microaggressions are often committed by well-intentioned people, who may not be consciously aware of the impact of their words or behaviors. In this section, we explore how microaggressions manifest in healthcare settings and how they may affect LGBT cancer patients and their families. Nadal and coauthors [49] described three major categories of microaggressions that we will use to structure this section, and supplement it with examples drawn from the literature about LGBT patient experiences as well as research on microagressions experienced in the mental health/therapy arena [50].

Micro-assaults include name-calling and more overt discrimination. This is the most blatant, and perhaps intentional of the varieties of microaggressions. Examples: a nurse refuses to care for an LGBT patient, a physician during rounds refers to the "faggot" with colon cancer, hospital staff rotate going to a patients' room to see the "freak" transgender patient, a patient's same-sex partner is told he is not welcome during visiting hours or must leave during health-care decision-making sessions. A nurse sends a chaplain to visit with an LGBT patient because he is concerned that the patient is "going to hell if she does not repent." These behaviors are all denounced by hospital patient rights policies and the Joint Commissions' charge for respectful quality care for all. Even though a minority of healthcare providers engage in these damaging behaviors, if others do not stand up and challenge them, they can do great damage to the reputation of a clinic, hospital, or other healthcare setting.

Micro-insults include rudeness, condescension, and insensitivity, and may reflect ignorance rather than intentional differential treatment, or may reflect discomfort when working with patients/clients/coworkers who are different. Examples: not using the patient's preferred name and pronouns (e.g., calling a transgender woman, "he"), disrespecting or ignoring a partner of a patient, or implying that one's sexuality or gender are choices. Sometimes micro-insults might be based on believing stereotypes about LGBT people, such as thinking that all gay men are hypersexual or all older lesbians are asexual, or believing that bisexual people are confused about their sexuality, or that transgender people are mentally ill. A common assumption that many healthcare providers make is that LGBT identity is associated with disease or disorder, particularly sexually transmitted infections, or that the patient's sexuality or gender identity is the root of every health problem with which the LGBT patient presents. Sometimes micro-insults are conveyed in body language rather than in overt comments or behaviors. A subtle distancing or reluctance to touch a patient, a hesitant tone of voice, or lack of eye contact may signal to patients that the healthcare provider is uncomfortable with them.

Micro-invalidations include denials of discrimination, trivializing of one's worries about differential treatment, and dismissal of past experiences as unimportant. Examples: No place to record one's same-sex partner on a form (invalidates the relationship); no place to record one's sexual orientation or gender identity on a form or in an oral history with a healthcare provider (invalidates the importance of the identity); statements such as "Now that this state has legalized same-sex marriage, there is no more discrimination against LGBT people," or "How dare you compare your issues to racial civil rights," or "we are here to discuss your cancer treatment; your sexual orientation is irrelevant." Another example is telling victims of a hate crime or discrimination that they are being "too sensitive." Some LGBT people have been told that their "blatant" appearance or behavior was the cause of the violence or discrimination. Telling someone who says, "I think I might be transgender," that they are just going through a phase invalidates the enormous courage it takes to reveal such personal information. Another way that healthcare providers might invalidate a patient's experience is to say that their clinic or hospital is inclusive because they have one openly LGBT employee.

Consequences of Microaggressions

Several studies have shown that the stress resulting from discrimination and harassment, whether overt or subtle, intentional or from well-meaning sources, affect both physical and mental health over time [51, 52]. They result in a perceived need for hyper-vigilance in healthcare settings. Dealing with visiting policies, sharing of information and decision-making, and just being physically located in a setting where one stands out, requires much energy (stigma management) from the LGBT patient. That degree of monitoring of one's environment is physically and mentally taxing to the patient who must also deal with painful, tiring, uncomfortable cancer treatments. Cancer patients should not have to waste precious energy worrying how their partner or family is being treated.

Recommendations

Individual Healthcare Providers

In one study a transgender man [53] described what health care providers need to do: "you need to prepare yourself for different types of people walking in your office" and "the last thing I wanted was to be a training case for a practitioner who has never provided care for a transgender person before" (p. 26). Vulnerable patients who are dealing with their own mortality should not be placed in the role of primary educator for their healthcare providers. There are many resources available now for healthcare provider education, as shown in Tables 12.1 and 12.2. Reygan and D'Alton [54] reported on a brief (50 min) training for healthcare providers who were involved with oncology and palliative care, and showed that even this brief introduction to terminology, healthcare issues, and oncology/palliative care issues of LGB patients resulted in significant shifts in comfort with terminology, confidence in providing LGB care, and increased knowledge. Perhaps the most important things that healthcare providers can do is to (1) examine their own belief systems and consider how they might impact their patients; (2) inquire compassionately about sexual and gender identities and family structures as part of comprehensive

Table 12.1 Web-based resources for educating healthcare providers about LGBT care

Centers for Disease Control and Prevention	http://www.cdc.gov/lgbthealth/
Eliason MJ, Dibble SL, DeJoseph JF, Chinn	*LGBTQ cultures: What health care professionals need to know and sexual and gender diversity.* 2009. Available at http://www.nursingcenter.com/lnc/static?pageid=928987
Fenway Health	http://www.fenwayhealth.org
Gay & Lesbian Medical Association (GLMA)	*Guidelines for care of lesbian, gay, bisexual, and transgender patients.* Available at http://www.glma.org/_data/n_0001/resources/live/GLMA%20guidelines%202006%20FINAL.pdf
Joint Commission	*Advancing effective communication cultural competence and patient-and family-centered care for the lesbian, gay, bisexual, and transgender (LGBT) community: A field guide.* November 8, 2011. Available at http://www.jointcommission.org/lgbt/
Lavender health—LGBTQ Resource Center	http://lavenderhealth.org/education/preparation/. This site has an LGBT 101 health powerpoint and a list of case studies and other classroom or continuing education discussion questions and activities
World Professional Association for Transgender Health	http://www.wpath.org

Table 12.2 Recent books for educating healthcare providers about LGBT care

American College of Physicians (ACP): *The Fenway guide to lesbian, gay, bisexual, and transgender health*. Philadelphia: ACP, 2008
Dibble SL, Robertson PA. (Eds.) *Lesbian health 101: A clinician's guide*. San Francisco: UCSF Nursing Press, 2010
Institute of Medicine: *The health of lesbian, gay, bisexual, and transgender people: Building a foundation for better understanding*. Washington, DC: National Academies Press, 2011
Meyer IH, Northridge ME. (Eds.) *The health of sexual minorities: Public health perspectives on lesbian, gay, bisexual and transgender populations*. New York: Springer Science + Business Media, 2010
Substance Abuse and Mental Health Services Administration. *Top health issues for LGBT populations information & resource kit*. HHS Publication No. (SMA) 12–4684. Rockville, MD: Substance Abuse and Mental Health Services Administration, 2012
Witten TM, Eyler AE (Eds). Lesbian, gay, bisexual, and transgender aging: Research and clinical perspectives. Baltimore: Johns Hopkins University Press, 2012

patient-centered care; (3) do not make assumptions that sexual or gender identities are related to any specific health or sexual behaviors; and (4) learn how to take a sexual history without judgment or discomfort. Some issues that need to be addressed in a sexual history include sexual and gender identities, sexual abuse history, contraception when necessary, current and history of risky sexual activities, and current concerns about sexual functioning. If recreational drugs have been linked with sexual activities, this is important to consider, as it may affect pharmacological treatments and may require treatment for both the sexual and drug dependence. For those who are hesitant about taking a full sexual history, a simple question/comment such as "Many patients undergoing cancer treatment (or some specific treatment) have questions about how this might affect their sexual lives or relationships with partners. Do you have any concerns about this that we should discuss?" For more guidance on sexual history taking, see the CDC (http://www.cdc.gov/STD/treatment/SexualHistory.pdf).

During a physical assessment, it is important for healthcare providers to tell patients what they are going to do before they start doing it. It is important to let patients know that if they feel uncomfortable, the provider will stop. In particular, touching a patient near the genitals or breasts, can be stressful and traumatic. Being careful about talking through what will happen in the physical exam and why will be helpful for many patients, including any who have experienced any kind of sexual abuse or traumas related to the body.

Education of Healthcare Professionals

Currently, healthcare education contains little information about LGBT patient care. Most of the research to date has urged that more content be infused into medical and allied health professional programs, but until certification or licensing exams include this content, it is a hard sell. Oncology residency programs and other specialty training also needs content on LGBT healthcare as part of a larger cultural sensitivity emphasis. Ways to shift the climate in educational programs from one where LGBT students and faculty are at best invisible and at worst, discriminated against, to one that is welcoming and inclusive, will require changes in curricula, hiring and retention practices, employee benefits and rights, student rights, and other policies and institutional activities [55]. In many programs, LGBT-related research is not encouraged or valued in the ways that other forms of diversity are accepted. Highlighting the work of LGBT health scholars and mentoring students to do LGBT health research are critical for preparing the next generation of educators and clinicians. Snowden [55] suggests many concrete ways to improve the climate for LGBT students and employees in health professional schools.

Healthcare Delivery Systems

There are now several guides to transforming healthcare systems to become welcoming and inclusive of LGBT patients and communities. The Joint Commission's [56] field guide offers concrete suggestions for changing written forms and data collection systems, modifying policies and procedures, and educating healthcare providers. The Health Equality Index (HEI) from the Human Rights Campaign [57] also highlights how hospitals and clinics across the U.S. are addressing equity for their LGBT patients. In the latest version of the HEI available at this writing (2013), 718 healthcare facilities had participated in the project. Their "Core Four" criteria include:

- Patient non-discrimination policy includes sexual orientation and gender identity; and the policy is readily accessible to patients
- Visitation policies grant equal rights to LGBT patients and their visitors (and broaden definitions of family)
- Employment nondiscrimination policies include sexual orientation and gender identity
- Training on LGBT patient-centered care is provided to key staff members (we propose that all staff members with patient contact have basic training and key clinical staff members receive more advanced training).

In conclusion, LGBT patients with cancer face some of the same trials and tribulations in healthcare settings and in interaction with healthcare providers as they experience in the outside world. However in the outside world, patients might not have to repeatedly subject themselves to these challenging interactions. These experiences of overt discrimination and more subtle microaggressions are the source of a great deal of stress. This stress could be vastly reduced by simple changes in healthcare delivery structures, such as prominently displaying and enforcing nondiscrimination policies, and by training in cultural sensitivity for all healthcare providers and support staff. All patients deserve the right to focus their energy on healing and coping with challenges presented by a cancer diagnosis, not defending themselves from a hostile or uninformed provider or system of care.

References

1. Brennan AM, Barnsteiner J, Siantz ML, Cotter VT, Everett J. Lesbian, gay, bisexual, transgendered, or intersexed content for nursing curricula. J Prof Nurs. 2012;28(2):96–104.
2. Obedin-Maliver J, Goldsmith E, Stewart L, White W, Tran E, Brenman S, et al. LGBT-related content in undergraduate medical education. JAMA. 2011;306:971–7.
3. Beagan BL. Neutralizing differences: producing neutral doctors for (almost) neutral patients. Soc Sci Med. 2000;51:1253–65.
4. Eliason MJ, Dibble SL, Robertson PA. Lesbian, gay, bisexual, and transgender (LGBT) physicians' experiences in the workplace. J Homosex. 2011;58(10):1355–71.
5. Dhaliwal JS, Crane LA, Valley MA, Lowenstein SR. Student perspectives on the diversity climate at a U.S. medical school: the need for a broader definition of diversity. BMC Res Notes. 2013;6:154.
6. Sanchez, .F, Rabatin J, Sanchez JP., Hubbard S, Kalet A. (2006). Medical students' ability to care for LGBT patients. Fam Med. 2006;38(1):21–7.
7. Eliason MJ, Dibble S, DeJoseph J. Nursing's silence on lesbian, gay, bisexual, and transgender issues: the need for emancipatory efforts. ANS Adv Nurs Sci. 2010;33(3):206–18.
8. Eliason MJ, Dibble SL, De Joseph JF, Chinn P. LGBTQ Cultures: What healthcare professionals need to know about sexual and gender diversity. Philadelphia: Lippincott; 2009.
9. Hardacker CT, Rubinstein B, Hotton A, Houlberg M. Adding silver to the rainbow: the development of the nurses' health education about LGBT elders (HEALE) cultural competency curriculum. J Nurs Manag. 2013;22(2):257-66.
10. Lim FA, Bernstein I. Promoting awareness of LGBT issues in aging in a baccalaureate nursing program. Nurs Educ Perspect. 2012;33(3):170–5.
11. Lim FA, Brown DV Jr, Jones H. Lesbian, gay, bisexual, and transgender health: fundamentals for nursing education. J Nurs Educ. 2013;52(4):198–203.
12. Randall CE (1989). Lesbian phobia among BSN educators: a survey. J Nurs Educ. 1989;28(7):302–6.
13. Eliason MJ, Randall CE. Lesbian phobia in nursing students. West J Nurs Res. 1991;13(3): 363–74.
14. Eliason MJ, Donelan C, Randall C. Lesbian stereotypes. Health Care Women Int. 1992;13(2): 131–44.
15. Eliason MJ, Raheim S. Experiences and comfort with culturally diverse groups in undergraduate pre-nursing students. J Nurs Educ. 2000;39(4):161–5.
16. Dinkel S, Patzel B, McGuire MJ, Rolfs E, Purcell K. Measures of homophobia among nursing students and faculty: a Midwestern perspective. Int J Nurs Educ Scholarsh. 2007;4 (1): 1–12.
17. Blackwell CW. Belief in the "free choice" model of homosexuality: a correlate of homophobia in registered nurses. J LGBT Health Res. 2007;3:31–40.
18. Sirota T. Attitudes among nurse educators toward homosexuality. J Nurs Educ. 2013;52(4): 219–27.
19. Dorsen C. An integrative review of nurse attitudes towards lesbian, gay, bisexual, and transgender patients. Can J Nurs Res. 2012;44(3):18–43.
20. Röndahl G, Innala S, Carlsson M. Nurses' attitudes towards lesbians and gay men. J Adv Nurs. 2004;47(4):386–92.
21. Eliason MJ, DeJoseph JF, Dibble SL, Deevey S, Chinn PL. LGBTQ nurses' experiences in the workplace. J Prof Nurs. 2011;27(4):237–44.
22. Rounds KE, McGrath BB, Walsh E. Perspectives on provider behaviors: a qualitative study of sexual and gender minorities regarding quality of care. Contemp Nurse. 2013;44(1):99–110.
23. Katz A. Gay and lesbian patients with cancer. Oncol Nurs Forum. 2009;36(2):203–7.
24. Durso LE, Meyer IH. Patterns and predictors of disclosure of sexual orientation to healthcare providers among lesbians, gay men, and bisexuals. Sex Res Social Policy. 2013;10(1):35–42.
25. Eliason MJ, Schope R. Does "don't ask, don't tell" apply to health care? Lesbian, gay, and bisexual people's disclosure to health care providers. J Gay Lesbian Med Assoc. 2001;5(4):125–34.

26. Steele LS Tinmouth JM Lu A. Regular health care use by lesbians: a path analysis of predictive factors. Fam Pract. 2006;23(6):631–6.
27. Dibble SL, Roberts SA. A comparison of breast cancer diagnosis and treatment between lesbian and heterosexual women. J Gay Lesbian Med Assoc. 2002;6(1):9–17.
28. Boehmer U, Case P. Sexual minority women's interactions with breast cancer providers. Women Health. 2006;44(2):41–58.
29. Fobair P, O'Hanlan K, Koopman C, Classen C, Dimiceli S, Drooker N, et al. Comparison of lesbian and heterosexual women's response to newly diagnosed breast cancer. Psychooncology. 2001;10(1):40–51.
30. Harding R, Epiphaniou E, Chidgey-Clark J. Needs, experiences, and preferences of sexual minorities for end-of-life care and palliative care: a systematic review. J Palliat Med. 2012;15(5):602–11.
31. Lambda Legal. When health care isn't caring: lambda legal's survey of discrimination against LGBT people and people with HIV (New York: Lambda Legal, 2010). www.lambdalegal.org/health-care-report. Accessed 23 Feb 2015.
32. McGregor BA, Carver CS, Antoni MH, Weiss S, Yount SE, Ironson G. Distress and internalized homophobia among lesbian women treated for early stage breast cancer. Psychol Women Q. 2001;25:1–9.
33. Boehmer U, Linde R, Freund KM. Sexual minority women's coping and psychological adjustment after a diagnosis of breast cancer. J Womens Health. 2005;14:214–24.
34. Sinding C, Grassau P, Barnoff L. Community support, community values: the experiences of lesbians diagnosed with cancer. Women Health. 2006;44(2):59–79.
35. Ebin J. Why bisexual health? J Bisex. 2012;12:168–77.
36. Fredriksen-Goldsen K, Kim H, Barkan S, Balsam KF, & Mincer SL. Disparities in health-related quality of life: a comparison of lesbians and bisexual women. Am J Public Health. 2010;100(11):2255–61.
37. Boehmer U, Glickman M, Winter M, Clark MA. Lesbian and bisexual women's adjustment after a breast cancer diagnosis. J Am Psychiatr Nurses Assoc. 2013;19(5):280–92
38. Boehmer U, Glickman M, Winter M. Anxiety and depression in breast cancer survivors of different sexual orientations. J Consult Clin Psychol. 2012;80:382–95.
39. Arena PL, Carver CS, Antoni MH, Weiss S, Ironson G, Duran RE. Psychosocial responses to treatment for breast cancer among lesbian and heterosexual women. Women Health. 2006;44(2):81–102.
40. Boehmer U, Glickman M, Milton J, Winter M. Health-related quality of life in breast cancer survivors of different sexual orientations. Qual Life Res. 2012;21:225–36.
41. Jabson JM, Donatelle RJ, Bowen DJ. Relationship between sexual orientation and quality of life in female breast cancer survivors. J Womens Health. 2011;20(12):1819–24.
42. Thomas C, Wootten VA, & Robinson P. The experiences of gay and bisexual men diagnosed with prostate cancer: results from an online focus group. Eur J Cancer Care Care. 2013;22(4):522–9.
43. Koester KA, Collins SP, Fuller SM, Galindo GR, Gibson S, Steward WT. Sexual healthcare preferences among gay and bisexual men: a qualitative study in San Francisco, CA. PLoS One. 2013;8(8):e71546. doi: 10.1371/journal.pone.0071546.
44. Dewey JM. Knowledge legitimacy: how trans-patient behavior supports and challenges current medical knowledge. Qual Health Res. 2008;18(10):1345–55.
45. Kosenko K, Rintamaki L, Raney S, Maness K. Transgender patient perceptions of stigma in health care contexts. Med Care. 2013;51(9):819–22.
46. Joint Commission. Patient-centered communication standards for hospitals. R^3 report: requirement, rationale, reference. February 9, 2011 Issue 1. 2011. http://www.jointcommission.org/assets/1/18/R3%20Report%20Issue%201%2020111.PDF. Accessed 20 Feb. 2014.
47. Herek GM, Cogan JC, Gillis JR. Victim experiences in hate crimes based on sexual orientation. J Soc Issues. 2002;58(2):319–39.
48. Sue DW, Capodilupo CM, Torino GC, Bucceri JM, Holder AM, Nadal KL, et al. Racial microaggressions in everyday life: implications for clinical practice. Am Psychol. 2007;62(4):271–86.

49. Nadal KL, Wong Y, Issa M, Meterko V, Leon J, Wideman M. Sexual orientation microaggressions: processes and coping mechanisms for lesbian, gay, and bisexual individuals. J LGBT Issues Couns. 2011;5:21–46.
50. Shelton K, Delgado-Romero EA. Sexual orientation microaggressions: The experience of LGBT and queer clients in psychotherapy. J Couns Psychol. 2011;58(2):210–21.
51. Frost D, Lehavot K, Meyer IH. Minority stress and physical health among sexual minority individuals. J Behav Med. 2015;:38(1):1–8.
52. Meyer IH. Prejudice, social stress, and mental health in lesbian, gay, and bisexual populations: conceptual issues and research evidence. Psych Sex Orient Gend Divers. 2013;1(S):3–26.
53. Poteat T, German D, Kerrigan D. Managing uncertainty: a grounded theory of stigma in transgender healthcare encounters. Soc Sci Med. 2013;84:22–9.
54. Reygan F, D'Alton P. A pilot training programme for health and social care professionals providing oncological and palliative care to lesbian, gay, and bisexual patients in Ireland. Psychooncology. 2013;22:1050–4.
55. Snowden, S. Recommendations for enhancing the climate for LGBT students and employees in health professional schools. Washington, DC. GLMA: Health Professionals Advancing LGBT Equality; 2013.
56. Joint Commission. Advancing effective communication cultural competence and patient-and family-centered care for the lesbian, gay, bisexual, and transgender (LGBT) community: a field guide. 2011. http://www.jointcommission.org/lgbt/. Accessed 8 Nov. 2011.
57. Human Rights Campaign. About the Healthcare Quality Index. http://www.hrc.org/hei/about-the-hei#.VouvdlqPSRM. Accessed 23 Feb 2015.

Chapter 13
Needs of LGBT Cancer Survivors

Liz Margolies and Charles Kamen

Abstract Lesbian, gay, bisexual, and transgender (LGBT) cancer survivors in the United States have unique needs that may go unaddressed in cancer care. Many of these needs center around deciding whether or not to disclose LGBT identity and how to include diverse supportive others in the medical decision making and treatment experience. Others arise from disparities that impact the LGBT community at large and that may be further complicated by a diagnosis of cancer. In this chapter, we outline several specific needs, including: acceptance of identity disclosure, respect for unique social support systems, understanding of LGBT sexuality, and reduction of gender expectations. We underscore these needs by including quotes from LGBT survivors describing their experiences receiving a cancer diagnosis and seeking cancer treatment. We also discuss tailored and LGBT-friendly support services, cultural competence in providing cancer care, and interventions to address specific disparities that impact LGBT survivors. We close with recommendations for future service development and research.

Introduction

Between 420,000 and 1,000,000 lesbian, gay, bisexual, and transgender (LGBT) cancer survivors are estimated to live in the United States [1, 2]. LGBT survivors are comparable in number to other subgroups of cancer survivors that have been the target of specific research and clinical attention, [3, 4] and yet they have remained invisible in psychosocial cancer research and in oncology clinics for decades [5]. National databases and epidemiological surveys do not routinely collect information on sexual orientation and gender identity, and assessments of cancer survivors' needs have remained relatively mute on the specific needs of LGBT survivors [6].

L. Margolies (✉)
National LGBT Cancer Network, New York, NY, USA
e-mail: liz@cancer-network.org

C. Kamen
Department of Surgery, University of Rochester Medical Center, Rochester, NY, USA

U. Boehmer, R. Elk (eds.), *Cancer and the LGBT Community*,
DOI 10.1007/978-3-319-15057-4_13

In this chapter we will outline what little research exists on the needs of LGBT survivors. We will also summarize existing services aimed at addressing these needs, and provide suggestions and recommendations for tailoring future services to this underserved and underrepresented population. Throughout, we will examine findings about the LGBT population in general through the lens of cancer survivorship, theorizing ways in which needs of the LGBT community broadly may manifest in the specific context of cancer survivorship.

We will also interweave findings from a qualitative study of LGBT cancer survivors into our discussion. The study's principal investigator, Marilyn Smith-Stoner from California State University San Bernardino, worked with Liz Margolies, LCSW, the Executive Director of the National LGBT Cancer Network. A total of 311 self-identified lesbian, gay, bisexual, or transgender cancer survivors (with a range of cancer types) participated in the study. Data are included below from qualitative responses to two open ended survey questions: "If you were to give a class to healthcare workers, focused on cancer care, what would you tell them about being LGBT and being diagnosed with cancer?" and "Is there anything else you'd like us to know about your experience of cancer?" [7, 8]. We will move from the needs of survivors generally, to the needs of LGBT survivors as a group, to the experiences of specific survivors to frame this issue.

Overarching Needs of LGBT Survivors

Receiving a diagnosis of cancer is a frightening and stressful experience [9]. The process of seeking cancer treatment and supportive care only compounds this stress. Cancer survivors are bombarded with clinical data and clinical options, asked to make complex medical decisions, and confronted with myriad uncertainties and unanswered questions. Their loved ones and care partners also experience considerable stress as they (often invisibly) support the cancer survivor through treatment and its side effects and into long-term survivorship [10].

The cancer experience takes a toll not only on the patient's physical body, but on mental health as well. Almost all patients experience some distress and between 15 and 40 % of cancer patients will develop clinical anxiety and/or depression [11]. Distress and clinical anxiety and depression may persist for years post diagnosis [12]. The risk for distress is less related to cancer type than to psychosocial factors, such as being younger, non-white, female and/or having a history of depression [13].

How, then, is the experience of cancer survivorship similar or different for LGBT survivors and their partners? The NCI website does not list sexual orientation or gender identity in their inventory of factors that affect coping, but identifies multiple conditions that are more prevalent and problematic in this population, such as "whether the patient is able to get into treatment," "the number of stressful life events the patient has had in the last year," and "whether the patient gets support from friends and family." As a group, LGBT people are less likely to have adequate health insurance, [14] more likely to have experienced stressful discrimination based on their gender identity and/or sexual orientation, [15] and more likely to be alienated from their families of origin [16].

For many LGBT cancer survivors, therefore, the stress inherent in cancer diagnosis and treatment is greatly magnified by pre-existing disparities. Disparate factors can result in increased distress among LGBT survivors over the course of treatment, as well, and critical questions about treatment options and recovery may be followed immediately by concerns about social stigma. While every new patient wonders "Will I survive this?" LGBT patients may also experience concerns about their safety, such as, "Can I come out to my doctor?", "Will I be treated differently if I do?" ,"Will my chosen family be welcome?" and "Will I be offered the information I need to know to take care of my relationship, my sexuality, my fertility, and my family?" LGBT survivors face potential discrimination within the healthcare system. Their questions about sexual side effects may be left unanswered due to discomfort, lack of knowledge, or lack of cultural competence on the part of providers. Their families of choice may be invisible or unwelcome. This latter issue is particularly problematic, as multiple studies that examined quality of life (QOL) after a breast cancer diagnosis found a relationship between social support and mental health [17–24]. Taken together, these factors make navigation of the cancer experience considerably more challenging for LGBT survivors and their care partners than for their heterosexual counterparts.

We discuss below the unique facets of LGBT survivorship, including issues of disclosure, differences in social support systems, sexuality concerns, and the impact of cancer on gender identity. Providers and social service organizations need to be aware of these needs and skilled in addressing them in order to deliver quality care.

Acceptance of Identity Disclosure

One potential need of LGBT cancer survivors is the need to disclose their LGBT identities to providers. Research on LGBT patients seeking medical treatment in general has highlighted the difficulty many LGBT persons experience in disclosing their identity [25]. Studies have also shown that disclosure of identity, and acceptance of this disclosure on the part of the medical care team, is linked with better health outcomes on the part of the patient. While little research has examined this issue in the context of cancer care, the need to and importance of disclosing is likely to apply to oncology and supportive care clinics as well. A participant in the internet-based study perhaps put it best by saying, "Healthcare providers also need to be aware that homophobia and the closet are the biggest obstacles to LGBT healthcare. Many [LGBT patients] don't go because of homophobia they've experienced from doctors, or they don't get the proper care because they can't disclose that they're LGBT (which might figure into a diagnosis). A healthcare provider should be a safe space for everyone, because healthcare is so important to individual and community health."

Why is identity disclosure so critical to LGBT patients? The answer to this question is rooted in the concept of "patient centered care." An increasing body of research on patient centered care suggests that patients' assessment of the *quality* of their own healthcare is more predictive of health outcomes than provider ratings or blood work or scans [26]. Patients who are the most satisfied with their healthcare tend to stay healthier. In this model, how patients feel about medical decisions, as well as a perception of equitable treatment by providers, blends together to create the best possible health outcomes. The patient centered care model suggests that cancer survivors will have better health outcomes when they can bring their whole selves to treatment, rather than having to hide their sexual orientation and gender identity.

LGBT patients must repeatedly weigh the benefits of disclosure with the risks of coming out, as this is not a one-time activity. Cancer care involves dozens of health and social service providers, from oncologists to phlebotomists, MRI technicians, clerical staff, nurses and social workers. Patients will have to decide multiple times whether it feels safe to disclose themselves and their partners. Having a potentially life threatening illness, coupled with limited provider options, makes the stakes even higher, thereby dramatically increasing the vulnerability and cancer stress for most LGBT patients. As a result, in the internet-based study described above, some people who were out in the rest of their lives chose to stay in the closet during cancer treatment, leaving their partners completely out of the hospital and doctors' offices. In many cases, concern may be warranted. Some patients have reported homophobic or transphobic responses from their providers. If possible, when confronted with these responses, they changed doctors.

Most patients are treated in medical centers near their homes and many do not have a choice in their healthcare team, either because of limited/no insurance or because there is only one cancer treatment center within driving distance. Sometimes, the only option is a hospital or clinic with a reputation for discrimination against LGBT patients. Safety is not guaranteed and few facilities, either private or public, make a point of broadcasting their welcome to LGBT people. Perceived safety is a guiding light for many LGBT people, and in navigating cancer care, that light may be difficult to find.

As one survivor stated, "Although my doctor knew all about me, each encounter with new people—with blood draws, ultrasound, breast x-ray, etc.—had the basic anxiety of the procedure and layered on to that, the possibility of homophobia and having to watch out for myself."

Another wrote, "My partner did not come to the hospital because the only good hospital around was a Catholic hospital and I didn't want my treatment compromised by them finding out about my 'sinful lifestyle'. An anti-gay surgeon could easily 'accidentally' miss one of the many small lesions of the cancer or not take out an infected lymph node. An anti-gay nurse could take longer to give pain medicine. Being discovered as a lesbian in a Catholic hospital can be lethal when having cancer."

A transgender man added, "My oncologist, who, still, after almost 2 years of seeing him every 3 months, continues to refuse to understand what being transgender means. I have an incredibly difficult and uncomfortable relationship with this doctor and no way to get out of it. The lack of respect for me is unbelievable."

A positive story: "I was lucky and had a very positive experience. My partner was involved in every aspect of my care and wasn't treated any differently, nor was she excluded from any decisions or information that was given to me."

As these quotes highlight, the decision about whether or not to disclose identity to providers is primary for LGBT survivors. Disclosure can directly affect the care they receive and, equally importantly, their perception of that care. LGBT survivors need a cancer care environment that invites disclosure of identity and promotes acceptance of disclosures when they are offered.

Respect for Unique Social Support Systems

As stated earlier, support systems are a critical aspect of cancer treatment and can have a profound impact on recovery and health outcomes. While many cancer patients rely on their family for support, it is not uncommon for LGBT people to be alienated from their family of origin because of their gender identity and/or sexual orientation [27]. LGBT support teams may therefore differ from the mainstream and may be invisible to healthcare providers who do not know how to ask about or recognize the importance of key players. These supportive others, crucial for healing, may be inadvertently excluded from providing care or assisting with medical decision making. Rather than, or in addition to, family members, LGBT people may rely on their partner (who may be a legal stranger in the eyes of 39 states in the US), their ex-lovers, and their friends to provide support [28]. To underscore this point, in the internet-based survey, 77 % of the LGBT respondents reported that friends were a part of their personal and emotional support system during cancer diagnosis and treatment. This was higher than the percentage reporting that their partner (62 %) or their parents (40 %) and siblings (40 %) were part of their support system. By contrast, heterosexual and cisgender cancer patients are most likely to name a spouse as their primary source of personal and emotional support [29, 30].

Acknowledgement and welcome of these diverse care partners is a need, not only of the LGBT cancer survivor, but of the care partner. In general, care partners of cancer survivors tend to experience distress and burden, [30, 31] and this stress may be exacerbated by lack of acknowledgement by the cancer care team. Including diverse care partners in the sharing of clinical data and the making of medical decisions can improve outcomes for LGBT survivors and care partners alike. While no studies have specifically examined the needs of LGBT survivors' care partners, research on the LGBT community in macrocosm has shown that support is just as important to LGBT adults as it is to heterosexual and cisgender adults, if not more so [32]. Social policies that overtly refuse to acknowledge LGBT support systems and relationships have a negative impact on the health and wellbeing of LGBT persons [33]. These same trends are undoubtedly replicated, and perhaps magnified, in the microcosm of the cancer clinic.

As one survivor wrote, "My lover at the time and my ex bonded together to support me for over 2 years. My friends and community and doctors wrapped themselves around me." A gay man concurred: "My partner IS MY FAMILY and when they treat him as such my outcomes are much better. He is my advocate and can remember everything I can't. Good outcomes depend on his involvement as does my emotional well being." By contrast, a lesbian survivor added, "She (my partner) was generally welcomed but treated as a 'friend' not a 'spouse' and care-taker. She was never really offered emotional support by the treatment team as I noted other (straight) patient's partners and care-givers were. She was never offered access to caregiver's supports or resources."

A transgender survivor told us, "My support system, many of whom are trans and gender variant people, were made to feel very uncomfortable by my doctors and medical staff due to disregard for pronoun use, sideways glances, and overall awkward responses. My friends comprised my entire support system and were critical to my care. The reluctance to respectfully interact and, in some cases, communicate clearly with my friends was extraordinarily difficult for me and lead to much added stress. I already felt so alone without my family."

Acceptance, welcoming, and respect for these diverse care partners is a strong need of LGBT survivors. In addition, few services are tailored to the needs of diverse care partners. Same sex partners may feel excluded from support groups and other services that include primarily spouses of cancer survivors. Friends or ex-partners, similarly, may feel they do not belong in such settings. Couples services that target married heterosexual couples may not be able to address the needs of same-sex couples. There is a need for additional services for these diverse care partners.

Understanding of LGBT Sexuality

Cancer treatment, including surgery, radiation and chemotherapy, has an impact on both sexual functioning and interest. Unfortunately, healthcare providers have little training and often less comfort in addressing the sexual concerns of their patients [34]. Printed educational materials may be offered instead of frank discussion. Most of these booklets assume marriage and heterosexuality, though this trend is beginning to change and the word "partner" is being used more often in printed and online documents. LGBT sexuality is not identical to heterosexual sexuality, however. A simple change in partner pronoun fails to capture this complexity. Many LGBT people engage in sexual practices that may not be addressed in printed materials and may be beyond the scope of knowledge or comfort of oncology medical and social service providers. For example, prostate cancer treatment often compromises erectile functioning and healthcare providers may be competent in discussing the options for vaginal penetration post treatment [35]. But a gay survivor may not be able to find information about anal penetration, which requires a firmer erection, even if he is willing to be out to his provider and ask direct questions [36]. Similarly, the gay survivor who engages in receptive anal intercourse needs specific information about his options.

As a survivor told us, "I think we might be able to discuss more openly how sex and sensuality can be an important part of coping/healing/recovery processes. I thought this aspect was underplayed and even stigmatized in most environments, but to me it was one of the reasons I fought to survive." Another, however, said, "Luckily my radiologist could talk about how the treatment might affect my sex life and used terms and concepts that indicated an understanding of gay men's sexual behavior (for example he asked who was the top and who was the bottom etc)."

The need here is twofold. On the one hand, healthcare providers must be willing and able to discuss sexuality post-cancer without falling back on heterosexual assumptions. This will require first that providers feel comfortable discussing patients' and survivors' sex lives, and second, that they know their patients' sexual and gender identities. In addition, healthcare providers must possess information about LGBT sexuality that they can impart to patients and survivors. This will require more research, better guidelines, and diverse materials that can be offered to LGBT patients and survivors concerned about the sexual side effects of treatment.

Information About Cancer's Impact on Fertility and Families

Younger LGBT cancer patients are concerned, as most patients of childbearing age are, about the impact of treatment on their fertility. Reliable information about this topic is seldom conveyed to survivors of any sexuality. The information that is available, whether through printed materials, oncology social workers, or doctors, often assumes that childbearing will only be a concern for legally married, heterosexual patients. When they are out to their providers, it is often assumed that LGBT survivors will, therefore, not want fertility information, even though LGBT people often use alternative forms of insemination and surrogacy. A lesbian, for example, may want to freeze her eggs. One survivor said it clearly: "Please offer us fertility options."

Reduction of Gender Expectations in Cancer Care

Cancer care contains many unexamined gender expectations and these can be off-putting to LGBT people, especially for those who are gender nonconforming. This is seen most often in breast cancer treatment settings, where the expectation remains strong that a survivor will elect to have breast reconstruction after a mastectomy [37]. Many lesbians have had to repeatedly explain their decision to not do so, which can lead to additional stress in an already difficult time [38]. Some transgender men with breast cancer have used the disease as an opportunity to have gender-confirming surgeries, but may also confront questioning of their decision to have male, rather than female, chest reconstruction by their surgeons and care providers.

Also in the context of breast cancer, pink ribbons and pink paraphernalia may not be viewed as healing by lesbian, bisexual, and gender nonconforming patients, but as one more instance of forced femininity. It may leave such patients feeling that the structures that exist to support patients with breast cancer are not welcoming of their sexual and gender identities. For transgender men with breast cancer, this “pinking” is particularly painful and alienating.

The metaphor of cancer as a battle and the patient as a warrior may be viewed as unhelpful by many men, who may feel pressured to adopt masculine roles of stoicism and emotional guardedness as a result [39]. This metaphor may seem particularly off-putting to gay men, for whom traditionally masculine gender roles may feel irrelevant. Gay men who do seek to discuss their emotional concerns or ask for help dealing with psychological distress may have their needs dismissed due to the gender expectation that men “tough it out” and do not disclose vulnerability and “softer” emotions.

As one survivor told us: “I really resented assumptions about my priorities. There’s a hell of a lot of emphasis in the breast cancer awareness movement and in group oncology practices about helping women look stereotypically feminine. I personally have no interest in breast reconstruction, and it irked me that I was automatically referred to a plastic surgeon at the time of my mastectomy. It irked me that reconstruction was so pushed in the patient ed materials…” A trans survivor said: “Well, I had one positive thing happen to me because of my breast cancer experience. To wit, I was given a total, bilateral mastectomy with male chest reconstruction as a part of my treatment. This was definitely a silver lining and if you can avail your patient of something positive that can come from [this] situation, be sure to make every effort to do so. It meant the world to me.”

Gender expectations are deeply engrained in American society, and these societal expectations are perpetuated in cancer care. LGBT survivors have a need to feel welcomed and not to feel alienated by overt gendering of care; to the extent that gender expectations can be reduced in cancer clinics, LGBT survivors will feel both more accepted and more comfortable.

Needs Within Specific Cancer Types

The needs of breast and prostate cancer survivors have been perhaps better described than those of other cancer survivors in both heterosexual and LGBT populations [40]. While LGBT survivors of all types of cancer would benefit from the opportunity to disclose, support for care partners, sexuality information and reduced gender expectations, specific needs may emerge in the context of certain cancer types. Below, in the absence of research on diverse cancer diagnosis groups, we speculate on the form these needs might take.

Lung Cancer Rates of lung cancer are increasing among certain LGBT subgroups, particularly gay and bisexual men who are living with HIV [41, 42]. Unfortunately, the lack of data from large national databases, such as the SEER registry, restricts our ability to estimate prevalence rates for lung cancer among LGBT adults outside of the context of HIV. However, higher prevalence of lung cancer is likely due to high rates of tobacco use in the LGBT community, [43] as discussed earlier in this book. LGBT cancer survivors may also be more likely to continue smoking post-cancer diagnosis than their heterosexual counterparts [44]. There is a need for culturally competent tobacco cessation treatment tailored to LGBT persons and to LGBT cancer survivors in particular [45]. Such treatments may mobilize support networks to aid the cancer survivor in quitting smoking, [46] and may use the teachable moment of cancer diagnosis with an LGBT-centric framework to guide the intervention.

Lymphoma and Blood Cancers Lymphomas are often co-morbid with HIV, and so the experience of HIV in the LGBT community has directly influenced the experience of this cancer type [47, 48]. In the internet-based survey, one patient with lymphoma reported, "I have told everyone about my cancer that was diagnosed last year but I still haven't told anyone other than my husband about my HIV diagnosis from 7 years ago. I am almost grateful for the cancer to allow me to be at least a little more open and honest about my health without actually disclosing my HIV status." Another patient reported, "I now do presentations in regards to Cancer and HIV, since I have been living with HIV for over 27 years." Whether patients were open about their HIV status or not, living with HIV shaped their experience of cancer.

Support and Intervention for LGBT Cancer Survivors and Care Partners

Given the lack of research attention paid to LGBT survivors, it is not surprising that few interventions and support services have been designed to address the specific and additional needs of LGBT survivors [49]. The tacit assumption has been, and continues to be, that sexual orientation and gender identity do not play a role in treatment and supportive care for cancer. Many LGBT patients may also feel that their LGBT identity has little bearing on cancer care. As one patient from the online study put it, "I don't think being labeled as LGBT helped or hindered…we are all human beings first." Another said, "I don't feel as if I've been denigrated because I'm LGBT or even that it was an issue before, during, or after my diagnosis," and a third added, "The environment in which I received my care was extremely heteronormative. I never would have felt comfortable enough to be out at that time. Also, I was fighting for my life, so sexual orientation didn't seem so important at the time." Support groups typically operate under this assumption and use a one-size-fits-all model, thereby attempting to parse messages to a common denominator and introduce topics that will be of relevance to all survivors with a specific cancer type or stage on the cancer continuum, regardless of sexual and gender identity.

However, a growing body of knowledge indicates that LGBT identity does affect cancer care [50–53]. The majority of LGBT survivors echo this perspective, saying, for example, "As an alone, aging senior, I am also dealing with fear of rejection by being "out" even though I was very "out" when younger and in a partnership. There is a big part of the "cancer" experience that never gets shared with the care givers or service providers when you are not comfortable letting them know who you really are!" and "I can say I have had mixed experiences going through cancer as a lesbian, compared to my original diagnosis when straight." One participant stated, "My LGBT status… as someone who is not quite cis-gender and who is definitely without a doubt QUEER… doesn't really affect much in terms of my attitude and my experience," but then went on to add, "Another strange thing is that it is REALLY HARD to find information about getting very small implants or implants appropriate for a male appearing chest. So, in this regard, I guess that my LGBT status comes to play… because everything is centered on this society's "ideal" breast size." Even LGBT survivors who might initially perceive their identity as unimportant to their cancer care can think of ways in which the system of care was not responsive to their particular needs. Below, we offer reflections on the types of services that currently exist, and how they meet or do not meet the needs of LGBT survivors outlined above. We also provide recommendations for increasing support services for LGBT survivors at the clinic level.

Advantages and Disadvantages of Mainstream Support Groups and Services

Given the stress and psychological distress experienced and reported by LGBT cancer survivors, providers are likely to refer these survivors to support groups or other supportive services. Research suggests that support groups and services can positively impact quality of life and influence health outcomes in individuals with cancer [54]. However, services provided must be perceived as supportive by those who access them [55]. Given the lack of attention paid to LGBT-specific issues, LGBT survivors are likely to be referred to general groups of survivors. These groups and services are likely to be unresponsive to the six LGBT-specific needs discussed above, and may therefore be of limited use to LGBT survivors.

There is limited empirical data on the experience of LGBT cancer survivors seeking supportive services. One study of lesbian/bisexual breast cancer survivors found that they were more likely to have had histories of discrimination, but that they were also more likely to have attended a cancer support group or mental health counseling [56]. In the LGBT community more broadly, 99 % of therapy providers report seeing an LGBT client in their practice, [57] and gay men have been shown to be more likely than heterosexual men to seek care for psychological distress [58]. If LGBT individuals are seeking supportive services more often than their heterosexual counterparts, and if this tendency continues in the context of cancer care, are they able to find culturally competent service providers who also understand the needs of cancer survivors and who welcome them into treatment?

Extant research findings are inconsistent. In general, LGBT persons who have sought supportive services in the community do appear to benefit from these services [59, 60]. However, the current model of social support groups for cancer patients and survivors is not always welcoming to LGBT survivors. Lesbian, gay, bisexual, transgender and gender nonconforming survivors may find that they are the only member of the group with their specific identity and set of concerns, and most facilitators have not received LGBT cultural competence training [61]. For example, the language of "husbands" in breast cancer support groups and the talk about vaginal intercourse in prostate cancer support groups can be alienating to lesbian and gay survivors. Simply switching the gender of the partner is not the same as understanding the impact of cancer on LGBT relationships [62]. Similarly, the same-sex partner who seeks support may be the only man or woman in a care partner support group. Many transgender people have been actively excluded from support groups, like transgender men who are not welcome in a breast cancer group [63]. Even if accepted, being the only LGBT person in a group is isolating and defeats the purpose of healing through shared experiences. There is little chance for support and mutual sharing about the issues mentioned previously; heterosexual survivors may not be able to relate to the experience of disclosing a marginalized identity to providers and dealing with secrecy and discrimination, for example. As one lesbian breast cancer survivor put it, "I ended up going to a support group where I was the only queer woman. They were great people and my being out wasn't a problem, but I missed having that support. The local LGBT health org did not have an active support group at the time for queer women going through cancer treatment. Very unfortunate. Ironically, my partner had a support group to go to at this place, but I didn't." From another: "The support group I was offered was the one provided at the hospital. I was the only queer person in the room and while the leaders were very well-meaning, there were moments of alienation (I spoke up but still) especially when the topic of sex and cancer came up."

Advantages and Disadvantages of Targeted LGBT Support Groups and Services

As this discussion of limitations highlights, there is an overwhelming need for services that can specifically address the needs of LGBT cancer survivors. Targeted groups for LGBT cancer survivors were the most requested service by the survivors themselves in the internet-based study described above. There are very few such groups in the entire country. They require not only a skilled facilitator, but a critical mass of eligible and interested group members, all available on the same day/time and within driving distance. Outside of the largest urban areas, it can be difficult to find enough people to start a group. Survivors who are not out to their providers will not be offered referrals to LGBT groups and the treatment center may not be aware that they have sufficient numbers to start their own. To successfully form an LGBT support group requires collaboration between community groups and cancer facilities.

These limitations often mean that LGBT support group members will be at different points on the cancer continuum, a less-than-ideal situation according to literature on support group formation [54]. People who have been newly diagnosed have different needs than those who are post treatment or dealing with metastatic disease. Similarly, people with different cancer types might be grouped together in LGBT-specific services, and the needs of a colorectal cancer patient, for example, may be very different than those of a head and neck cancer patient. As one participant said, "I found discrimination in entering existing LGBT groups, both older members versus newer members (older members bonding among their past experiences) and regarding different types of cancers…" LGBT groups focused on particular cancer types would be ideal, as highlighted by this participant: "Having a gay male support group was the best thing that happened to me. I feel very lucky to be able to discuss both feelings and sensations without any inhibition at all in the company of other gay men who also had prostate cancer." However, such groups would suffer from extremely small participation rates in most areas in the US, assuming that LGBT survivors interested in forming such a group could find a suitable clinician.

Web-based/online LGBT support groups offer some advantages over the in-person format. First, in-person groups are becoming increasingly hard to fill across both heterosexual and LGBT cancer populations [64]. This shift is due in part to the large numbers of survivors who now keep their jobs during and after treatment, but then lack the time and energy to participate in an evening group. Online groups offer people the opportunity to get support while at home. Second, online groups permit geographically isolated individuals an opportunity to participate with other survivors. The third benefit of online support services is that they are accessible and welcoming for cancer survivors with physical, visual, hearing, cognitive or communication disabilities. Research confirms that a web-based support group can be useful in reducing depression and cancer-related trauma, as well as perceived stress, among women with primary breast carcinoma [65]. These online groups may still suffer from the problem of small numbers, as reported by one survivor: "Even online the LGBTQ support groups are hard to find and if found, there is never any activity in them. Reassurance or comfort in this arena has been impossible to find."

Other Tailored Support Services and Interventions

Though few services target LGBT survivors directly, many educational materials and interventions may be still applicable to them and address their questions about cancer treatment and outcomes. Shallow and deep tailoring approaches [66] could ensure that the message of these materials reaches and resonates with the LGBT population. Shallow tailoring could simply involve including pictures of same-sex couples and LGBT individuals, or testimonials from LGBT survivors, into materials aimed at providing general information about cancer. The LIVESTRONG brochure on "Coming Out with Cancer," for example, used similar information as was used in the LIVESTRONG brochure for heterosexual survivors; however, this information was interspersed with images and testimonials from LGBT survivors [2]. Once tailored, the information may need to use specialized outreach to access the LGBT survivors who could most benefit from the information.

Some interventions may need to undergo deep tailoring, however, before they will be applicable to LGBT survivors. For example, therapies aimed at addressing sexuality concerns for breast and prostate cancer survivors may need to account for the experiences of LGBT patients in this domain [36, 64, 67]. Supportive care for anal cancer among gay and bisexual men may need to address sexual side effects of this type of cancer, which may not be relevant for heterosexual survivors [68]. New interventions may be needed to address specific disparities noted in LGBT populations, such as disparities in rates of psychological distress and substance use.

Targeted and tailored support services could take many forms. In addition to LGBT-specific support groups and educational materials, peer networks could also assess and match on sexual orientation. These may take the form of "buddy" programs or patient navigators. These networks could be administered locally, through a cancer center or community organization, or they could exist virtually and match LGBT cancer survivors to one another nationwide. At present, networks such as the Colon Cancer Alliance (ccalliance.org) match newly diagnosed colorectal cancer patients with colorectal cancer survivors who can provide support and share their experiences of diagnosis and treatment. Survivors are matched on "stage of diagnosis, age, gender, and primary concerns." Cultural competence in LGBT colon cancer needs is not guaranteed. LGBT survivors, however, may feel most comfortable and most supported when talking to another LGBT survivor who shares their concerns and experiences. A participant echoed this recommendation by saying, "Without knowing other lesbians who had had breast cancer who helped me through the process, I am not sure how I would have fared."

Cultural Competence and LGBT Friendliness in the Oncology Clinic

Thus far, we have discussed ways in which ancillary services could be tailored to the needs of LGBT survivors. However, many aspects of the system of cancer care as a whole need to adapt in order to meet the most basic needs of LGBT survivors from the moment of first contact with the medical system. As a result of stigma, and of real and expected discrimination by medical institutions, many LGBT individuals avoid or delay receiving medical care [69]. Receiving a diagnosis of cancer renders coping by avoidance untenable, however, forcing LGBT cancer survivors to engage routinely and intimately with numerous medical providers. This may lead to anxiety, vigilance, and increased stress on the part of LGBT survivors [70].

LGBT patients enter the healthcare system wary and scan for signs of welcome or discrimination. It is the responsibility of the providers and treatment facilities to broadcast their welcome. Well before they are face to face with a medical professional, LGBT survivors have received multiple messages that indicate whether or not they will be accepted. For example, LGBT patients and caregivers often look for posted nondiscrimination signs that include mention of sexual orientation and gender identity. They notice the art on the walls, the printed materials in the waiting room, and they may look to see if there are images that reflect themselves. Is there a rainbow sticker or a Safe Space symbol? Is there a gender-neutral bathroom? Does the intake form offer options that reflect LGBT gender identities and relationship status?

To ameliorate the impact of stigma, LGBT survivors have a need to feel welcomed into cancer treatment settings. This need is shared by all cancer survivors, and by patients in general; however, for minority and underserved patient populations, gestures of welcome may need to be made overt and active. Studies have shown that up to 52% of African American patients have experienced discrimination in the context of seeking medical care, including allowing White patients to be seen before them, White patients being seen without an appointment, and condescending behavior by providers [71]. Latino/a patients, similarly, experienced discrimination including moving their children out of the patient room into the hall, limiting their family visits to one person at a time, and ignoring the needs of family members [72]. Further underscoring this point, In a large national survey of transgender people, a full 19% reported being refused healthcare, solely because of their transgender or gender nonconforming status. The numbers were even higher for transgender people of color [73].

Active welcoming of LGBT survivors may involve posting symbols, such as the Safe Space symbol, to indicate openly that the clinic and its providers support the LGBT community. It may also involve statements and gestures by providers and staff to indicate inclusiveness of LGBT patient perspectives. These gestures may include use of non-heterosexist, gender-inclusive language when dealing with patients, positive response to LGBT survivors' disclosures, and welcoming of LGBT survivors' care partners. As one participant said, "It would have gone much better if there was some indicated awareness that as a patient I had a sexual orientation that they cared to know about and that I could be assured of being accepted and treated with the same quality of care as anyone."

Visible advertisement of a clinic's welcoming stance toward LGBT survivors must go beyond the treatment facility itself. Collaboration and networking with LGBT community organizations can help to spread the word that a particular clinic or set of providers is non-discriminatory and LGBT affirming. Such networking may include advertisements in LGBT newspapers, presence at LGBT health fairs, or simply communicating with local LGBT community leaders. Advertisement of a welcoming environment can be underscored by introduction of a clinic non-discrimination policy that includes LGBT identity. Making this policy explicit to providers and staff will reinforce the importance of treating all patients with respect and dignity, regardless of sexual orientation and gender identity.

These outward signals of a clinic's openness must be paired with culturally competent care in order for the clinic environment to be truly welcoming. Training in cultural competence for LGBT specific issues is not currently part of most medical education, nor is LGBT-specific cultural competence emphasized in oncology practice [74, 75]. Perhaps most importantly, providers and all clerical staff must be trained to welcome disclosure and then respond in a culturally competent manner when a cancer survivor reveals an LGBT identity. Cultural competence also involves not making heterosexual or gendered assumptions that could prevent or force individuals to disclose. In the internet-based survey, 58 % of participants who had come out did so to correct a heterosexual or gendered assumption made by their provider. This underscores the importance of having a culturally competent and welcoming environment where LGBT patients are invited to disclose in safety.

To facilitate disclosure to cancer care providers, clinics might consider including items on their intake forms specifically assessing partnership and gender, broadly defined. Questions asking more specifically about sexual orientation and gender identity may need to be piloted, or run by a community advisory board that includes LGBT advisors, before being included in standard clinic paperwork. In the study described above, only 19 % of LGBT participants who had come out to their providers did so because an intake form specifically asked about identity.

Once survivors have disclosed their identity, continuing an open dialogue about sexuality, gender, and partnership issues with providers is critical [25]. Even in clinics where it is not feasible to include items assessing these issues on intake forms, providers can be trained and prepared to converse with patients about them, enhancing the aura of welcoming described above. In the internet-based study, 17 % of participants reported that they disclosed their identity because they were directly asked by a provider.

In the words of a participant in the internet-based study, "There are still doctors and others of different cultural and religious backgrounds that have negative feelings towards LGBT individuals. As a result, it is very difficult to openly discuss one's sexual orientation for fear of rejection and non-interest in one's health matters." By contrast, another participant stated, "We live in New York City—in a very gay neighborhood and my treatment was at a very 'gay hospital.' Being an out lesbian in a serious monogamous relationship was not particularly an issue nor was the presence of my partner in the hospital or during my treatment." The welcoming stance, or lack thereof, of the cancer care facility can thus have a pervasive effect on LGBT survivors' experience of care.

Interventions for Specific Issues Among LGBT Survivors

Much of what is known about the behavior change needs of LGBT cancer survivors is based on findings regarding behavior change in the LGBT population in general. Health and behavioral disparities that affect individuals within the LGBT community at large are likely to continue to affect LGBT cancer survivors [44, 76]. Behavior change interventions targeting LGBT survivors must acknowledge and work from these disparities, while also capitalizing on areas of community and individual resilience. Specific disparities in need of behavioral intervention include psychological distress, substance use, obesity, and physical activity.

Psychological Distress

As described above, rates of psychological distress are highly disparate among LGBT survivors. In the context of cancer and cancer care, the National Comprehensive Cancer Network (NCCN) defines distress as any unpleasant emotional, psychological, or social experience associated with cancer diagnosis or treatment [9]. Psychological distress can range from mild sadness and fear to significant mental health difficulties, such as diagnosable mood and anxiety disorders. Approximately one-third of all oncology patients will experience clinically diagnosable levels of psychological distress, [77] making this one of the most ubiquitous side effects of cancer treatment [78] and a primary target for intervention [79]. Psychological distress can persist for years after diagnosis and may have a profound impact on a cancer survivor's well-being and quality of life [80].

Studies have consistently shown that LGBT adults have 1.5 to 3.0 times higher rates of psychological distress than their heterosexual counterparts [58, 76, 81]. This high prevalence of distress, as discussed earlier in the book, is likely due to the impact of minority stress on LGBT persons. Chronic exposure to and expectation of discrimination and prejudice can lead to hypervigilance, chronic worry, negative attributions about the self, and eventually to diagnosable anxiety and depression among LGBT persons [76].

While data are limited regarding rates of psychological distress among LGBT cancer survivors, those data that do exist highlight significant disparities. Boehmer and colleagues demonstrated that lesbian and bisexual women with a cancer history experience significantly worse self-reported health than their heterosexual counterparts [53]. Similarly, Kamen and colleagues found that gay men who had been diagnosed with cancer reported a higher number of days of poor mental health per month than their heterosexual counterparts [44]. These studies used large datasets to estimate prevalence, but focused exclusively on lesbian/bisexual women and gay men, respectively, and were limited by the fact that national surveys do not specifically recruit LGBT cancer survivors and so have relatively small sample sizes [53]. However, these findings do highlight a general disparity in psychological distress and the need for interventions specifically targeting psychological distress in a range of LGBT individuals.

The NCCN recommendations state that all cancer patients should be screened for distress during their initial visit, and in future visits as clinically indicated [9]. Knowing that a survivor is LGBT may emphasize the importance of screening for psychological distress, and may add measurably to the process of screening. NCCN recommendations also state that screening processes should assess the level and nature of a survivor's distress. Understanding the psychosocial factors that may influence distress, including minority stress and LGBT identity issues, are therefore an important part of this screening process.

Substance Use

The minority stress model, as discussed earlier also provides a sociological basis for understanding increased rates of substance use in the LGBT community. LGBT adults are on average two times more likely to report use of tobacco, alcohol, and other substances than their heterosexual counterparts [60, 81]. As with psychological distress, this increased prevalence in the community at large likely plays out among cancer survivors in specific.

Tobacco Use Tobacco use among cancer survivors is a major public health concern. Rates of lifetime and of continued use are highest among lung [82] and head and neck [83] cancer patients. Given the strong link between smoking and both of the aforementioned types of cancer, continued tobacco use post-cancer diagnosis gives rise to concerns about problematic clinical course, poor treatment response, and cancer recurrence [84]. Tobacco has also been linked to increased risk, and risk of recurrence, of many other types of cancers [85].

Given this risk, and the increased prevalence of tobacco use in the LGBT community, there is a need for targeted interventions to reduce tobacco use among LGBT survivors. Such interventions could engage directly with the LGBT community to emphasize the importance of tobacco use cessation, particularly for LGBT survivors [43]. Interventions could be nested as a component of a tobacco cessation media campaign aimed directly at the LGBT community, again highlighting the impact of smoking on cancer incidence and recurrence [46]. Interventions and media about these interventions should be designed with input from LGBT survivors, who can speak directly to what worked, what did not work, and what might work better in encouraging LGBT community members affected by cancer to stop smoking. Training of cancer care providers and LGBT community leaders should also involve emphasizing the importance of tobacco cessation and provide culturally competent approaches to screening and referral for cessation services.

Alcohol Use Alcohol use has been linked with increased risk of several kinds of cancer, including head and neck, stomach, colorectal, and liver cancers [86]. As with tobacco use, continued excessive use of alcohol post-cancer diagnosis has been linked with risk of cancer recurrence, poor clinical outcome, and comorbidity [87].

While behavioral interventions have been developed to reduce alcohol consumption among LGBT subgroups in the context of HIV and sexual risk behavior, [88] no interventions have yet been developed to address this issue among LGBT cancer survivors. There is a need for interventions that can address psychosocial factors increasing risk for continued alcohol use in those who have undergone cancer treatment, with a specific focus on alcohol abuse and dependence. Tailored interventions for LGBT cancer survivors would likely address the role of the bar in the gay community, [89] social network and peer influences that perpetuate alcohol use, and the impact of minority stress on substance use [90].

Other Substance Use While rates of other substance use disorders are also consistently higher among LGBT persons than their heterosexual peers, even fewer studies have been conducted on behavior change interventions to address these disparities than on interventions to address smoking and alcohol use. Nearly all of the interventions have been conducted in the context of sexual risk behavior and HIV [91]. It is unclear how use of substances other than tobacco and alcohol might be linked to development, exacerbation, and recurrence of cancer; how existing interventions could be tailored to LGBT cancer survivors; and hence, what the needs are of LGBT cancer survivors who have a comorbid substance use disorder. Further research on these topics is needed. At present, assessing for substance use in screening procedures and keeping LGBT-friendly substance use referrals on hand are recommended.

Obesity, Physical Activity, and Energy Balance

Physical inactivity, obesity, and associated metabolic issues are major cancer risk factors for all people. Breast; cervical; ovarian; colon and rectal; endometrial; esophageal; thyroid; gallbladder; kidney; and pancreatic cancers are all directly linked to obesity [92]. Obese and overweight cancer patients tend to respond poorly to surgical, radiation, and chemotherapy treatment, and have higher risk of cancer recurrence and mortality post-diagnosis and treatment than patients and survivors who are of normal weight [93]. The cancer-related risk associated with overweight and obesity is estimated to approach that associated with tobacco use [94].

Rates of obesity and engagement in physical activity vary across subgroups of the LGBT community. In general, studies have shown that lesbian and bisexual women have higher rates of obesity and lower rates of physical activity than heterosexual women, [95] while gay and bisexual men tend to have lower rates of obesity and higher rates of physical activity than heterosexual men [96]. Data on trans persons are lacking [97]. Other studies have indicated that while gay men report greater concern about their body image than heterosexual men, these concerns do not necessarily translate into higher rates of engagement in physical activity [98]. Very few studies have examined how these rates in the LGBT community as a whole may apply to LGBT cancer survivors. The teachable moment of cancer may inspire LGBT survivors to engage in physical activity at rates equivalent to heterosexual counterparts; however, additional research is needed to firmly establish prevalence of obesity and physical activity in this population.

In terms of behavior change needs for LGBT survivors related to physical activity, existing exercise interventions for cancer survivors have not been targeted or tailored to the LGBT community. In particular, exercise interventions that have included care partners have typically included only heterosexual marital partners or family members [29]. As highlighted above, LGBT cancer survivors may have non-marital, non-familial support systems that may feel alienated from these interventions. Designing exercise programs that include a range of care partners could address this need.

The experiences of lesbian cancer survivors in the internet-based qualitative study highlighted the difficulties experienced by sexual minority women who are also obese: "I went to UCSF for radiation and got treated but there was an attitude I did not like. I think it had to do with my size, I am fat…more than being a lesbian. This did not bother me that much at the time I was focused on getting well. Later on it bothers me some." Tailored messages about risk of recurrence associated with obesity in lesbian and bisexual women could encourage sexual minority women to increase their physical activity, lose weight, and improve their health post-cancer diagnosis.

Body Image Concerns While only tangentially related to obesity and physical activity, body image concerns are another major issue at play in the health and psychosocial needs of LGBT cancer survivors. Gay and bisexual male survivors, in particular, may feel that their value as a sexual partner has diminished as a result of the physical changes brought on by cancer. Lesbian women have complex reactions to mastectomy and other physical changes, as highlighted by quotes from the internet-based survey. Some women said, e.g., "As a lesbian I have a good body image. The decision to have a mastectomy was easy," while another said, "It was hard to come to terms with my sexuality…as a newly realized femme queer after a bilateral mastectomy in the already judgmental queer/lesbian community." A tailored and culturally competent exercise intervention could begin to address some of these concerns by incorporating body esteem messages with physical exercises designed to address some of the physical and body image related side effects of cancer and its treatment.

Recommendations and Future Directions

Based on the literature reviewed above and the experiences shared by LGBT survivors, we close by reiterating five recommendations:

1. **Ensure cultural competence in all staff**: Providers, clerical staff and healthcare management should take steps to become educated about the stigma-related stress many LGBT people carry into treatment, as well as strategies to reduce such stress, including means for inviting LGBT patients/clients to come out to their providers and welcoming their care partners. In addition, providers need to be educated in how to speak about sex and sexuality to LGBT patients and how to ask about their social support groups.
2. **Protect the needs of LGBT staff**: Culturally competent behavior should be extended beyond staff members' interactions with patients to include safe treatment for LGBT staff. Leadership of the healthcare institutions and offices must

actively convey that LGBT-welcoming behavior is a core expectation of all workers and cultivate protection for LGBT workers.

3. **Collect referral lists for LGBT-welcoming providers, including local mental health providers**: Understanding that many culturally competent services are offered outside of the oncology clinic, it is important to develop a referral list of providers and services that are LGBT welcoming.
4. **Broadcast LGBT welcome through collaborations with community based organizations and media**: After setting up this foundation, healthcare institutions and offices need to broadcast their LGBT-welcoming policies and training to potential and current patients. This is best accomplished both within and outside of the facility.
5. **Review and revise social support programs**: To ensure LGBT welcome and usefulness, social support programs need to be reviewed using the six additional challenges for LGBT cancer survivors outlined earlier as a framework.

In addition to these clinical and policy recommendations, we also recommend additional research on the needs of LGBT cancer survivors. Such research could begin with an examination of the issues: symptoms LGBT survivors find most troubling, services they lack, behavior change needs, and the needs of care partners. Once these needs have been delineated and described, research must move into development, testing, and dissemination of interventions. Merely highlighting the issues is not sufficient; the field must also begin to address disparities and gaps in service for LGBT survivors and their care partners, thereby improving the health and well-being of this underserved and underrepresented population.

References

1. Gates G. How many people are lesbian, gay, bisexual, and transgender? Los Angeles: The Williams Institute, UCLA School of Law; 2011.
2. LIVESTRONG Foundation. Coming out with cancer. Austin: LIVESTRONG Foundation; 2010.
3. Mariotto AB, Rowland JH, Yabroff KR, et al. Long-term survivors of childhood cancers in the United States. Cancer Epidemiol Biomarkers Prev. 2009;18(4):1033–40.
4. Howlader N, Ries LA, Mariotto AB, Reichman ME, Ruhl J, Cronin KA. Improved estimates of cancer-specific survival rates from population-based data. J Natl Cancer Inst. 2010;102(20):1584–98.
5. Boehmer U. Twenty years of public health research: inclusion of lesbian, gay, bisexual, and transgender populations. Am J Public Health. 2002;92(7):1125–30.
6. Sell RL, Becker JB. Sexual orientation data collection and progress toward healthy people 2010. Am J Public Health. 2001;91(6):876–82.
7. Margolies L, Scout NFN. LGBT patient-centered outcomes: cancer survivors teach us how to improve care for all: national LGBT cancer network; April 2013.
8. Kamen C, Margolies L, Smith-Stoner M, et al. Correlates and outcomes of Lesbian, Gay, Bisexual, and Transgender (LGBT) identity disclosure to cancer care providers. Multinational Association of Supportive Care in Cancer. Miami, FL; 2014.
9. Holland JC, Bultz BD, National comprehensive Cancer N. The NCCN guideline for distress management: a case for making distress the sixth vital sign. J Natl Compr Cancer Netw. 2007;5(1):3–7.

10. Jepson C, McCorkle R, Adler D, Nuamah I, Lusk E. Effects of home care on caregivers' psychosocial status. Image J Nurs Sch. 1999;31(2):115–20.
11. Parle M, Jones B, Maguire P. Maladaptive coping and affective disorders among cancer patients. Psychol Med. 1996;26(4):735–44.
12. Sheard T, Maguire P. The effect of psychological interventions on anxiety and depression in cancer patients: results of two meta-analyses. Br J Cancer. 1999;80(11):1770–80.
13. Lerman C, Kash K, Stefanek M. Younger women at increased risk for breast cancer: perceived risk, psychological well-being, and surveillance behavior. J Natl Cancer Inst Monogr. 1994(16):171–6.
14. Buchmueller T, Carpenter CS. Disparities in health insurance coverage, access, and outcomes for individuals in same-sex versus different-sex relationships, 2000–2007. Am J Public Health. 2010;100(3):489–95.
15. Herek GM. Hate crimes and stigma-related experiences among sexual minority adults in the United States: prevalence estimates from a national probability sample. J Interpers Violence. 2009;24(1):54–74.
16. Ryan C, Russell ST, Huebner D, Diaz R, Sanchez J. Family acceptance in adolescence and the health of LGBT young adults. J Child Adolesc Psychiatr Nurs. 2010;23(4):205–13.
17. Ganz PA, Desmond KA, Leedham B, Rowland JH, Meyerowitz BE, Belin TR. Quality of life in long-term, disease-free survivors of breast cancer: a follow-up study. J Natl Cancer Inst. 2002;94(1):39–49.
18. Kornblith AB, Herndon JE, 2nd, Zuckerman E, et al. Social support as a buffer to the psychological impact of stressful life events in women with breast cancer. Cancer. 2001;91(2):443–54.
19. Kornblith AB, Ligibel J. Psychosocial and sexual functioning of survivors of breast cancer. Semin Oncol. 2003;30(6):799–813.
20. Low CA, Stanton AL, Thompson N, Kwan L, Ganz PA. Contextual life stress and coping strategies as predictors of adjustment to breast cancer survivorship. Ann Behav Med. 2006;32(3):235–44.
21. Mehnert A, Koch U. Psychological comorbidity and health-related quality of life and its association with awareness, utilization, and need for psychosocial support in a cancer register-based sample of long-term breast cancer survivors. J Psychosom Res. 2008;64(4):383–91.
22. Baider L, Andritsch E, Uziely B, et al. Effects of age on coping and psychological distress in women diagnosed with breast cancer: review of literature and analysis of two different geographical settings. Crit Rev Oncol Hematol. 2003;46(1):5–16.
23. Boehmer U, Freund KM, Linde R. Support providers of sexual minority women with breast cancer: who they are and how they impact the breast cancer experience. J Psychosom Res. 2005;59(5):307–14.
24. Boehmer U, Linde R, Freund KM. Sexual minority women's coping and psychological adjustment after a diagnosis of breast cancer. J Women's Health. 2005;14(3):214–24.
25. Durso LE, Meyer IH. Patterns and predictors of disclosure of sexual orientation to healthcare providers among lesbians, gay men, and bisexuals. Sex Res Social Policy. 2013;10(1):35–42.
26. Stewart M, Brown JB, Donner A, et al. The impact of patient-centered care on outcomes. J Fam Pract. 2000;49(9):796–804.
27. Savin-Williams RC. Verbal and physical abuse as stressors in the lives of lesbian, gay male, and bisexual youths: associations with school problems, running away, substance abuse, prostitution, and suicide. J Consult Clin Psychol. 1994;62(2):261–9.
28. Grossman AH, Daugelli AR, Hershberger SL. Social support networks of lesbian, gay, and bisexual adults 60 years of age and older. J Gerontol. 2000;55(3):171–9.
29. Badger T, Segrin C, Dorros SM, Meek P, Lopez AM. Depression and anxiety in women with breast cancer and their partners. Nurs Res. 2007;56(1):44–53.
30. Northouse L, Williams AL, Given B, McCorkle R Psychosocial care for family caregivers of patients with cancer. J Clin Oncol. 2012;30(11):1227–34.
31. Given BA, Given CW, Sherwood PR. Family and caregiver needs over the course of the cancer trajectory. J Support Oncol. 2012;10(2):57–64.

32. Kamen C, Burns M, Beach SR. Minority stress in same-sex male relationships: when does it impact relationship satisfaction? J Homosex. 2011;58(10):1372–90.
33. Hatzenbuehler ML, Keyes KM, Hasin DS. State-level policies and psychiatric morbidity in lesbian, gay, and bisexual populations. Am J Public Health. 2009;99(12):2275–81.
34. Ida DJ. Cultural competency and recovery within diverse populations. Psychiatric Rehabilitation J. Summer 2007;31(1):49–53.
35. Knight SJ, Latini DM. Sexual side effects and prostate cancer treatment decisions: patient information needs and preferences. Cancer J. 2009;15(1):41–4.
36. Blank TO. Gay men and prostate cancer: invisible diversity. J Clin Oncol. 2005;23(12):2593–96.
37. Al-Ghazal SK, Sully L, Fallowfield L, Blamey RW. The psychological impact of immediate rather than delayed breast reconstruction. Eur J Surg Oncol. 2000;26(1):17–9.
38. Boehmer U, Linde R, Freund KM. Breast reconstruction following mastectomy for breast cancer: the decisions of sexual minority women. Plast Reconstr Surg. 2007;119(2):464–72.
39. Hoyt MA, Stanton AL, Irwin MR, Thomas KS. Cancer-related masculine threat, emotional approach coping, and physical functioning following treatment for prostate cancer. Health Psychol. 2013;32(1):66–74.
40. Davies NJ, Kinman G, Thomas RJ, Bailey T. Information satisfaction in breast and prostate cancer patients: implications for quality of life. Psychooncology. 2008;17(10):1048–52.
41. Palacios R, Pascual J, Cabrera E, Lebrón JM, Guerrero-León MA, del Arco A, Santos J. Lung cancer in HIV-infected patients. Int J STD & AIDS. 2013. 0956462413499317.
42. Hou W, Fu J, Ge Y, Du J, Hua S. Incidence and risk of lung cancer in HIV-infected patients. J Cancer Res Clin Oncol. 2013;139(11):1781–94.
43. Matthews AK, Li CC, Kuhns LM, Tasker TB, Cesario JA. Results from a community-based smoking cessation treatment program for LGBT smokers. J Environ Public Health. 2013;2013:984508.
44. Kamen C, Palesh O, Gerry A, et al. Disparities in health risk behavior and psychological distress among gay versus heterosexual cancer survivors. (In submission).
45. Eliason MJ, Dibble SL, Gordon R, Soliz GB. The last drag: an evaluation of an LGBT-specific smoking intervention. J Homosex. 2012;59(6):864–78.
46. Johns MM, Pingel ES, Youatt EJ, Soler JH, McClelland SI, Bauermeister JA. LGBT community, social network characteristics, and smoking behaviors in young sexual minority women. Am J Commun Psychol. 2013;52(1–2):141–54.
47. Holly EA, Lele C Non-Hodgkin's lymphoma in HIV-positive and HIV-negative homosexual men in the San Francisco Bay Area: allergies, prior medication use, and sexual practices. J Acquir Immune Defic Syndr Hum Retrovirol. 1997;15(3):211–22.
48. Gopal S, Patel MR, Yanik EL, et al. Association of early HIV viremia with mortality after HIV-associated lymphoma. AIDS. 2013;27(15):2365–73.
49. Jabson JM, Blosnich JR. Representation of lesbian, gay, and bisexual people in clinical cancer trials. Ann Epidemiol. 2012;22(11):821–3.
50. Katz A. Gay and lesbian patients with cancer. Oncol Nurs Forum. 2009;36(2):203–7.
51. Boehmer U, Glickman M, Milton J, Winter M. Health-related quality of life in breast cancer survivors of different sexual orientations. Qual Life Res. 2012;21(2):225–36.
52. Boehmer U, Cooley TP, Clark MA. Cancer and men who have sex with men: a systematic review. Lancet Oncol. 2012;13(12):e545–e53.
53. Boehmer U, Miao X, Ozonoff A Cancer survivorship and sexual orientation. Cancer. 2011;117(16):3796–804.
54. Carmack Taylor CL, Kulik J, Badr H, et al. A social comparison theory analysis of group composition and efficacy of cancer support group programs. Soc Sci Med. 2007;65(2):262–73.
55. Ussher JM, Kirsten L, Butow P, Sandoval M. A qualitative analysis of reasons for leaving, or not attending, a cancer support group. Soc Work Health Care. 2008;47(1):14–29.
56. Boehmer U, Glickman M, Winter M, Clark MA. Lesbian and bisexual women's adjustment after a breast cancer diagnosis. J Am Psychiatr Nurses Assoc. 2013;19(5):280–92.

57. Garnets L, Hancock KA, Cochran SD, Goodchilds J, Peplau LA. Issues in psychotherapy with lesbians and gay men. A survey of psychologists. Am Psychol. 1991;46(9):964–72.
58. Cochran SD, Mays VM, Sullivan JG. Prevalence of mental disorders, psychological distress, and mental health services use among lesbian, gay, and bisexual adults in the United States. J Consult Clin Psychol. 2003;71(1):53–61.
59. Willging CE, Salvador M, Kano M. Brief reports: unequal treatment: mental health care for sexual and gender minority groups in a rural state. Psychiatr Serv. 2006;57(6):867–70.
60. Berg MB, Mimiaga MJ, Safren SA. Mental health concerns of gay and bisexual men seeking mental health services. J Homosex. 2008;54(3):293–306.
61. Price M, Butow P, Kirsten L. Support and training needs of cancer support group leaders: a review. Psychooncology. 2006;15(8):651–63.
62. Margolies L Families of choice; Sources of support for LGBT cancer survivors. LIVESTRONG Foundation Blog: LIVESTRONG Foundation; 2013.
63. Corliss HL, Belzer M, Forbes C, Wilson EC. An evaluation of service utilization among male to female transgender youth: qualitative study of a clinic-based sample. J LGBT Health Res. 2007;3(2):49–61.
64. Thomas C, Wootten A, Robinson P. The experiences of gay and bisexual men diagnosed with prostate cancer: results from an online focus group. Eur J Cancer Care. 2013;22(4):522–9.
65. Winzelberg AJ, Classen C, Alpers GW, et al. Evaluation of an internet support group for women with primary breast cancer. Cancer. 2003;97(5):1164–73.
66. Resnicow K, Baranowski T, Ahluwalia JS, Braithwaite RL. Cultural sensitivity in public health: defined and demystified. Ethn Dis. Winter 1999;9(1):10–21.
67. Chambers SK, Ferguson M, Gardiner RA, Aitken J, Occhipinti S. Intervening to improve psychological outcomes for men with prostate cancer. Psychooncology. 2013;22(5):1025–34.
68. Palefsky J. Human papillomavirus and anal neoplasia. Curr HIV/AIDS Rep. 2008;5(2):78–85.
69. Brotman S, Ryan B, Cormier R. The health and social service needs of gay and lesbian elders and their families in Canada. Gerontologist. 2003;43(2):192–202.
70. Institute of Medicine. The health of lesbian, gay, bisexual, and transgender people: building a foundation for better understanding. Washington, DC; 2011.
71. Rankin KM, David RJ, Collins JW Jr. African American women's exposure to interpersonal racial discrimination in public settings and preterm birth: the effect of coping behaviors. Ethn Dis. Summer 2011;21(3):370–6.
72. Davies B, Larson J, Contro N, Cabrera AP. Perceptions of discrimination among Mexican American families of seriously ill children. J Palliat Med. 2011;14(1):71–6.
73. Grant JM, Mottet LA, Tanis J. National transgender discrimination survey: report on health and health care. Washington, DC: National Center for Transgender Equality; October 2010.
74. McNair R. Outing lesbian health in medical education. Women Health. 2003;37(4):89–103.
75. Gonser PA. Culturally competent care for members of sexual minorities. J Cult Divers. 2000 Fall;7(3):72–5.
76. Meyer IH. Prejudice, social stress, and mental health in lesbian, gay, and bisexual populations: conceptual issues and research evidence. Psychol Bull. 2003;129(5):674–97.
77. Stanton AL. Psychosocial concerns and interventions for cancer survivors. J Clin Oncol. 2006;24(32):5132–37.
78. Deimling GT, Bowman KF, Sterns S, Wagner LJ, Kahana B. Cancer-related health worries and psychological distress among older adult, long-term cancer survivors. Psychooncology. 2006;15(4):306–20.
79. Hamer M, Chida Y, Molloy GJ. Psychological distress and cancer mortality. J Psychosom Res. 2009;66(3):255–8.
80. Schwartz CL. Long-term survivors of childhood cancer: the late effects of therapy. Oncologist. 1999;4(1):45–54.
81. Cochran SD, Mays VM. Burden of psychiatric morbidity among lesbian, gay, and bisexual individuals in the California quality of life survey. J Abnorm Psychology. 2009;118(3):647–58.

82. Hecht SS. Tobacco smoke carcinogens and lung cancer. J Natl Cancer Inst. 1999;91(14):1194–210.
83. Marron M, Boffetta P, Zhang ZF, et al. Cessation of alcohol drinking, tobacco smoking and the reversal of head and neck cancer risk. Int J Epidemiol. 2010;39(1):182–96.
84. Ostroff JS, Jacobsen PB, Moadel AB, et al. Prevalence and predictors of continued tobacco use after treatment of patients with head and neck cancer. Cancer. 1995;75(2):569–76.
85. Talamini R, Bosetti C, La Vecchia C, et al. Combined effect of tobacco and alcohol on laryngeal cancer risk: a case-control study. Cancer Causes Control. 2002;13(10):957–64.
86. Bagnardi V, Blangiardo M, Vecchia C L, Corrao G. A meta-analysis of alcohol drinking and cancer risk. Br J Cancer. 2001;85(11):1700–5.
87. Kwan ML, Kushi LH, Weltzien E, et al. Alcohol consumption and breast cancer recurrence and survival among women with early-stage breast cancer: the life after cancer epidemiology study. J Clin Oncol. 2010;28(29):4410–6.
88. Wong FL, Rotheram-Borus MJ, Lightfoot M, et al. Effects of behavioral intervention on substance use among people living with HIV: the healthy living project randomized controlled study. Addiction. 2008;103(7):1206–14.
89. Jones-Webb R, Smolenski D, Brady S, Wilkerson M, Rosser BR. Drinking settings, alcohol consumption, and sexual risk behavior among gay men. Addict Behav. 2013;38(3):1824–30.
90. Lindley LL, Walsemann KM, Carter JW Jr. The association of sexual orientation measures with young adults' health-related outcomes. Am J Public Health. 2012;102(6):1177–85.
91. Mimiaga MJ, Reisner SL, Vanderwarker R, et al. Polysubstance use and HIV/STD risk behavior among Massachusetts men who have sex with men accessing Department of Public Health mobile van services: implications for intervention development. AIDS Patient Care STDS. 2008;22(9):745–51.
92. Renehan AG, Tyson M, Egger M, Heller RF, Zwahlen M Body-mass index and incidence of cancer: a systematic review and meta-analysis of prospective observational studies. Lancet. 2008;371(9612):569–78.
93. Litton JK, Gonzalez-Angulo AM, Warneke CL, et al. Relationship between obesity and pathologic response to neoadjuvant chemotherapy among women with operable breast cancer. J Clin Oncol. 2008;26(25):4072–77.
94. Calle EE, Thun MJ. Obesity and cancer. Oncogene. 2004;23(38):6365–78.
95. Fogel S, Young L, Dietrich M, Blakemore D. Weight loss and related behavior changes among lesbians. J Homosex. 2012;59(5):689–702.
96. Conron KJ, Mimiaga MJ, Landers SJ. A population-based study of sexual orientation identity and gender differences in adult health. Am J Public Health. 2010;100(10):1953–60.
97. Fredriksen-Goldsen KI, Cook-Daniels L, Kim HJ, et al. Physical and mental health of transgender older adults: an at-risk and underserved population. Gerontologist. 2014;54(3):488–500.
98. Kaminski PL, Chapman BP, Haynes SD, Own L. Body image, eating behaviors, and attitudes toward exercise among gay and straight men. Eat Behav. 2005;6(3):179–87.

Chapter 14
Challenges and Recommended Solutions to End of Life Care for Lesbian, Gay, Bisexual and Transgender Patients Diagnosed with Cancer with a Life-Limiting Prognosis

Ronit Elk

Abstract There is a sizeable LGBT population for whom end of life care services are required. However, over and above the tremendous challenges that most people face at end of life, there are several significant additional obstacles that LGBT patients at end of life encounter, barriers that often prevent them from receiving appropriate end of life care.

There remains a paucity of research that focuses specifically on understanding the needs, preferences, and perspectives of LGBT patients with life-limiting cancers or other terminal illnesses at end of life, and how their preferences and those of their partners and families of choice influence their end of life care decisions. This gap in turn limits our ability to design evidence-based LGBT-focused palliative care and end of life programs. Lack of sensitivity to, or respect for, cultural and social differences may compromise end of life care for LGBT patients and yet care is provided within a healthcare system where staff are often uncomfortable with, or even discriminate against, LGBT patients, their life partners, and families of choice. Despite significant recent legal changes in terms of visitation of a loved one in the hospital and acting as a proxy when an LGBT patient is no longer able to, legal and enforcement barriers remain; while heterosexual, married couples have the right to make medical decisions for a partner who is incapacitated, this is not automatically a right for LGBT couples.

Implications for future research, program development and policy development and enforcement are discussed.

R. Elk (✉)
College of Nursing, University of South Carolina, Columbia, SC, USA
e-mail: ELK@mailbox.sc.edu

U. Boehmer, R. Elk (eds.), *Cancer and the LGBT Community*,
DOI 10.1007/978-3-319-15057-4_14

Need for End of Life Care for LGBT Elders Diagnosed with Cancer

The risk of developing cancer increases with age, with about 77% of all cancers diagnosed in people aged 55 and older [1]. Although the exact number of the gay elderly population is not known, the National Gay and Lesbian Task Force Policy Institute estimates that 1.4–3.8 million US Americans over 65 are LGBT based on a range of 5−10% of the US population. They project that this population will expand and reach between 3.6 and 7.2 million by 2030 [2].

The risk of life-threatening illness, including cancer, among lesbians, gay men and transsexuals is unfortunately high. The risks of smoking and alcohol abuse are higher among LGBT people [3–11], which in turn are associated with higher risk of some cancers [12–14]. Lesbians also have a higher lifetime risk of breast, cervical, uterine and ovarian cancer than heterosexual women [15, 16]. Gay men have a much higher risk of anal cancer [17] as well as HIV-related cancers [18–24]. There is a greater risk of HIV, breast and prostate cancer for male to female transgender people [14, 25, 26], and of ovarian, breast and cervical cancer for female to male transgender people [26].

There are factors that contribute to poorer prognosis and outcome in patients with cancer; for example, if the cancer is detected at a later stage, obesity (excess body weight contributing to one out of five cancer-related deaths) [27], or low socioeconomic background [28], are all factors that may contribute to poorer prognosis in lesbian women. Although their overall risk doesn't differ from heterosexual women, women in same-sex relationships have three times greater age-adjusted risk of dying from breast cancer [29]. For a more detailed discussion of these factors please see Fredriksen-Goldsen et al. (Chap. 4).

Recent studies have found that almost 75% of lesbian and gay seniors live alone, which places them at increased risk of isolation [30, 31], often translating into not having a caregiver. While adult children and other family members are frequently the caregivers for elders facing an illness that has a poor prognosis, studies have found [32] that lesbian and gay seniors are less likely to have children to care for them at times of illness. While it is well recognized that lesbian and gay elders more often rely on friends and informal caregivers, "families of choice", than birth families as do their heterosexual peers [33], the sizeable increase in LGBT people who are aging and nearing the end of life will place considerable strain on these families of choice.

Based on the projected numbers of LGBT seniors, the significant number of LGBT people being diagnosed with advanced cancers, as well as those who may not have immediate family to care for them as they age, it is clear that there is a sizeable LGBT population for whom end of life care services are required.

Receiving a Diagnosis with a Life-Limiting Prognosis

Receiving a diagnosis with a life-limiting prognosis is one of life's most arduous trials. People often experience physical suffering, psychological anguish and spiritual distress, resulting in strain on both the patient and caregivers [34, 35]. There are many challenges that the patient and his/her loved ones have to face including deliberating treatment options, choosing the appropriate treatment facilities to receive care in, deciding where to spend one's last days, making legal choices such as writing wills, and determining who will make treatment choices when one is no longer able to do so [36]. Relationships with family, friends, and spiritual communities may shift, and communication with the healthcare team becomes central to the care received [37]. However, over and above the tremendous challenges that most people face at end of life, there are several significant additional obstacles that LGBT elders at end of life encounter, barriers that often prevent them from receiving appropriate end of life care.

End of life Care Takes into Consideration the Patient's Life Context

> I ask people to look inside themselves, and I ask them, 'do you love somebody? If you do, can you imagine being denied access to them at the end of life, when love is most needed?'[1]
> C.M.

The most common kinds of care provided to those at end of life are palliative care (provided to patients with serious illnesses, including, but not limited to, at end of life) and hospice care (provided to patients at the end of life.) The goals of both palliative and hospice care are to prevent and alleviate suffering, and enhance the patient's quality of life by closely attending to the patient's physical, psychological, social and spiritual needs. Care is provided by a team of professionals including a doctor, nurse, social worker, chaplain, occupational therapist and a wide range of complementary therapists, and includes attention to the patient's medical needs as well as the patient and the family's psychological, psychosocial, legal, and spiritual needs. Most importantly, care is patient-and-family/caregiver focused, and tailored to the specific patient and family's unique wishes. Usually a patient is referred to the palliative care team by their treating physician, and palliative care is provided in tandem with the ongoing medical care the patient is receiving. Delivery of palliative care has been shown to reduce symptoms, alleviate suffering, improve the coordination of care, enhance doctor-patient communication, and result in the patient's and family's satisfaction with the care provided [34, 38–52].

In providing end of life care, consideration of the patient's culture and life context is essential; both culture and life context strongly influence the patient and their loved ones' response to the diagnosis and illness, the discussion and decisions the patient and loved one have about treatment preferences, and their deliberations and choices about the end of life care, including information and health communication methods that they prefer [53–55]. Lack of sensitivity to, and lack of respect for cultural and social differences may compromise end of life care for racial/ethnic

---

[1] Quotes from C.M. are from an interview of the author with Chris MacLellan [Name used with permission] who cared for his life partner, Richard Schiffer, throughout his illness and death. For full information on their story go to: *http://interactive.sun-sentinel.com/lgbt-dying-couple/index.html*.

minority [56] and sexual minority patients. Most of the early studies of patients at end of life in the US focused on white patients, but in recent years there have been a wide range of studies focusing on the attitudes, values, beliefs and access to end of life care of racial and ethnic minorities [56–66], confirming that there are in fact differences in beliefs and perspectives between divergent groups. Studies have found that race, religion, ethnicity, gender, age, and culture strongly influence (a) end of life-sustaining measures [67–74], (b) end of life care preferences [75], (c) type of information patients would like to receive [76, 77], and (d) preferred health communication methods [78, 79]. It is therefore logical that sexual and gender identity are also important factors in determining needs and preferences of patients.

Paucity of Research on LGBT Elders' End of life Care Needs and Preferences

In order to deliver person-centered palliative care to LGBT patients, an in-depth understanding of the unique needs of LGBT patients with life-limiting illness, as well as their perspectives and care preferences, is essential. However, there remains a paucity of research that focuses specifically on understanding the needs, preferences, and perspectives of LGBT individuals at end of life, and how their preferences and those of their partners influence their end of life care decisions [80–83]. Other than the literature focusing on those with HIV and AIDS, there have only been a handful of studies focusing on (a) the experiences of LGBT people at end of life (e.g. [82, 84–92]) and a few focusing on (b) their anticipated future plans [88, 93, 94].

Harding et al. [80] conducted a systematic review, of the existing literature focusing on the needs, preferences, views, and experiences of LGBT people on end of life care, and were only able to find 12 studies. The majority of the studies focused on lesbian women or gay men, only a few included bisexual individuals, and none examined the needs or preferences of transgender individuals. A few common themes emerged: (a) *Partners in Healthcare Decision-Making:* In two studies of cancer patients, lesbians with cancer [95] and lesbians and gay men with cancer [84] said they wanted to have their partners included in decision making and treatment planning. However, after making this request to their provider, many patients experienced a lack of sensitivity and/or support by their provider in honoring their request. (b) *Providers, Palliative Care and Physician Assisted Suicide:* In one of the few studies that assessed preferences at end of life in a community sample [96], several findings emerged: (I) A large proportion of lesbians and gay men wanted their health care provider to know of their wishes if they became incapacitated. However, the majority had not discussed this with their provider. (ii) The majority preferred a focus on pain relief even if it shortened their life, rather than on efforts to extend life. (iii) More than two-thirds of the sample supported physician assisted suicide (PAS), a significantly higher proportion than the acceptance of PAS by heterosexuals. (c) *Views of Hospice Care:* In a study of lesbian and heterosexual women [83], both groups reported positive views of hospice care, with lesbians holding more positive views. Significantly more heterosexual women preferred life-sustaining efforts than lesbians. The authors concluded that lesbians might not be as hesitant to engage with end of life care services as previously thought. (d) *Spirituality:* Only one study [97], of lesbians with cancer, examined the role of spirituality in LGBT patients at end of life. They reported that women found spiritual support as a way to cope with cancer. (e) *Advance Care Planning:* (I) Although there was a high rate of knowledge about living wills and health care proxies among lesbians, less than half had completed either one of these. [96]. (ii) In a study of lesbians and gay men who were providing care to their same-sex partners [93], the majority had advance directives, primarily to protect the caregiver from family members who did not approve of the relationship. Despite these legal protections, most participants remained concerned that their wishes would not be respected. (iii) In a study of heterosexual and lesbian and bisexual women [88], lesbians and bisexual women were found to have adopted long-term care legal planning strategies (e.g., naming a health care proxy) as well as either executing a will, naming a health care proxy, purchasing long term care insurance or discussing living arrangements with family members. A further study by this group [94] examined the effect of social support on the likelihood of advance care planning, and found that lesbian women whose support person was their partner were seven times more likely to have named a health care proxy than heterosexual women without a partner.

The paucity of research on understanding the needs, preferences, and perspectives of LGBT people at end of life, and how their preferences and those of their partners influence their end of life care decisions, currently limits our ability to design evidence-based LGBT-focused palliative care and end of life programs for patients whose cancer prognosis is poor.

Health Care within a System that May Not Understand LGBT Patients

> When he was admitted into the ER the doctors didn't acknowledge me; when I said 'I might be able to give you more of the full story', they said, 'And who are you?' I identified myself as his partner and caregiver. A straight couple wouldn't have had to do that. C.M.

End of life care usually takes place within healthcare systems such as hospitals, nursing homes, and hospices. There is often a significant lack of cultural sensitivity or training for taking care of LGBT patients among health care professionals [95, 98–101]. Professionals often feel uncomfortable, unprepared or untrained to take care of their LGBT clients. In a recent paper [102], the authors, both of whom are social workers, wrote about being caught "off guard" about a gay or lesbian patient at the end of life, and when discovering they were not heterosexual, being ill-equipped to provide adequate care due to lack of sufficient training. Healthcare providers may also be completely unaware that their patient may be LGBT [82, 92, 103], and not recognize or acknowledge their patient's partner, nor engage the partner in decision-making, a major omission during end of life, when family members, or in the case of many LGBT patients, families of choice [104], are integral to the process, often serving as the primary caregivers. Family members or family of choice members become key participants in the healthcare-patient-family team that works together to help the patient's journey be one that aligns with the values and beliefs of the patient and his/her loved ones. Lack of understanding about, or lack of acknowledgement and recognition of the ones closest to the LGBT patient can result in a significant and preventable increase in stress and anxiety in both the patient and loved ones. In certain parts of the country, especially where same-sex marriage is still illegal and strongly stigmatized, LGBT people may be treated with disdain. This carries through to the healthcare system. There is documented evidence that some healthcare providers have strong biases against sexual and gender minorities that prevent them from providing quality care to their LGBT patients [105], and that some discriminate against their patients who are not heterosexual [85, 99, 103, 106, 107].

Fear of such discrimination often results in caution or even dread in coming out to healthcare providers, and further distances LGBT elders from seeking medical care. In a study of lesbian women with cancer [95], patients felt their care was being compromised because of heterosexist bias that prevented them from revealing their sexuality. All 24 patients perceived their medical establishment as hostile towards them. In the same study, although the majority of patients wanted their partners to be part of their treatment decision-making and treated as spousal equivalents, partners were often ignored by the health care providers and excluded from treatment planning. In a later study of lesbian and bisexual women with breast cancer [86], the majority disclosed their sexual orientation, as they felt safe in doing so; however, the physician's neutral reaction was perceived as negative. In a study of older LGBT people [108] almost a quarter reported that they often do not disclose their sexuality, as they have little or no confidence that healthcare professionals will treat them with dignity and respect in their later years. In another study, researchers [96] found that over a third of older respondents did not disclose their sexual orientation to their providers due to their serious concern about a negative response or even poor treatment as a result of provider bias. In a more recent study of gay and lesbian patients over 60 by the same group of researchers [101], this finding was once again confirmed. Over half the respondents were afraid of coming out to their health care providers on whose care they were dependent, and they expressed fear of being mistreated by a healthcare professional who was prejudiced or homophobic. A recent study of older lesbians [92] found that more than one-tenth did not reveal their orientation to any of their providers and more than 10 % reported perceived discrimination in a healthcare setting. Whether due to actual or perceived discrimination, or due to fears of discrimination based on prior experiences or observing discrimination or bad treatment of others by health care providers, homophobia and heterosexism remain significant barriers in lack of communication with health care providers [82].

One of the most haunting and painful aspects of end of life among the LGBT community is the suffering from "disenfranchised grief" [92, 99, 103]. This term was coined in 1989 and is defined as grief that is experienced when "individuals incur a loss that is not or cannot be openly acknowledged, publicly mourned or socially supported" [109]. When an LGBT person loses a life partner and is unable to share it with others or is not accorded the same societal and community acknowledgement and support provided to those who lose a heterosexual spouse, the partner feels disenfranchised and risk of suffering such grief is high, although not universal [99]. At times, the bereaved partner may have to simultaneously deal with death of a partner and coming out at the same time. If the family of the loved one who has passed is not supportive of the relationship, the remaining partner may be left out of funeral and future arrangements. In instances where the family is supportive but the church and broader community are not, the family too may experience disenfranchised grief.

Recent Programmatic Developments

Within the last few years several training programs (e.g., "No Need to Fear, No Need to Hide" created by SAGE [110]) have been developed for healthcare professionals, and have been demonstrated to be effective in enhancing understanding of LGBT patients. Similar programs in other countries [111] have proved equally successful. Although extremely significant, these programs do not focus on the unique needs and challenges that arise *during end of life* care. To the best of our knowledge, to date, there has been a lack of any specific attention to programs that provide LGBT-friendly end of life or palliative care [82].

Legal Protection and Barriers That Impact End of Life Care for LGBT Couples

> Our green folder [with the health care proxy and the power of attorney] went everywhere with us; it was our lifeline. I was always worried about an emergency where we'd have to interact with medical care staff who didn't know about us, so our green folder went everywhere with us. C.M.

Since 2010, three major legal changes have taken place that have the possibility of substantially improving end of life care for LGBT couples in a same-sex marriage. The end of life care implications of each are described below.

1. *Presidential Memorandum 20511 of 2010* Prior to this mandate, partners of LGBT patients who were unconscious or not coherent could have been prevented by the hospital from (a) visiting their partners in hospitals, or (b) acting as health care surrogates for partners who were incapacitated, including at end of life [98]. This changed this on April 15th, 2010 when President Obama signed a landmark Presidential Memorandum regarding (a) hospital visitations and (b) health decision-making for same-sex partners. (a) *Hospital Visitations*:

The President directed the Department of Health and Human Services (HHS) to address these issues and in response, the Centers for Medicare and Medicaid (CMS), an HHS agency, amended its rules. Hospitals that accept Medicaid and Medicare must respect patients' Advance Directives and are also prohibited from denying visitation privileges based on, inter alia, sexual orientation. This means that in all states and in all hospitals that accept Medicaid and Medicare, the LGBT patient has the legal right for his/her loved one to visit in the hospital. The Department of Health and Human Services has released a guidance letter to ensure that hospitals that participate in Medicaid and Medicare programs have established written policies to implement these regulations. The letter also clarifies that visitations rights be granted without requiring documentation of those relationships in the majority of cases, and in the few circumstances in which documentation is required, the hospital cannot ask for documentation from LGBT couples other than what they would ask of heterosexual couples. This major change came about in the wake of the nationally known case of Janice Langbehn who was denied the right to visit her partner, Lisa Pond, who suddenly collapsed while the family was on vacation in Florida. President Obama presented Ms. Langbehn the Presidential Citizens Medal for her fight for hospital visitation rights for same-sex couples. Unfortunately, despite this change in federal law, there are documented cases in which partners have been denied the right to visit their partner, or even forcibly removed from the loved one's bedside, even after sharing their documentation, proving that they have the legal right to be at their loved one's bedside.

(b) *Acting as Health Care Surrogates* An advance directive is a document by which a person records how they wish to be treated should they become too ill or unable to make health care decisions themselves. Often this includes a living will or last will and testament as well as a health care proxy (or Durable Power of Attorney for Health Care) that indicates who will make healthcare decisions if the person becomes too ill or incapacitated. Unlike in visitation of LGBT partners where federal law governs, in the case of an advance care directive, state law governs. If an LGBT patient has not executed an advance directive granting rights to their same-sex partner, state health care surrogacy laws take over; the state selects a legal guardian based on a hierarchy of relatives, starting with a spouse, then adult children, parents, then other biological family members. This means that a biological family member can take over decision-making such as whether or not to continue treatment or decide whether or not to remove a loved one from a ventilator or other healthcare decisions so critical to end of life care, and they can do so regardless of the wishes of the same-sex spouse. Whether this can happen or not is determined by the state's legal perspective towards same-sex marriage. (I) If the state permits same-sex unions, the same-sex s If the state prohibits same-sex unions pouse becomes the patient's health care surrogate. This is the best-case scenario, but even here some hospitals don't follow the law, and don't allow same-sex partners to make health care decisions, even if the partners have a legal advance care document. (ii) If the state prohibits same-sex unions, the partner of the dying patient cannot become a health care surrogate *unless* the patient has a legal advance directive and has appointed his same-sex spouse as a health care proxy. It is therefore extremely important that same-sex couples execute an advance directive and appoint one another as health care surrogates, especially in states where same-sex marriage is prohibited.

2. *Repeal of DOMA* In a turning point decision in June 2013, the US Supreme Court struck down the discriminatory Defense of Marriage Act (DOMA), affirming that all couples who are married deserve equal legal respect and treatment from the federal government. As affirming as this ruling is for same-sex couples, it does not change any of the discriminatory state laws that exclude same-sex couples from state-conferred marriage rights, an aspect that has direct implications for the end of life care of a partner of an LGBT person. For example, receipt of a same-sex spouse's Medicare benefits (health benefits provided to someone over the age of 65) is only possible if she/he is married under the law of the state where he/she is living at the time of filing for benefits.
3. *The Affordable Care Act (ACA)* also has a nondiscrimination provision, Section 1557, which includes sex-based protection on the basis of gender identity and sex stereotypes. Although the scope of Section 1557's protection for same-sex couples is less clear, many courts are considering this to include nondiscrimination against same-sex couples. Therefore if a hospital discriminates against same-sex couples, this Section of the ACA can be used in court for the Department of Health and Human Services to investigate the hospital. Fighting a hospital in court for discrimination (e.g., for illegally removing a same-sex partner from the patient's bedside) is challenging in normal circumstances, but when one's partner is so ill, close to death or has passed away, it often becomes too overwhelming to pursue.

The expansion of Medicaid, as well as Medicare/Medicaid dual eligibility (for those who are both elderly and low income or disabled), has the potential to greatly improve the care of LGBT elders who are of low socioeconomic status (who are also likely to be minority women) [98]. However, since the implementation of the Affordable Care Act (ACA) is governed by state laws, only LGBT individuals who live in states where there is Medicaid expansion can benefit from this.

However, even with these significant improvements, legal barriers remain for those LGBT couples living in states where marriage is not considered legal. While heterosexual couples have the right to make medical decisions for a partner who is incapacitated, this is not automatically a right for LGBT couples [112–115].

Implications for Research, Practice, and Policy

The paucity of research on understanding the needs, preferences, and perspectives of LGBT people at end of life currently limits our ability to design evidence-based LGBT-focused palliative care and end of life programs for all patients including those with cancer. Large-scale research is a priority [80]. It is only through this process that we can gather the information needed to design evidence-based programs tailored to the unique needs of the LGBT community.

In order to provide patient-centered palliative and end of life care and services to LGBT patients and their families, it is essential that the physical, psychological, social, cultural, and spiritual needs of these patients are recognized, understood, and to the fullest extent possible, met. This includes: (a) *Recognition and Acceptance of Sexual Orientation* and identity and all that it entails [80, 92]. This means that the partner must be recognized and involved in the care and decision-making process, and all care must be delivered in an environment that is nonjudgmental and understanding [80, 101]. In a recent article on vulnerable populations in healthcare, Waisel [116] wrote that too often the care and treatment of an 'unfamiliar' patient is impeded because physicians are unfamiliar with or suspicious of patients they are not familiar with. He called on all physicians whom he claimed "have a collective obligation to improve healthcare for vulnerable populations" (p. 191).

Results of large-scale research studies will provide the evidence needed to design such evidence-based programs. (b) *Training of Health Care Staff:* Training of all staff involved, from management to the allied health professional, is essential [80]. Such training needs to include such aspects as understanding of LGBT needs, as well as a recognition of the provider's personal bias [103], and removal of heterosexual assumptions [99]. Equally important is understanding and enforcing the legal rights of patients within that county and state, as well as federal rights. Training programs that enhance LGBT cultural proficiency among elder care staff have been developed. These include, for example, "No Need to Fear, No Need to Hide", created by Services and Advocacy for Gay, Lesbian, Bisexual and Transgender Elders [117] and the Brookdale Center on Aging in New York [110], as well as " Project Visibility", created by the Boulder Country, Colorado Aging Services [118], and "Opening Doors", created by Age Concern England in London [119]. These important programs have been demonstrated to be effective in enhancing understanding of LGBT patients. Similar programs in other countries [111] have proved equally successful. A broader implementation of such programs across healthcare settings will enhance the cultural competency of healthcare staff.

Significant legal changes have been implemented in the last few years that have the potential to greatly improve end of life care for LGBT patients and their loved ones. However, even with these significant improvements, legal barriers remain for those LGBT couples living in states where marriage is not considered legal, most especially not having the automatic right to make medical decisions for a partner who is incapacitated. Expansion of decision-making capabilities for same-sex partners is a right which will continue to be fought for in the courts. Legal changes need to be enforced by the appropriate governing bodies. Organizations such as the Joint Commission, that accredits and certifies more than 20,000 health care organizations and programs in the US, could further enhance stronger enforcement of LGBT-inclusive cultural competency requirements in its accrediting process, and not provide accreditation to hospitals that have discriminated against LGBT patients (as they have done). Further inclusion of some of the proposals included in the field guide [120], and making LGBT cultural competency an integral and specific part of accreditation, rather than optional, and holding facilities to a higher standard in which all patients are served equally [115], should be the goals. Two recent national training programs for hospitals and healthcare settings, one by the Joint Commission [120], the other by the Human Rights Campaign [121], are training and certification processes (HEI) by which hospitals who wish to demonstrate optimal care for LGBT patients can receive training and certification to ensure that they meet legal, CMS, and Joint Commission requirements for LGBT patient-centered care. A report released in 2013 indicates which organizations have participated in training, and which are recognized as "Leaders in Healthcare Equality." Finally, such agencies must take action to enforce visitation and proxy rights, to ensure that hospital personnel are trained in all legal matters that pertain to LGBT patients, and provide care to all patients without discrimination.

References

1. American Cancer Society. Cancer facts & figures 2014. Atlanta, GA; 2014.
2. Grant JM. Outing age 2010. Washington, DC: National Gay and Lesbian Task Force Policy Institute; 2009.
3. Burgard SA, Cochran SD, Mays VM. Alcohol and tobacco use patterns among heterosexually and homosexually experienced California women. Drug Alcohol Depend. 2005;77(1):61–70.
4. Gruskin EP, et al. Patterns of cigarette smoking and alcohol use among lesbians and bisexual women enrolled in a Large Health Maintenance Organization. Am J Public Health. 2001;91(6):976–9.
5. Heffernan K. The nature and predictors of substance use among lesbians. Addict Behav. 1998;23(4):517–28.
6. McCabe SE, et al. Sexual orientation, substance use behaviors and substance dependence in the United States. Addiction. 2009;104(8):1333–45.
7. Ryan CM, Huggins J, Beatty R. Substance use disorders and the risk of HIV infection in gay men. J Stud Alcohol. 1999;60(1):70–7.
8. Ryan H, et al. *Smoking among lesbians, gays, and bisexuals: a review of the literature*. Am J Prev Med. 2001;21(2):142–9.
9. Stall RD, et al. Cigarette smoking among gay and bisexual men. Am J Public Health. 1999;89(12):1875–8.
10. Tang H, et al. Cigarette smoking among lesbians, gays, and bisexuals: how serious a problem? (United States). Cancer Causes Control. 2004;15(8):797–803.
11. Valanis BG, et al. Sexual orientation and health: comparisons in the women's health initiative sample. Arch Fam Med. 2000;9(9):843–53.
12. Hughes C, Evans A. Health needs of women who have sex with women. BMJ (Clinical Research Ed.). 2003;327(7421):939–40.
13. Mayer KH, et al. Sexual and gender minority health: what we know and what needs to be done. Am J Public Health. 2008;98(6):989–95.
14. O'Hanlan KA. Health policy considerations for our sexual minority patients. Obstet Gynecol. 2006;107(3):709–14.
15. Brown JP, Tracy JK. Lesbians and cancer: an overlooked health disparity. Cancer Causes Control. 2008;19(10):1009–20.
16. Dibble SL, Roberts SA, Nussey B. Comparing breast cancer risk between lesbians and their heterosexual sisters. Women's Health Issues. 2004;14(2):60–8.
17. Anderson JS, Vajdic C, Grulich AE. Is screening for anal cancer warranted in homosexual men? Sex Health. 2004;1(3):137–40.

18. Biggar RJ, Rosenberg PS, Coté T. Kaposi's sarcoma and non-Hodgkin's lymphoma following the diagnosis of AIDS. Multistate AIDS/Cancer match study group. Int J Cancer. 1996;68(6):754–8.
19. D'Souza G, et al. Incidence and epidemiology of anal cancer in the multicenter AIDS cohort study. J Acquir Immune Defic Syndr (1999). 2008;48(4):491–9.
20. Jacobson LP, Armenian HK. An integrated approach to the epidemiology of Kaposi's sarcoma. Curr Opin Oncol. 1995;7(5):450–5.
21. Katz MH, et al. Temporal trends of opportunistic infections and malignancies in homosexual men with AIDS. J Infect Dis. 1994;170(1):198–202.
22. Palefsky JM, et al. Prevalence and risk factors for human papillomavirus infection of the anal canal in human immunodeficiency virus (HIV)-positive and HIV-negative homosexual men. J Infect Dis. 1998;177(2):361–7.
23. Palefsky JM, Shiboski S, Moss A. Risk factors for anal human papillomavirus infection and anal cytologic abnormalities in HIV-positive and HIV-negative homosexual men. J Acquir Immune Defic Syndr. 1994;7(6):599–606.
24. van der Snoek EM, et al. Human papillomavirus infection in men who have sex with men participating in a dutch gay-cohort study. Sex Transm Dis. 2003;30(7):639–44.
25. Clements-Nolle K, et al. HIV prevalence, risk behaviors, health care use, and mental health status of transgender persons: implications for public health intervention. Am J Public Health. 2001;91(6):915–21.
26. Feldman JL, Goldberg JM. Transgender primary medical care. Int J Transgend. 2007;9(3–4): 3–34.
27. American Cancer Society. Does body weight affect cancer risk? American Cancer Society.
28. Simon S. American Cancer Society report: breast cancer death rates decline, but more slowly among poor. 3 Oct 2011.
29. Cochran SD, Mays VM. Risk of breast cancer mortality among women cohabiting with same sex partners: findings from the national health interview survey, 1997–2003. J Women's Health (15409996). 2012;21(5):528–33.
30. Adelman M, et al. Openhouse: community building and research in the LGBT aging population, in lesbian, gay, bisexual, and transgender aging: research and clinical perspectives. In: Kimmel D, Rose T, David S, editors. New York: Columbia University Press; 2006. pp. 247–64.
31. Rosenfeld D. Identity work among lesbian and gay elderly. J Aging Stud. 1999;13(2):121.
32. de Vries B. Aspects of life and death, grief and loss in lesbian, gay, bisexual, and transgender communities. In: Doka K, Tucci AS, editors. Living with grief: diversity and end-of-life care. Washington, DC: Hospice Foundation of America; 2009. pp. 243–57.
33. Project, L.M.A. and SAGE. Improving the lives of LGBT older adults. New York: Authors; 2010.
34. Morrison RS, et al. Palliative care consultation teams cut hospital costs for medicaid beneficiaries. Health Aff. 2011;30(3):454–63.
35. Kamal AH, et al. Palliative care needs of patients with cancer living in the community. J Oncol Pract. 2011;7(6):382–8.
36. Silveira MJ, et al. Patients' knowledge of options at the end of life. JAMA. 2000;284(19):2483.
37. Steinhauser KE, et al. Factors considered important at the end of life by patients, family, physicians, and other care providers. JAMA. 2000;284(19):2476.
38. Lagman R, et al. Acute inpatient palliative medicine in a cancer center: clinical problems and medical interventions—a prospective study. Am J Hosp Palliat Med. 2007;24(1):20–8.
39. Bakitas M, et al. The project ENABLE II randomized controlled trial to improve palliative care for rural patients with advanced cancer: baseline findings, methodological challenges, and solutions. Palliat Support Care. 2009;7(1):75–86.
40. Bakitas M, et al. Effects of a palliative care intervention on clinical outcomes in patients with advanced cancer: the project ENABLE II randomized controlled trial. JAMA. 2009;302(7):741–9.
41. O'Hara RE, et al. Impact on caregiver burden of a patient-focused palliative care intervention for patients with advanced cancer. Palliat Support Care. 2010;8(4):395–404.

42. Manfredi PL, et al. Palliative care consultations: how do they impact the care of hospitalized patients? J Pain Symptom Manage. 2000;20(3):166–73.
43. Morrison RS, Meier DE. The National Palliative Care Research Center and the Center to Advance Palliative Care: a partnership to improve care for persons with serious illness and their families. J Pediatr Hematol Oncol. 2011. 33(Suppl 2):S126–S131.
44. Penrod JD, et al. Hospital-based palliative care consultation: effects on hospital cost. J Palliat Med. 2010;13(8):973–9.
45. Higginson IJ, et al. Do hospital-based palliative teams improve care for patients or families at the end of life? J Pain Symptom Manage. 2002;23(2):96–106.
46. Higginson IJ, et al. Is there evidence that palliative care teams alter end-of-life experiences of patients and their caregivers? J Pain Symptom Manage. 2003;25(2):150–68.
47. Bailey FA, et al. Improving processes of hospital care during the last hours of life. Arch Intern Med. 2005;165(15):1722–7.
48. Bascom PB. A hospital-based comfort care team: consultation for seriously ill and dying patients. Am J Hosp Palliat Care. 1997;14(2):57–60.
49. Abrahm JL, et al. The impact of a hospice consultation team on the care of veterans with advanced cancer. J Pain Symptom Manage. 1996;12(1):23–31.
50. Kuin A, et al. Palliative care consultation in The Netherlands: a nationwide evaluation study. J Pain Symptom Manage. 2004;27(1):53–60.
51. Morrison RS, et al. Cost savings associated with US hospital palliative care consultation programs. Arch Intern Med. 2008;168(16):1783–90.
52. Casarett D, et al. Do palliative consultations improve patient outcomes? J Am Geriatr Soc. 2008;56(4):593–9.
53. Ersek M, et al. Multicultural considerations in the use of advance directives. Oncol Nurs Forum. 1998;25(10):1683–90.
54. Kagawa-Singer M, Blackhall LJ. Negotiating cross-cultural issues at the end of life: "You got to go where he lives". JAMA. 2001;286(23):2993–3001.
55. Searight HR, Gafford J. Cultural diversity at the end of life: issues and guidelines for family physicians. Am Fam Physician. 2005;71(3):515–22.
56. Krakauer EL, Crenner C, Fox K. Barriers to optimum end-of-life care for minority patients. J Am Geriatr Soc. 2002;50(1):182–90.
57. Adams CE, Horn K, Bader J. Hispanic access to hospice services in a predominantly Hispanic community. Am J Hosp Palliat Med. 2006;23(1):9–16.
58. Blackhall LJ, et al. Ethnicity and attitudes towards life sustaining technology. Soc Sci Med. 1999;48(12):1779–89.
59. Bonham VL. Race, ethnicity, and pain treatment: striving to understand the causes and solutions to the disparities in pain treatment. J Law Med Ethics. 2001;29(1):52–68.
60. Born W, et al. Knowledge, attitudes, and beliefs about end-of-life care among inner-city African Americans and Latinos. J Palliat Med. 2004;7(2):247–56.
61. Bullock K. Promoting advance directives among African Americans: a faith-based model. J Palliat Med. 2006;9(1):183–95.
62. Francoeur RB, et al. Palliative care in the inner city. Cancer (0008543X). 2007;109(2):425–34.
63. Johnson KS, Kuchibhatla M, Tulsky JA. What explains racial differences in the use of advance directives and attitudes toward hospice care? J Am Geriatr Soc. 2008;56(10):1953–8.
64. Kwak J, Haley WE. Current research findings on end-of-life decision making among racially or ethnically diverse groups. Gerontologist. 2005;45(5):634–41.
65. Reese DJ, et al. Hospice access and use by African Americans: addressing cultural and institutional barriers through participatory action research. Soc Work. 1999;44(6):549–59.
66. Barker JC. Lesbian aging: an agenda for social research. In: Herdt G, de Vries B, editors. Gay and lesbian aging: research and future directions. New York: Springer; 2004. pp. 29–72.
67. Johnson KS, et al. Racial differences in hospice revocation to pursue aggressive care. Arch Intern Med. 2008;168(2):218–24.
68. Kwak J, Haley WE. Current research findings on end-of-life decision making among racially or ethnically diverse groups. Gerontologist. 2005;45(5):634–41.

69. True G, et al. Treatment preferences and advance care planning at end of life: the role of ethnicity and spiritual coping in cancer patients. Ann Behav Med. 2005;30(2):174–9.
70. Johnson KS, Elbert-Avila KI, Tulsky JA. The influence of spiritual beliefs and practices on the treatment preferences of African Americans: a review of the literature. J Am Geriatr Soc. 2005;53(4):711–9.
71. Shrank WH, et al. Focus group findings about the influence of culture on communication preferences in end-of-life care. J Gen Intern Med. 2005;20(8):703–9.
72. Torke AM, et al. Medical care at the end of life: views of African American patients in an urban hospital. J Palliat Med. 2005;8(3):593–602.
73. Braun UK, et al. Voices of African American, Caucasian, and Hispanic surrogates on the burdens of end-of-life decision making. J Gen Intern Med. 2008;23(3):267–74.
74. Mazanec PM, Daly BJ, Townsend A. Hospice utilization and end-of-life care decision making of African Americans. Am J Hosp Palliat Med. 2010;27(8):560–6.
75. Blendon RJ, Szalay US. Should physicians aid their patients in dying? JAMA. 1992;267 (19):2658.
76. Searight HR, Gafford J. Cultural diversity at the end of life: issues and guidelines for family physicians. Am Fam Physician. 2005;71(3):515–22.
77. Shrank WH, et al. Focus group findings about the influence of culture on communication preferences in end-of-life care. J Gen Intern Med. 2005;20(8):703–9.
78. Jenkins C, et al. End-of-life care and African Americans: voices from the community. J Palliat Med. 2005;8(3):585–92.
79. Zapka JG, et al. Care at the end of life: focus on communication and race. J Aging Health. 2006;18(6):791–813.
80. Harding R, Epiphaniou E, Chidgey-Clark J. Needs, experiences, and preferences of sexual minorities for end-of-life care and palliative care: a systematic review. J Palliat Med. 2012;15(5):602–11.
81. Cartwright C. Ethical challenges in end-of-life care for GLBTI individuals. J Bioeth Inq. 2012;9(1):113–4.
82. Cartwright C, Hughes M, Lienert T. End-of-life care for gay, lesbian, bisexual and transgender people. Cult Health Sex. 2012;14(5):537–48.
83. June A, et al. Views of hospice and palliative care among younger and older sexually diverse women. Am J Hosp Palliat Med. 2012;29(6):455–61.
84. Katz A. Gay and lesbian patients with cancer. Oncol Nurs Forum. 2009;36(2):203–7.
85. Price E. Coming out to care: gay and lesbian carers' experiences of dementia services. Health Soc Care Community. 2010;18(2):160–8.
86. Boehmer U, Case P. Physicians don't ask, sometimes patients tell: disclosure of sexual orientation among women with breast carcinoma. Cancer. 2004;101(8):1882–9.
87. Boehmer U, Linde R, Freund KM. Sexual minority women's coping and psychological adjustment after a diagnosis of breast cancer. J Women's Health (15409996). 2005;14(3):214–24.
88. Clark MA, et al. Planning for future care needs: experiences of unmarried heterosexual and sexual minority women. Women Health. 2010;50(7):599–617.
89. Fobair P, et al. Comparison of lesbian and heterosexual women's response to newly diagnosed breast cancer. Psychooncology. 2001;10(1):40–51.
90. Curtis JR, et al. The quality of patient-doctor communication about end-of-life care: a study of patients with advanced AIDS and their primary care clinicians. Aids. 1999;13(9):1123–31.
91. Matthews A, et al. A qualitative exploration of the experiences of lesbian and heterosexual patients with breast cancer. Oncol Nurs Forum. 2002;29(10):1455–62.
92. Averett P, Yoon I, Jenkins CL. Older lesbians: experiences of aging, discrimination and resilience. J Women Aging. 2011;23:216–32.
93. Hash KM, Netting FE. Long-term planning and decision making among midlife and older gay men and lesbians. J Soc Work End Life Palliat Care. 2007;3(2):59–77.
94. Boehmer U, Clark M, Sullivan M. Advance care planning by unmarried women of different sexual orientations: the importance of social support. J Women Aging. 2010;22(4):306–20.

95. Matthews AK. Lesbians and cancer support: clinical issues for cancer patients. Health Care Women Int. 1998;19(3):193–203.
96. Stein GL, Bonuck KA. Attitudes on end-of-life care and advance care planning in the lesbian and gay community. J Palliat Med. 2001;4(2):173–90.
97. Varner A. Spirituality and religion among lesbian women diagnosed with cancer: a qualitative study. J Psychosoc Oncol. 2004;22(1):75–89.
98. Auldridge A, Espinoza R. Health equity and LGBT elders of color: recommendations for policy and practice. New York: SAGE (Services and Advocacy for GLBT Elders); 2013.
99. Fenge L-A. Developing understanding of same-sex partner bereavement for older lesbian and gay people: implications for social work practice. J Gerontol Soc Work. 2013:1–17.
100. Kim Y, Loscalzo M, Clark K. Sexual minority health in psycho-oncology. In: Holland J, et al., editors. Psycho-oncology. New York: Oxford University Press; 2015.
101. Stein GL, Beckerman NL, Sherman PA. Lesbian and gay elders and long-term care: identifying the unique psychosocial perspectives and challenges. J Gerontol Soc Work. 2010;53(5):421–35.
102. Aldredge PA, Conlon A. Reflections: gay men and lesbians at end-of-life. J Soc Work End Life Palliat Care. 2012;8(2):113–8.
103. Smolinski KM, Colon Y. Silent voices and invisible walls: exploring end of life care with lesbians and gay men. J Psychosoc Oncol. 2006;24(1):51–64.
104. Stein GL, Almack K, editors.Care near the end of life. The concerns, needs and experiences of LGBT elders. In: Ward R, Rivers I, Sutherland M, editors. Lesbian, gay, bisexual and transgender ageing: biographical approaches for inclusive care and support. London: Jessica Kingsley Publishers; 2012.
105. Association, G.a.L.M. Healthy people 2010: companion document for lesbian, gay, bisexual and trasgender (lgbt) health: San Francisco: CA; 2001.
106. Röndahl G, Innala S, Carlsson M. Nursing staff and nursing students' attitudes towards HIV-infected and homosexual HIV-infected patients in Sweden and the wish to refrain from nursing. J Adv Nurs. 2003;41(5):454–61.
107. Vermette L, Godin G. Nurses' intentions to provide home care: the impact of AIDS and homosexuality. AIDS Care. 1996;8(4):479–88.
108. Institute, M.M.M. Out and aging the metlife study of lesbian and gay baby boomers 2006: Westport, CT.
109. Doka KJ. Disenfranchised grief: Recognizing hidden sorrow. Disenfranchised grief: recognizing hidden sorrow. Lexington: Lexington Books/D. C. Heath and Com; 1989.
110. SAGE and Brookdale Center on Aging. No need to fear no need to hide: a training program about inclusion and understanding of lesbian, gay, bisexual and transgender elders for long-term care and assisted living facilities. New York. 2004.
111. Reygan FCG, D'Alton P. A pilot training programme for health and social care professionals providing oncological and palliative care to lesbian, gay and bisexual patients in Ireland. Psychooncology. 2013;22(5):1050–4.
112. Mollon L. The forgotten minorities: health disparities of the lesbian, gay, bisexual, and transgendered communities. J Health Care Poor Underserved. 2012;23(1):1–6.
113. Hernandez JO. Gay rights one baby-step at a time: protecting hospital visitation rights for same-sex partners while the lack of surrogacy rights lingers comment on "ethical challenges in end-of-life care for GLBTI individuals" by Colleen Cartwright. J Bioeth Inq. 2012;9(3):361–3.
114. www.lamdalegal.org. Lamda legal: making the case for equality. 2014. www.lamdalegal.org.
115. www.americanprogress.org. Moving the needle: the impact of the affordable care act on LGBT communities. 2014. https://www.americanprogress.org/issues/lgbt/report/2014/11/17/101575/moving-the-needle/.
116. Waisel DB. Vulnerable populations in healthcare. Curr Opin Anesthesiol. 2013;26(2):186–92.
117. LGBT Movement Advancement Project & SAGE, Improving the lives of LGBT older adults. 2010. http://sageusa.org/uploads/Advancing%20Equality%20for%20LGBT%20Elders%20[Final%20COMPRESSED].pdf].

118. Boulder County Aging Services. Evaluation of project visibility training: outcome and satisfaction. Boulder; 2006.
119. England, A. C. Opening doors: working with older lesbians and gay men. 2001, Age Concern England: London, UK. http://www.ageconcern.org/uk/Ageconcern/Documents/Opening_Doors_resource_pack.pdf.
120. The Joint Commission, Advancing effective communication, cultural competence, and patient- and family-centered care for the lesbian, gay, bisexual and transgender (lgbt) community: a field guide. Oak Brook: The Joint Commission; 2011.
121. Snowdon S. Healthcare equality index 2013: promoting equitable & inclusive care for lesbian, gay, bisexual and transgender patients and their families. Washington, DC: Human Rights Campaign; 2013.

Part IV
Cancer at the Intersection

Chapter 15
Cancer Care Needs of Transgender, Transsexual, and Other Gender Nonconforming Populations

Emilia Lombardi and Swagata Banik

Abstract Experiences of cancer among trans people is a neglected area of study and requires greater time and resources in order to provide them better care. Trans people's experience with cancer is greatly influenced by their own experiences of discrimination in society and health care. In addition, the use of exogenous hormones could influence the production of various cancers. This chapter will outline the many factors that can impact the production of cancer and how social factors can affect trans people's ability to seek treatment and recover. The chapter will also identify important recommendations that would benefit trans people in identifying and treating cancer. Overall, greater attention is needed on chronic health issues like cancer. Clearly, more research is needed in understanding the findings within many case studies of trans people and cancer. Health professionals will also need greater education in order to build up their cultural competency in treating trans people.

Background

Research focused on trans (individuals who have a different sex, gender identity, and/or gender expression than the one assigned to them at birth, often using hormones and surgery, to live as another gender. They are also referred to as transgender, transsexual, or gender nonconforming) populations' health needs have

E. Lombardi (✉)
Department of Public Health, Baldwin Wallace University, Berea, OH, USA
e-mail: elombard@bw.edu

S. Banik
Department of Public Health, Baldwin Wallace University, Berea, OH, USA

U. Boehmer, R. Elk (eds.), *Cancer and the LGBT Community*,
DOI 10.1007/978-3-319-15057-4_15

been primarily focused on HIV/AIDS, mental health, and substance use issues. The existing body of literature clearly indicates that trans people frequently face a multiplicity of challenges to their health and well-being contributed by social and institutional factors [1] that lead to challenges to accessing relevant health care services [2, 3]; social services such as homeless shelters, addictions services, and sexual assault [4, 5]. Accessibility and relevance issues have also been documented in relation to harm reduction and HIV prevention work [6, 7]. Trans people often experience direct harassment and discrimination in institutional and broader social contexts [8, 9].

Current Research on Trans Health

Although, less emphasis have been made on other health issues like cancer, extrapolating data from social determinants of trans health, one would anticipate the severity of health impact due to lack of access [10]. There has been studies examining the morbidity and mortality of trans people to see if hormone therapy is related to greater health risks and they generally found little health risks (including cancer) primarily associated with hormone use. However, the primary objectives of these studies were not to investigate cancer but to examine the prevalence of health problems resulting from hormone use [11–13] studies examining cancer among trans populations may underreport outcomes and may hide a higher incidence over time as their exposure to hormones increases [14].

Additional information is needed on understanding the issues trans people face in regards to cancer. The Institute of Medicine report identified the lack of research regarding cancer among transgender populations other than a small number of case studies examining the relationship between hormone therapy and hormone sensitive cancers (breast, ovaries, and prostate) [15]. But cancer is one of many issues in need of examination; trans people have reported many problems accessing health care which would exacerbate any health problem. Discrimination or the fear of discrimination would prevent trans people from seeking important health screenings that can identify cancers early.

Thus, there is very little information regarding transgender people's experience with cancer. Additionally, it is important to understand how being trans can influence people's experiences with cancer risk and cancer related health care rather than their overall risk for a diagnosis of cancer. The chapter will focus on these issues and develop a better understanding of the research and health care needs of trans populations.

The Impact of Hormone Replacement Therapy and Trans Status upon the Risk for Cancer

The concern regarding hormone replacement therapy (HRT) and the health of trans people is that many cancers are sensitive to hormones. Many cancers have androgen and estrogen receptors that respond in the presence of hormones, and the concern was that providing large dosages of hormones could increase the manifestation and growth of hormone dependent cancers (i.e. breast, prostate, ovaries). Although the Standards of Care (SOC) published by the World Professional Association of Transgender Health (WPATH) generally identified various cancers associated with estrogen and testosterone use as “inconclusive or no increased risk” [16]. While the findings of studies examining the prevalence of cancer among those receiving HRT have been small and attributed to other factors like tobacco use [11–13]. These clinical samples provide limited understanding of predominantly race and ethnic homogenous groups of trans people. Differences in outcomes due to demographic characteristics such as age, race, ethnicity, and clinical characteristics such as length of hormone treatment are not addressed by these cases.

Studies examining the morbidity and mortality of trans people who have been receiving hormone therapy in the Netherlands and Belgium found trans women to have a slightly higher risk of mortality due to lung cancer and leukemia, while trans men’s cancer mortality was not different from the general population [11–13]. The explanation given for the difference in lung cancer may have been due to greater smoking among transgender populations. Cancer prevention approaches need to examine the underlying health behaviors among this population. It is also imperative to understand the social context of the disease.

Hormone therapy for the purpose of changing secondary sex characteristics requires higher dosage compared to what is given to cisgender (one’s gender identity is congruent with one’s sex assigned at birth) people for other reasons and this is the reason why many are concerned about the use of hormones among trans people [17]. While trans men are no longer exposed to high levels of estrogens, testosterone itself has been found to be associated with risk for breast and cervical cancers [18, 19], but studies did not find an increased prevalence of these cancers among trans men [11–13]. An important distinction, however, lies in the amount of time trans people have been utilizing exogenous hormones compared to their cisgender counterparts. For example, trans women may only be exposed to estrogen for a smaller percentage of their life compared to many of their cisgender counterparts (who do not have any medical issues that many require exogenous hormones). An additional issue that has not been discussed is the age where a person may stop taking or reducing their dosage. Currently, there is no consensus nor there is any solid evidence base on for a specific time span for hormone use, and many people may begin their transition much later in life when their endogenous hormones may be already diminishing. Time exposed to hormones may be an important factor needing greater investigation in understanding the hormone/cancer link among trans populations. This is especially important as more people begin their transition at younger ages and will have a longer time period using exogenous hormones.

The clinical studies provide a starting point in examining the hormone use of a homogenous group of trans people who are receiving care. Other studies have identified populations of trans people who utilize hormones from nonmedical sources [20, 21]. So we know that hormones when prescribed and obtained from medical sources have not been found to increase cancer risks [11–13], we do not know what the effect hormones taken without medical supervision and with varying dosage and quality [22].

Further complication that requires investigation when examining the relationship between hormone therapy and cancer among trans people. Health care providers who are not aware of a patient's anatomical inventory regarding the presence or absence of specific organs may not consider gender-specific disorders even if the patient presents with its symptoms (e.g. prostate cancer in a male-to-female patient, or cervical cancer in female-to-male patient). This lack of awareness could lead to a delay in diagnosis and treatment.

Case Studies of Cancer in Trans Men and Women

Some trans men who are on hormonal testosterone therapy may still be exposed to low levels of estrogen still being produced by their bodies or by having testosterone converted into estradiol by aromatase enzymes. Until a transman undergoes oophorectomy, the body may still continue to produce some estradiol. However, there are questions regarding why some trans men are diagnosed with it when they were receiving testosterone therapy as part of their transition.

Case studies investigating ovarian cancers among trans men were focused on whether these cancers had androgen receptors. One study found a sample that was found to have abundant androgen receptors (tumors were sensitive to androgens like testosterone) [23]. Another case study discussed finding ovarian cancer in two trans men after many years on testosterone, while another study reported finding uterine and cervical cancer on a trans men while performing sex reassignment surgery (SRS), and another finding vaginal cancer 18 years after receiving SRS [24, 25]. These case studies made a point to indicate that it is important to remove all their reproductive organs and associated structures. In important detail discussed is the men's lack of gynecological care that could identify such problems early. A study by Peitzmeier et al (2014) found that compared to cisgender patients, trans men were more likely to have an inadequate Pap test (10.8 % vs. 1.3 % of tests) [26]. Their reasoning referred to a combination of physical changes induced by testosterone therapy and provider/patient discomfort with the exam. The implication of these case studies is that the specific experiences and medical care of trans people can impact important primary and secondary prevention activities regarding screening and early intervention.

A white trans woman who had genital surgery was found to have a stage III B anal cancer that required extensive surgery and reconstruction [27]. Additionally, the surgeon discussed the need to redo the vaginoplasty due to the importance to the patient. While anal cancer is not associated with any of the procedures related to transitioning from one gender to another, the perspective of the trans woman made this into a trans issue. The author stated that it was important for them to maintain the original surgery for the benefit of the patient. The experiences of trans patients can influence how they will respond to a diagnosis and treatment options.

Sometimes the people's perception of cancer and their trans status may cause them and others to minimize their risk for cancer. A study discussed finding prostate cancer in a trans woman 31 years after SRS and use of conjugated estrogens [28]. The assumption was that castration would prevent the growth of prostate cancers. In regards to this case, two thoughts were discussed by the authors. The first was the possibility of the existence of cancer cells prior to castration, (the trans woman had her surgery at age 45). Since many trans women do not begin their transition prior to 45 years of age they may already be within the window of risk for prostate cancer (especially if they have other risk factors). A large community sample found 37% of their sample of trans women to have transitioned (began to live full time as their identified gender) after 45 years of age [29]. Statistics for prostate cancer shows that greater risk is found for those 50 years of age and older (in 2010 the incidence for prostate cancer was 9.5/100,000 for those under 49 years of age and increases to 289.5/100,000 for those 50–65 years of age, and increases to 807,75/100,000 for those 65–74 years of age) [30]. This does not account for when (and if) they have some form of SRS that removes their testes. Another issue discussed by the authors is the possibility that the androgen receptors of the cancer became hypersensitive and did not need a large amount of androgens to be activated. One other case study made the same observation when they examined a trans woman with prostate cancer 41 years after initiating hormone therapy and had her testes removed 26 years prior [31]. Hormone therapy and SRS may not provide the protection against prostate cancer that it was once thought to provide to trans women.

A case study that exemplifies the concerns and fears trans people may have in regards to cancers that could affect their gendered appearance. An African-American trans woman was diagnosed with metastatic breast cancer [32]. Previous visits to her primary care doctor identified a lump in her left breast, but she declined mammography and biopsy. Her decisions to delay care until the cancer worsened was the result of numerous misconceptions and concerns regarding the procedure. She did not think she was at risk for cancer because she was trans, she described having "a male chest with hormones and silicone". She assumed the lump was the result of silicone. She also felt that she was not at risk for cancer because "men and women cancers are different". So being trans was in her mind protective against breast cancer. Additional issues included a preference for injectable hormones because the "pills can cause breast cancer", and misconceptions about cancer in general (cutting into the cancer will make it spread).

There are two issues to take from this case study. Physicians do need to take more time and identify the sociocultural beliefs of their patients. The author identified sample questions that physicians can use to better understand their perspective. Being trans added an additional factor in that the woman in question saw her body as being different from other women and that influenced her perception of risk. Cancers associated with one's breasts, prostate, and reproductive organs may prove to be very sensitive because of trans people's relationship between their bodies and their identities. Addressing care for trans people will require extra care for these issues, especially in providing health education.

HPV and Hepatitis

Reports on the prevalence and genotypes of HPV among trans populations are scarce in the literature. A recent study from Argentina reported 97.4 % HPV prevalence among 117 male to female transgender sex workers surveyed. High risk genotypes were detected in 82.5 % [33]. Two or more co-infecting HPV genotypes were found in 70.9 %. One case showed up to 10 different co-infecting types. The high HPV prevalence, the co-infection with multiple genotypes and the high frequency of high risk genotypes detected, together with the high HIV seroprevalence among trans women and extreme social marginalization, discrimination and stigmatization make this population extremely vulnerable to cancer risks [34]. Before planning long-term diagnostic and treatment strategies, it is imperative that we first address the issues of HPV awareness and willingness to participate in anal cancer screening for HIV positive trans people; thus, it is important to solicit perspectives of trans population community health advocates regarding anal cancer screening. Of course, these aspects need to be considered in the light of a major context in which social exclusion, limitations of the health system and STI-related stigma affect the access of trans populations to health care. Further, as a vulnerable population with a high HIV prevalence, HIV risk behaviors may place them at risk for hepatitis B and C and HPV, which have been found to be associated with various cancers [35–39].

Discrimination and Risk Behaviors

Both the Institute of Medicine and National Institutes of Health have identified the need for greater research about the health disparities of transgender people [15, 40]. What is known from existing research is that many transgender people have experienced some form of discrimination or harassment related to their gender nonconformity and that discrimination has been linked to many risk behaviors that could increase their cancer risks. What is also known is that many of them struggle with substance use [41–49]. However, tobacco and alcohol use among trans people is less well known. Studies examining the tobacco and alcohol use among Lesbian, Gay, Bisexual, and Transgender (LGBT) populations do not differentiate between the different groups [50–53]. Studies have found those with experiences of discrimination due to their gender identity to smoke and to use alcohol more often [29, 53]. There is reason to believe that trans people may utilize tobacco and alcohol as a form of coping due to their disadvantaged status, and lung and liver cancer risk associated with smoking and alcohol abuse, respectively, is well established [54]. In addition, the social factors related to discrimination can also influence their utilization and access to important health related resources [55–57].

Access to Care Issues Among Trans People

Discrimination can affect people's access to health resources (employment problems and health insurance), coping resources (social support), and mental and physical health problems (depression and substance use) [57–60]. Experiences or even the perception of discrimination by health care workers can have a significant impact on a range of health outcomes specifically by influencing their help seeking behavior.

Health care service providers have found that getting trans people the services they need (e.g. primary health care, substance use treatment, and housing) can be difficult for several reasons. Many trans adults are denied insurance coverage because of their use of hormone treatment and a diagnosis of gender identity disorder. Some providers may not want to work with trans clients [61]. Lack of sensitivity on the part of health care providers themselves may adversely influence whether trans people will access treatment and remain within it [43–45]. Trans people might resist seeking treatment because others have reported past discriminatory treatment on the part of service providers.

The National Transgender Discrimination Survey (NTDS) identified many problems identified by trans people regarding their experiences with and access to health care. Within their sample of 6450 transgender identified people, 19 % reported being refused treatment by a doctor or other provider because of their transgender or gender non-conforming status [29]. Additionally, 28 % of their participants reported verbal harassment within the doctor's office or other medical setting. Even more problematic, those who disclose their trans identity to their doctor were more likely to report being denied care (23 % vs. 15 %).

Even when trans people are able to access care, their provider may not have the information to properly care for them. Half of the study participants reported having to educate their provider on trans health issues. Among those most likely to report having to educate their providers were female to male trans people, those living full-time as their identified gender, and those on a public insurance program (Medicaid, etc.). The problems people experience with health care providers are not surprising, given the attitudes many physicians may have concerning trans people. Studies have found some physicians believe transsexual women to be emotionally disturbed or immoral [62]. Fortunately, there has been some improvement in physicians' attitudes over time [63].

Given these issues many trans people will choose to postpone needed health care. Within the same study, 28 % postponed or avoided needed medical treatment due to discrimination or disrespect from providers, and 33 % postponed preventive health care [29]. In regards to cancer care, this means that many trans people are not receiving important cancer screenings and possibly delay care to a point when their cancer becomes too serious to treat effectively. An example is presented in the documentary, Southern Comfort, which follows the last year in the life of Robert Eads, an FTM transsexual who died of ovarian cancer when his attempts to find a medical provider failed because the doctors in his community did not want to treat a trans patient [64].

Trans people's access to health insurance can also contribute to their postponement/avoidance of health care. Within the NTDS, 19 % reported not having health insurance, which is 4 % greater than that of the United States percentage (15 %) [65]. Many participants reported postponing needed medical care (48 %) and preventive care (50 %) because they could not afford it. Trans people's relationship with health insurance have been very problematic [61]. The need for trans specific care creates additional hardship for people. Even individuals with insurance may have trouble accessing primary and gender specific health care. Only a few doctors and clinics make hormones and related procedures available to patients (and may not accept Medicare or Medicaid). Very few insurance companies allow sex reassignment procedures under their plans, leaving even those who do have health insurance with few options in accessing gender related medical care. Much of their medical expenses come out of pocket, and many times they will have to search to find a doctor/clinic that will provide them the care they need even if that means having two sets of providers: One for their trans related services and another for their other health care. This creates a problem when physicians may not know of each other's existence and their ability to provide needed care to their trans patients.

While the reports above refer to the United States, these health care experiences are also common in European countries as well. In a report published by the International Lesbian and Gay Association (ILGA) approximately 20 % of the people they surveyed reported problems accessing non trans-related healthcare [66]. Follow-up reports that many people across Europe will avoid accessing any kind of healthcare due to the prejudicial treatment of healthcare professionals. The implication being that the problems faced by trans people is not unique to the US with its fee for service health care system, but also common within nations with state funded systems. The report also identified institutional-based systems for trans health care as providing poor care resulting from the power and control (the institutions have in regards to any form of trans health care) they exert over their trans patients. They concluded that health care providers do not have sufficient competency in treating trans individuals within their practice and require policies and procedures that will enhance their knowledge and prohibit discrimination.

Affordable Care Act and Trans Health

The Patient Protection and Affordable Care Act (ACA) enacted in 2010 has been designed to solve the major problems facing the United States health care system [67]. Its major goals are to improve people's access to health insurance and remove many of the actions that health insurance companies used to deny coverage to people (removing limitations on pre-existing conditions, etc). The law also provides citizens with access to preventive care that should help identify and improve health outcomes of many chronic diseases like cancer. What is most significant for trans people was not addressed directly by the legislation, but was addressed by the Dept. of Health and Human Services through its interpretation of that legislation. In a letter from the Dept.'s Office of Civil Rights it stated that they will consider discrimination based on gender identity and sex stereotypes as a form of sex discrimination under the Affordable Care Act [68]. The implication being that people will be protected under the ACA for discrimination resulting from their gender identity or expression, and that trans people should have better access to health care. The law's focus on preventive care means that trans people will potentially have better access to cancer screenings and subsequent care.

However, trans people may still experience discrimination regardless of the current administrative changes. An example, Jennifer Blair attempted to access a program to provide mammograms to low income women funded by the Centers for Disease Control and Prevention (CDC) and was denied because CDC guidelines did not include trans women as being eligible because they require their participants to be "genetically female" [69]. This policy was eventually changed by December, 2013 to include trans women, but there remain other challenges in regards to how trans people can access health care [70]. Many cancers, especially those found in reproductive organs, have attained a gendered aspect in that public perception and health programming become focused on people's gender rather than their body. The result are experiences like the above where someone was denied access to care because they did not fit a specific label, even though breast cancer is not just found within people who are "genetically female". Older trans women will require screening tests for breast and prostate cancers, as well as for testicular cancer if they still retain those organs. The gendered aspect of these cancers will likely mean that health insurance and other programs may deny them access to care because women "do not have prostates or testes" or in the case of Jennifer Blair not seen as women at all. Trans men will face the same problems in accessing gynecological care. So while the ACA could be very beneficial for trans people in regards to accessing affordable health care, we do not know at this time whether they will be able to access care that will encompass their entire biological status or limited to what is expected for their legal gender.

Recommendations

The primary issue needed in improving the health of trans people is to expand our knowledge beyond HIV, substance use, and violence as health issues. Not to say that these are not important, they are, but to focus solely on these does a disservice to trans populations by creating the image that trans people do not have other issues or by the lack of trans specific knowledge regarding cancer and other illnesses. The primary way to focus more attention on the diverse health issues facing trans populations is to improve and increase the health research on trans health issues.

Much of what is known regarding cancer risks and experiences in general is based upon the health surveillance done by the federal government. However, those studies do not include measures to identify trans populations or their unique risk factors (hormone use). One of the arguments made regarding the lack of inclusion within general population health studies was the lack of validated measures that can reliably identify trans populations and limit error and misunderstandings among cis populations. A report by the Williams Institute summarized potential measures that can be used within these types of studies to identify the health issues of trans individuals. One study found the use of a two question method was able to work within a population of college students [71]. Another methodological problem will be the sampling of sufficient numbers of trans people in order to conduct effective analysis.

A growing issue is the number of young people who are beginning their transition at younger ages. The result will be many trans people using exogenous hormones for most of their lives. The result could be that the later cancer risks of trans people who transition young could be similar to that of the general cis population in regards to hormone sensitive cancers (such as the case of breast cancer). The studies examining the impact of hormones among those transitioning from one gender to another primarily focused on people who began their transition later in life. Research must begin to focus on the health issues of young people transitioning in order to assess the health issues they are likely to experience in their later years. Another issue that can affect the experiences of young transitioning, trans people will be the age in which certain surgeries occur (removal of reproductive organs and other tissues sensitive to hormones) and how that can affect their risk for cancers of those organs.

Greater access to healthcare for preventive and more specific cancer treatments would greatly help trans populations. The activities around the Affordable Care Act have the potential to provide many trans people with health care they may not have been able to access otherwise. However, the inconsistent acceptance of the Medicaid Expansion will mean that many low income trans people will still not have access to health insurance within the United States. There are also other barriers in regards to trans people's access to health care, the primary issue are the many exclusions that are used to prevent trans people from accessing needed health care.

Anti-discrimination policies need to be developed and enforced that will prevent trans people from being discriminated against in their access to insurance or by the actions of health providers. Currently, policies are in place as part of the ACA that can protect trans people, but that protection could be dependent on what presidential administration is currently in place. Even within a relatively friendly administration, discriminatory policies can still persist [69]. The issue of discrimination is still an issue within many health settings when trans specific care is needed, such as the case of trans men needing pap smears and related services and trans women needing similar care requiring a sensitive and knowledgeable provider. Sometimes situations arise that can negatively impact the health care of trans people. A recent demand made by the American Board of Obstetrics and Gynecology for its members (who they require for their certification) to only treat women [72]. A Board representative stated that "the specialty of obstetrics and gynecology was specifically designed to treat problems of the female reproductive tract and was restricted to taking care of women". This policy was quickly changed [73], but it is another example of how policy can change regarding the provision of medical care that could potentially affect trans people. The issue regarding trans people was not discussed, but the question remains regarding how trans people are to be treated, and this is an example where health care providers require greater education on trans health issues.

The greater access to trans specific health care can be very important in protecting trans people from many cancers. The most specific is by removing potential organs that can become cancerous. However, the primary way trans specific care can aid in the prevention and treatment of cancers is by improving trans people's engagement with their provider and with their health care in general. This has been found to be the case in regards to HIV related services [74].

Providers and trans people alike can benefit from greater education regarding trans people's risks and issues regarding cancer. The sensitive nature regarding trans people's bodies requires providers and health programs to utilize cultural competent care and information. There is movement to incorporate trans specific issues within the education of health care providers and in developing programs for trans people [75–78]. Tobacco cessation programs have been very involved in developing programs specifically for trans (and lesbian, gay, and bisexual) populations [77]. These programs work to make sure program materials include trans relevant materials and that staff are knowledgeable about trans issues. The goal becomes to create resources that encompass the many issues faced by trans people in regards to cancer prevention and care. These resources will be able to benefit both trans patients and health care providers.

Conclusion

Compared to health issues like HIV/AIDS, there is still little known regarding the cancer risks and experiences of trans people. Identifying next steps falls into three goals: (1) to increase and improve health research regarding trans populations, (2) to prevent the discrimination of trans people within health care (including insurance), and (3) to improve the cultural competency of health care providers. All of these require a conscious effort on the part of governmental and private entities to change how they collect data and in how they treat trans people. To get there requires greater advocacy and education. We are at the point now regarding cancer and related health issues as we were regarding HIV/AIDS approximately 15 years ago. There is work being generated that is getting people's attention and it is improving the amount and kind of care trans people can expect, but there is still much that needs to be done.

Recommendations for Clinical Care

1. An important tool for health providers serving trans people include an anatomy inventory to help identify potential cancer screening needs. Additionally, electronic health records need to ensure that important information regarding trans people is collected [79].
2. Trans people need to be represented within all studies including prevention and epidemiologic studies.
3. The support of cancer survivors who are trans is an important issue to address. However, trans people's access to survivor groups is difficult, especially concerning cancers that are tied to specific genders. Trans men may have problems with support networks that consist primarily of cisgender women, and the same can be said regarding trans women and men's support networks. It is important to identify and even create trans competent cancer support networks.
4. There are many resources that can aid health providers in becoming more competent in regards to the care of trans people. The following organizations provide services and information in regards to the health of trans people.
   a. The Center of Excellence for Transgender Health, http://transhealth.ucsf.edu/. Is a long running program dedicated to increasing access to comprehensive, effective, and affirming health care services for trans and gender-variant communities.
   b. World Professional Association for Transgender Health (WPATH), www.wpath.org/. International multidisciplinary professional association promoting evidence based care, education, research, advocacy, public policy and respect in transgender health.
   c. GLMA: Health Professionals Advancing LGBT Equality http://www.glma.org/. Works to ensure equality in healthcare for lesbian, gay, bisexual and transgender (LGBT) individuals and healthcare providers.

Acknowledgements The authors wish to thank Henry Ng, MD, MPH (MetroHealth System and CWRU School of Medicine) and Don Allensworth-Davies, PhD, MSc (Cleveland State University) for their comments and suggestions on this chapter.

References

1. Bauer GR, Hammond R, Travers R, Kaay M, Hohenadel KM, Boyce M. I don't think this is theoretical; this is our lives: how erasure impacts health care for transgender people. J Assoc Nurses AIDS Care. 2009;20(5):348–61.
2. Xavier J, Honnold J, Bradford J. The Health, health-related needs, and lifecourse experiences of transgender Virginians. Virginia HIV Community Planning Committee and Virginia Department of Health. Richmond, VA: Virginia HIV Community Planning Committee and Virginia Department of Health; 2007.
3. Dewey JM. Knowledge legitimacy: how trans-patient behavior supports and challenges current medical knowledge. Qual Health Res. 2008;18(10):1345–55.
4. Nemoto T, Operario D, Keatley J, Nguyen H, Sugano E. Promoting health for transgender women: Transgender Resources and Neighborhood Space (TRANS) program in San Francisco. Am J Public Health. 2005;95(3):382–84.
5. Sperber J, Landers S, Lawrence S. Access to health care for transgendered persons: results of a needs assessment in Boston. Int J Transgenderism. 2005;8(2):75–91.
6. Bockting W, Robinson B, Rosser B. Transgender HIV prevention: qualitative evaluation of a model prevention education program. J Sex Educ Ther. 1998;23(2):125–33.
7. Cope A, Darke J. Trans accessibility project. Ontario: Violence Intervention and Education Workgroup; October 1999.
8. Hill SC, Daniel J, Benzie A, Ayres J, King G, Smith A. Sexual health of transgender sex workers attending an inner-city genitourinary medicine clinic. Int J STD AIDS. 2011;22(11):686–7.
9. Feinberg L. Trans health crisis: for us it's life or death. Am J Public Health. 2001;91(6):897–900.
10. Pittsburgh Transgender Health Research Summer Institute. Transgender health: a review and guidance for future research—Proceedings from the Summer Institute at the Center for Research on Health and Sexual Orientation, University of Pittsburgh. Int J Transgenderism. 2010;12(4):211–29.
11. Wierckx K, Mueller S, Weyers S, et al. Long-term evaluation of cross-sex hormone treatment in transsexual persons. J Sex Med. 2012;9(10):2641–51.
12. Wierckx K, Elaut E, Declerq E, et al. Prevalence of cardiovascular disease and cancer during cross-sex hormone therapy in a large cohort of trans persons: a case control study. Eur J Endocrinol. 2013;4:471–8.
13. Asscheman H, Giltay EJ, Megens JA, de Ronde WP, van Trotsenburg MA, Gooren LJ. A long-term follow-up study of mortality in transsexuals receiving treatment with cross-sex hormones. Eur J Endocrinol. 2011;164(4):635–42.
14. Mueller A, Gooren L. Hormone-related tumors in transsexuals receiving treatment with cross-sex hormones. Eur J Endocrinol. 2008;159(3):197–202.
15. Committee on lesbian g, bisexual, and transgender health issues and research gaps and opportunities; board on the health of select populations. The health of lesbian, gay, bisexual, and transgender people: building a foundation for better understanding. Washington DC: Institute of Medicine; 2011.
16. Coleman E, Bockting W, Botzer M, et al. Standards of care for the health of transsexual, transgender, and gender-nonconforming people, version 7. Int J Transgenderism. 2012;13(4):165–232.
17. Gooren LJ, Giltay EJ, Bunck MC. Long-term treatment of transsexuals with cross-sex hormones: extensive personal experience. J Clin Endocrinol Metab. 2007;jc.2007–1809.
18. Schover LR. Androgen therapy for loss of desire in women: is the benefit worth the breast cancer risk? Fertil Steril. 2008;90(1):129–40.
19. Dizon DS, Tejada-Berges T, Koelliker S, Steinhoff M, Granai CO. Ovarian cancer associated with testosterone supplementation in a female-to-male transsexual patient. Gynecol Obstet Invest. 2006;62(4):226–8.

20. Garofalo R, Deleon J, Osmer E, Doll M, Harper GW. Overlooked, misunderstood and at-risk: exploring the lives and HIV risk of ethnic minority male-to-female transgender youth. J Adolesc Health. 2006;38(3):230–6.
21. Sperber J, Stewart Landers JD, Lawrence M. Access to health care for transgendered persons: results of a needs assessment in Boston. In: Bockting W, Avery E, editors. Transgender health and HIV prevention: needs assessment studies from transgender communities across the United States. New York: Haworth Press; 2006. pp. 75–91.
22. Rhodes SD, Fernández FM, Leichliter JS, et al. Medications for sexual health available from non-medical sources: a need for increased access to healthcare and education among immigrant Latinos in the rural southeastern USA. J Immigr Minority Health. 2011;13(6):1183–6.
23. Dorff TB, Shazer RL, Nepomuceno EM, Tucker SJ. Successful treatment of metastatic androgen-independent prostate carcinoma in a transsexual patient. Clin Genitourin Cancer. 2007;5(5):344–6.
24. Urban RR, Teng NN, Kapp DS. Gynecologic malignancies in female-to-male transgender patients: the need of original gender surveillance. Am J Obstet Gynecol. 2011;204(5):e9–12.
25. Hage JJ, Dekker JJ, Karim RB, Verheijen RH, Bloemena E. Ovarian cancer in female-to-male transsexuals: report of two cases. Gynecol Oncol. 2000;76(3):413–5.
26. Peitzmeier SM, Reisner SL, Harigopal P, Potter J. Female-to-male patients have high prevalence of unsatisfactory Paps compared to non-transgender females: implications for cervical cancer screening. J Gen Intern Med. 2014;29:778–84.
27. Caricato M, Ausania F, Marangi GF, et al. Surgical treatment of locally advanced anal cancer after male-to-female sex reassignment surgery. World J Gastroenterol. 2009;15(23):2918–9.
28. Turo R, Jallad S, Prescott S, Cross WR. Metastatic prostate cancer in transsexual diagnosed after three decades of estrogen therapy. Can Urol Assoc J. 2013;7(7–8):E544–6.
29. Grant JM, Mottet LA, Tanis J, Harrison J, Hermon JL, Keisling M. Injustice at every turn: a report of the national transgender discrimination survey. Washington: National Center for Transgender Equality and National Gay and Lesbian task Force; 2011.
30. Surveillance Epidemiology and End Results (SEER) Program. SEER*Stat Database: Incidence—SEER 18 Regs Research Data, Nov 2011 Sub (1973–2010). Surveillance, Epidemiology, and End Results (SEER) Program 2013; 2014.
31. Miksad RA, Bubley G, Church P, et al. Prostate cancer in a transgender woman 41 years after initiation of feminization. JAMA. 2006;296(19):2316–7.
32. Dhand A, Dhaliwal G. Examining patient conceptions: a case of metastatic breast cancer in an African American male to female transgender patient. J Gen Intern Med. 2010;25(2):158–61.
33. dos Ramos Farias MS, Picconi MA, Garcia MN, et al. Human papilloma virus genotype diversity of anal infection among trans (male to female transvestites, transsexuals or transgender) sex workers in Argentina. J Clin Virol. 2011;51(2):96–9.
34. Miguez MJ, Burbano-Levy X, Rosenberg R, Malow R. The importance of HIV status and gender when designing prevention strategies for anal cancer. J Assoc Nurses AIDS Care. 2011;22(6):454–64.
35. Augustin G, Bruketa T, Korolija D, Milosevic M. Lower incidence of hepatic metastases of colorectal cancer in patients with chronic liver diseases: meta-analysis. Hepatogastroenterology. 2013;60(125):1164–9.
36. Damin DC, Ziegelmann PK, Damin AP. Human papillomavirus infection and colorectal cancer risk: a meta-analysis. Colorectal Dis. 2013;15(8):e420–8.
37. Li L, Wu B, Yang LB, Yin GC, Liu JY. Chronic hepatitis B virus infection and risk of pancreatic cancer: a meta-analysis. Asian Pac J Cancer Prev. 2013;14(1):275–79.
38. Shimakawa Y, Yan HJ, Tsuchiya N, Bottomley C, Hall AJ. Association of early age at establishment of chronic hepatitis B infection with persistent viral replication, liver cirrhosis and hepatocellular carcinoma: a systematic review. PLoS One. 2013;8(7):e69430.
39. Xu JH, Fu JJ, Wang XL, Zhu JY, Ye XH, Chen SD. Hepatitis B or C viral infection and risk of pancreatic cancer: a meta-analysis of observational studies. World J Gastroenterol. 2013;19(26):4234–41.

40. NIH LGBT Research Coordinating Committee. Consideration of the Institute of Medicine (IOM) Report on the Health of Lesbian, Gay, Bisexual, and Transgender (LGBT) Individuals. Washington DC: National Institutes of Health; 2013.
41. Lombardi EL, Wilchins RA, Priesing D, Malouf D. Gender violence: transgender experiences with violence and discrimination. J Homosex. 2001;42(1):89–101.
42. Reback CJ, Simon PA, Bemis C, Gatson B. The Los Angeles transgender health study: Community Report; 2001. West Hollywood.
43. Clements K. The transgender community health project: descriptive results. San Francisco: San Francisco Dept. of Public Health; 1999.
44. Moriarty H, Thiagalingam A. Audit of service to a minority client group: male to female transsexuals. Int J STD AIDS. 1998;9(4):238–240.
45. The transgender substance abuse treatment policy group of the San Francisco lesbian G, bisexual, and transgender substance abuse task force. Transgender protocol: treatment services guidelines for substance abuse treatment providers. San Francisco, Calif: Author; 1995.
46. GLBT Health Access P. Access to health care for transgendered persons in greater Boston. Boston: JSI Research and Training Institute, Inc.; 2000.
47. Reback CJ, Lombardi EL. HIV risk behaviors of male-to-female transgenders in a community-based harm reduction program. Int J Transgenderism. 1999;3(1 + 2). http://web.archive.org/web/20070423032342/http://www.symposion.com/ijt/hiv_risk/reback.htm. Accessed 3 March 2015.
48. Reback C, Simon P, Bemis C, Gatson B. The Los Angeles transgender health study: community report. Los Angeles: Van Ness Recovery House: Prevention Division; 2001.
49. Xavier JM. The Washington, DC Transgender needs assessment survey final report for phase two: tabulation of the survey questionnaires; presentation of findings and analysis of the survey results; and recommendations. Washington, DC August 24, 2000.
50. Clarke MP, Coughlin JR. Prevalence of smoking among the lesbian, gay, bisexual, transsexual, transgender and queer (LGBTTQ) subpopulations in Toronto–the Toronto Rainbow Tobacco Survey (TRTS). Can J Public Health. 2012;103(2):132–6.
51. Remafedi G. Lesbian, gay, bisexual, and transgender youths: who smokes, and why? Nicotine Tob Res. 2007;9(Suppl 1):S65–71.
52. Sell RL, Dunn PM. Inclusion of lesbian, gay, bisexual and transgender people in tobacco use-related surveillance and epidemiological research. J LGBT Health Res. 2008;4(1):27–42.
53. Newcomb ME, Heinz AJ, Mustanski B. Examining risk and protective factors for alcohol use in lesbian, gay, bisexual, and transgender youth: a longitudinal multilevel analysis. J Stud Alcohol Drugs. 2012;73(5):783–93.
54. Meyer IH, Schwartz S, Frost DM. Social patterning of stress and coping: does disadvantaged social statuses confer more stress and fewer coping resources? Soc Sci Med. 2008;67(3):368–79.
55. Ahmed AT, Mohammed SA, Williams DR. Racial discrimination & health: pathways & evidence. Indian J Med Res. 2007;126(4):318–27.
56. Bastos JL, Faerstein E. Conceptual and methodological aspects of relations between discrimination and health in epidemiological studies. Cad Saude Publica. 2012;28(1):177–83.
57. Johnston DW, Lordan G. Discrimination makes me sick! An examination of the discrimination-health relationship. J Health Econ. 2012;31(1):99–111.
58. Gee GC. A multilevel analysis of the relationship between institutional and individual racial discrimination and health status. Am J Public Health. 2002;92(4):615–23.
59. Hahm HC, Ozonoff A, Gaumond J, Sue S. Perceived discrimination and health outcomes a gender comparison among Asian-Americans nationwide. Womens Health Issues. 2010;20(5):350–8.
60. Todorova IL, Falcon LM, Lincoln AK, Price LL. Perceived discrimination, psychological distress and health. Sociol Health Illn. 2010;32(6):843–61.
61. JSI Research and Training Institute Inc. Access to health care for transgendered persons in greater Boston. Boston: Gay, Lesbian, Bisexual, and Transgender Health Access Project; 2000.

62. Green R, Stoller R, MacAndrew C. Attitudes toward sex transformation procedures. Arch Gen Psychiatry. 1966;15:178–82.
63. Franzini L, Casinelli D. Health professionals' factual knowledge and changing attitudes toward transsexuals. Soc Sci Med. 1986;22(5):535–9.
64. Southern Comfort [Documentory]: HBO Theatrical Documentary; 2001.
65. United States Census Bureau. HIB-1. Health Insurance Coverage Status and Type of Coverage–All Persons by Sex, Race and Hispanic Origin: 1999 to 2012. In: hihistt1B.xls, Editor. United States Census Bureau; 2012.
66. Whittle S, Turner L, Combs R, Rhodes S. Transgender EuroStudy. Brussels, Belgium: The European Region of the International Lesbian and Gay Association; 2008.
67. The Patient Protection and Affordable Care Act. Public Law 111–148. Title IV, x4207, USC HR. Vol 3590; 2010.
68. Rodriguez L. Guidance clarifying that sex-based discrimination includes discrimination on the basis of gender identity and sex stereotypes. 2012. Washington DC: Dept of Health and Human Services. http://www.hrc.org/files/assets/resources/HHSResponse8612.pdf.
69. Martin N. For transgender patients, a growing fight over health coverage. ProPublica. 2013 Oct 22.
70. Marie Molloy P. CDC reverses discriminatory breast cancer screening rule for trans people. The Advocate. 2013. http://www.advocate.com/politics/transgender/2013/12/23/cdc-reverses-discriminatory-breast-cancer-screening-rule-trans. Accessed 26. Dec. 2013.
71. Tate CC, Ledbetter JN, Youssef CP. A two-question method for assessing gender categories in the social and medical sciences. J Sex Res. 2012;50:767–76.
72. Grady D. Gynecologists run afoul of panel when patient is male. The New York Times. 2013 Nov 22.
73. Grady D. Gynecologists may treat men, board says in switch. The New York Times. 2013 Nov 27;A14.
74. Grimaldi J, Jacobs J. The HIV hormone bridge: connecting impoverished HIV+ transsexual sex workers to HIV medical care. [Database]. 1998. http://www.aegis.org/aidsline/1998/dec/m98c1575.html:http://www.aegis.org/aidsline/1998/dec/m98c1575.html. Accessed 29. Oct. 2003.
75. Lim FA, Brown DV, Jr, Jones H. Lesbian, gay, bisexual, and transgender health: fundamentals for nursing education. J Nurs Educ. 2013;52(4):198–203.
76. Rutherford K, McIntyre J, Daley A, Ross LE. Development of expertise in mental health service provision for lesbian, gay, bisexual and transgender communities. Med Educ. 2012;46(9):903–13.
77. Eliason MJ, Dibble SL, Gordon R, Soliz GB. The last drag: an evaluation of an LGBT-specific smoking intervention. J Homosex. 2012;59(6):864–78.
78. Obedin-Maliver J, Goldsmith ES, Stewart L, et al. Lesbian, gay, bisexual, and transgender-related content in undergraduate medical education. JAMA. 2011;306(9):971–7.
79. Deutsch MB, Green J, Keatley J, Mayer G, Hastings J, Hall AM. Electronic medical records and the transgender patient: recommendations from the World Professional Association for Transgender Health EMR Working Group. J Am Med Inform Assoc. 2013;20(4):700–3.

Chapter 16
The Needs of Racial/Ethnic LGBT Individuals Across the Cancer Care Continuum

Alicia K. Matthews, Natalie Ross, Meenhye Lee and Frances Aranda

Abstract In the past two decades there has been a proliferation of research, services and political and social advocacy for sexual minority individuals. Despite these gains, knowledge about sexual minorities of color remains quite limited. The majority of studies on LGBT and cancer are hindered by low representation of non-Whites and few studies have large enough samples of people of color to permit reliable statistical analyses and meaningful results. Smaller-scale studies that rely on volunteer samples often include larger proportions of race/ethnic minority women, but even studies that purposefully target these groups are limited by relatively small subgroup sample sizes, particularly for groups other than African American and Latina. At least part of the problem of recruitment of LGBT individuals of color relates to historical distrust of research and White researchers in communities of color. However, other factors likely include the lack of cultural competency of researchers, failure to utilize evidence-based and proven approaches to recruit and retain individuals of color, research protocols that include exclusion criteria that disproportionately impact participants of color, and the reluctance of some people to disclose a sexual- or gender-minority status, to name just a few challenges. Against this backdrop of limited empirical data, we provide an overview of the unique issues facing LGBT individuals of color, and provide a discussion of general and unique risk factors across the cancer control continuum.

Introduction

In the United States, cancer cases are expected to increase 45 % by 2030, becoming the leading cause of death in [1]. In 2012, it was estimated that nearly 1.6 million cases of cancer were diagnosed—790,740 cases for women in particular [2]. In 2013, another 1.7 million cases are expected to be diagnosed in the United States,

A. K. Matthews (✉) · M. Lee · F. Aranda
College of Nursing, University of Illinois, Chicago, IL, USA
e-mail: Aliciak@uic.edu

N. Ross
Howard Brown Health Center, Chicago, IL, USA

U. Boehmer, R. Elk (eds.), *Cancer and the LGBT Community*,
DOI 10.1007/978-3-319-15057-4_16

Table 16.1 Age-adjusted cancer incidence rates by race/ethnicity: United States, 2010*

Cancer site	All	African American/ Black	American Indian/Alaska Native	Asian/ Pacific Islander	Hispanic	White
Breast	118.7	117.2	61.2	85.8	86.1	119.5
Cervical	7.5	9.8	6.3	6.3	9.6	7.2
Colon-Rectum (Women)	35.4	42.6	27.0	28.5	29.4	34.4
Colon-Rectum (Men)	46.2	56.9	32.1	38.5	41.7	45.2
Age-Adjusted Cancer Death Rates by Race/Ethnicity: United States, 2010*						
Breast	21.9	30.2	11.4	11.7	14.3	21.3
Cervical	2.3	3.9	22	1.7	2.6	2.1
Colon-Rectum (Women)	13.0	17.6	9.7	9.8	9.4	12.6
Colon-Rectum (Men)	18.7	27.5	14.2	13.1	15.7	18.1

*Note: Rates are per 100,000 persons: U.S. Cancer Statistics Working group. United States Cancer Statistics: 1999–2010 Incidence and Mortality Web-based Report. Atlanta: U.S. Department of Health and Human Services, Centers for Disease Control and Prevention and National Cancer Institute; 2013. Available at: www.cdc.gov/uscs

and about 580,350 US Americans are expected to die of cancer this year. The toll exacted by cancer is not evenly distributed across U.S. populations, with demonstrated cancer disparities among subsections of the population based on a range of factors including socioeconomic status, race/ethnicity, residence, and sex. As shown in Table 16.1, among both men and women, racial and ethnic minorities—in particular African Americans are disproportionately burdened with cancer. To illustrate, breast cancer is the most common cancer in African American women [2]. Long-term survival rates for breast cancer among African Americans are significantly lower than their White counterparts despite a lower breast cancer incidence rate (78 vs. 90%). Similar disparities by race exist in cervical cancer incidence and mortality rates, with African American women having a 2.6% higher incidence than White women [2]. Moreover, cancer mortality rates are 7.7% higher in African American women than White women [2]. Among men, the patterns are similar with African Americans and Latinos experiencing the highest rates of cancer and mortality associated with cancers. Reasons for such inequities include a number of interrelated (i.e. sociocultural, linguistic, economic, structural) barriers to prevention and treatment [3]. There are other subpopulations who report even great risk for cancer rates specifically, the lesbian, gay, bisexual, and transgender (LGBT) populations.

Cancer Disparities and LGBT Populations

In response to the clear and persistent trends the elimination of cancer-related health disparities among racial/ethnic minorities has been a national public health priority. For the first time *Healthy People 2020*, the nation's roadmap for improving the health of US Americans, also includes sexual minorities as a priority. Although precise data on cancer rates among lesbians are lacking [4], evidence suggests that sexual minority status may contribute to excess risk for the development of certain types of cancers, including breast cancer [5, 6], anal cancer [7], lung cancer [8] and cancers associated with HIV/AIDS [9]. The causes of these disparities are complex and likely influenced by the same factors that drive cancer disparity rates among African American and other underserved populations. These factors include poor continuity of care [10]; socioeconomic factors, such as lack of adequate insurance coverage [11]; medical mistrust [12]; cultural and emotional factors [13]; and providers' unintentional bias and inadequate cultural competency [14].

To date, few cancer-related studies have been conducted with LGBT people of color. Until additional research is available, clinicians, researchers, and policy makers must extrapolate from the extant literature on race/ethnicity and sexual minorities in general. However, an intersectional analysis would suggest that neither literature will adequately capture the experiences of LGBT people of color [15]. Due to exposure to multiple interlocking systems of oppression, sexual orientation likely exacerbates existing racial/ethnic disparities among LGBT people of color [15].

At this point it is important to note that similar to the population at large, LGBT individuals of color will come from multiple and diverse communities, each with their own cultural norms, attitudes, behaviors, and beliefs. However, the experiences of belonging to two distinct identity groups—one based on race/ethnicity and the other based on sexual orientation and/or gender identity—may create some commonalities linking members of diverse LGBT communities of color based on shared experiences of oppression and discrimination. That being said, this chapter will not be a comprehensive review of each of the primary racial/ethnic groups residing in the U.S. nor, due to lack of data, will it be an adequate review of any one racial/ethnic group. Instead the purpose of this chapter is to describe the extant literature on cancer-related disparities across the cancer continuum in LGBT populations. Where possible, an emphasis will be placed on highlighting the unique needs and concerns of LGBT of color, aiming to improve the experiences and outcomes associated with cancer in these diverse communities.

Cancer and LGBT Communities of Color

In the past two decades there has been a proliferation of research, services and political and social advocacy for sexual minority individuals. Despite these gains, knowledge about sexual minorities of color remains quite limited. The majority of studies on LGBT and cancer are hindered by low representation of non-Whites and few studies have large enough samples of people of color to permit reliable statistical analyses and meaningful results. Smaller-scale studies that rely on volunteer samples often include larger proportions of race/ethnic minority women, but even studies that purposefully target these groups are limited by relatively small subgroup sample sizes, particularly for groups other than African American and Latinos. At least part of the problem of recruitment of LGBT of color relates to historical distrust of research and White researchers in communities of color [16]. However, other factors likely include the lack of cultural competency of researchers [17], failure to utilize evidence-based and proven approaches to recruit and retain individuals of color [18], research protocols that include exclusion criteria that disproportionately impact participants of color [19], and the reluctance of some people to disclose a sexual- or gender-minority status [20], to name just a few challenges. Against this backdrop of limited empirical data, we provide an overview of the unique issues facing LGBT of color, and provide a discussion of general and unique risk factors across the cancer control continuum.

LGBT Research Across the Cancer Control Continuum

In 2009, the Institute of Medicine (IOM) published a comprehensive review of racial and ethnic disparities in health care [14]. In this report, a model was presented that posited health care disparities arise from a complex interplay of economic, social, and cultural factors (see Fig. 16.1). The model also emphasized that disparities can occur at multiple phases along the cancer control continuum. As seen in Fig. 16.1, the cancer control continuum includes cancer prevention, early detection, diagnosis and treatment, survivorship and end-of life care. In the following sections, we discuss each phase of the cancer control continuum and briefly review the available literature on LGBT populations, and information specific to LGBT of color were available.

Prevention Behavioral and lifestyle factors have been identified as contributing to cancer disparities based on race/ethnicity [22]. In the general population, modifiable health risk behaviors with strong links to cancer include tobacco and alcohol

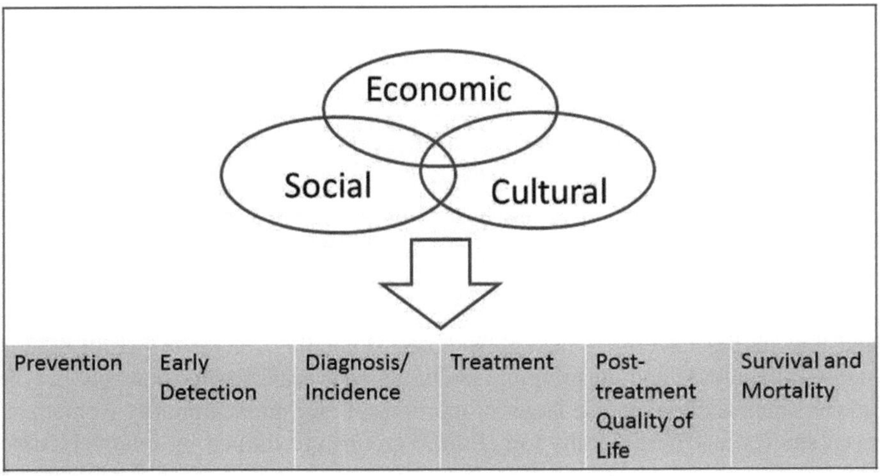

Fig. 16.1 Factors that influence health disparities. (Source [21]; Uses with Permission)

use, level of physical activity, and body weight status [23]. Sexual minority individuals have numerous behavioral risks for cancer including high rates of obesity, high rates of alcohol and tobacco use; and among women, reproductive risk factors such as nulliparity; lower rates of birth control use, and older age of first birth [24–30]. The negative impact of these factors may be compounded by the combined influences of a sexual minority status and a racial minority status. For example, 78.2 % of African American women meet criteria for being overweight and 49.6 % for obesity, while 61.2 % of White women meet the criteria for being overweight and 33.0 % for obesity [31]. A more recent study [32], found that compared with heterosexual women of the same race/ethnicity, White and African American sexual minority women had an increased likelihood of being overweight and maintaining that overweight status overtime. However, sexual minority status was unrelated to weight among Latinas and inconsistently linked to weight among Asian women. Among men, sexual minority status was protective against unhealthy weight among all major racial/ethnic groups examined.

The lack of behavioral interventions aimed at reducing cancer risk behaviors among sexual minority populations is another important barrier to improving cancer outcomes. HIV and STI prevention studies represent the highest proportion of behavioral and health promotion intervention involving LGBT participants [33]. Studies associated with tobacco cessation are emerging in the literature [34–36]. However, the available literature points to a clear need for additional research aimed at increasing physical activity, smoking cessation, and diet and nutrition. Studies examining the comparative benefit of culturally tailored versus non-tailored interventions remain a priority as well as studies that are specifically focused on LGBT communities of color [37].

Detection and Diagnosis Cancer screening behaviors may directly contribute to elevated risk for late-stage diagnosis and poor cancer outcomes. Primary among the target strategies for reducing cancer health disparities is increasing access to and participation in cancer screening by racial and ethnic minorities [38]. In the general population, racial/ethnic minorities are more likely to be diagnosed with more advanced stages of cancer compared to Whites [39]. Racial/ethnic minorities are also less likely to follow up on abnormal mammography results in a timely fashion, which leads to a decreased likelihood of being diagnosed at earlier stages of cancer formation [40]. Sexual minority women have also been identified as a population at risk for late-stage diagnosis of cancer [25]. Grindel et al. [41] found that among lesbians, rates of breast cancer screening in the past two years ranged from 58 to 84 %. Additionally, rates of cervical cancer screening continue to be lower than expected for women in the general population [42]. Charlton et al. [43] reported that compared to heterosexual women, sexual minority women (SMW) are significantly less likely to report past year and ever having cervical cancer screening. However, one review article found the literature to be mixed as to whether there are sexual orientation group disparities in mammographic screening [44]. In one of the few studies reporting on African American SMW, Ramsey et al. [45] found that 35 % of a sample of 1596 African American lesbians, age 18–70 years, reported they did not see a gynecologist regularly. Matthews et al. [42] reported on cancer risk and screening behaviors of African American SMW. Eighty-five percent of women over the age of forty reported ever having a mammogram and 69 % reported having been screened in the previous year. The majority of participants reported ever having a Pap test but reports of past year screening were low (68 %). A limitation of the two previous studies was the lack of a heterosexual comparison group. At least one study did not find differences based on sexual orientation in samples of women of color in having recent mammograms [46].

Despite consistent reports of lower screening rates, little is known about the factors contributing to the disparity. The research to date suggests that health care factors place SMW women at late stage detection and treatment of cancers including a lower likelihood of having medical insurance, poor access to health care services, the lack of culturally competent health care providers, and unmet medical needs [47]. Among heterosexual women, these factors have been directly related to lower screening rates. Although access to health care is a known barrier to cancer screening, Kerker et al. [48] found that SMW were less likely than heterosexual women to have had routine breast or cervical screening, even after controlling for health insurance coverage. One factor that may serve as a unique barrier to screening for SMW is homophobia and the lack of cultural competency of health care providers. Research suggests that SMW are less likely to engage in preventive health care [49]. This may be in part explained by communication barriers with health care providers arising from fears of homophobia or based on past negative experiences [48]. Perceived discrimination in health care settings has been associated with lower rates of cancer screening among SMW. Tracy et al. [50] found non-routine screeners were more likely to delay seeking healthcare and less likely to disclose sexual minority orientation to their primary care physician as a result of perceived discrimination. Further, health care providers frequently do not ask about sexual orientation or assume heterosexuality which also serves as a key barrier to appropriate health care [51].

Among gay and bisexual men, little is known about adherence to colorectal or prostate screening recommendations. However, more is known about anal cancers with research being conducted that examined knowledge and risk perception [52], studies examining uptake of anal cytology screening among HIV positive men who have sex with men (MSM) [53], barriers and facilitators to routine human papillomavirus (HPV) screening [54], and the psychological impact of anal cancer screening among HIV-infected MSM [55]. In a study examining uptake of HPV screening among MSM, D'Souza et al. [56] found that anal Pap screening was uncommon among a large sample of MSM with rates somewhat higher among HIV-infected MSM (10 % vs. 39 %). Most study participants expressed moderate or strong interest in screening (86 %) with high rates of uptake of screening when offered (85 %). Declining to have screening was associated with being African American suggesting a potential for HPV-related anal cancers among MSM secondary to lower rates of screening.

Treatment Individual experiences within the health care system influence attitudes about receipt of health care services and potentially also the utilization of health care services [57, 58]. The quality of the patient-provider interaction is one important component of a patient's experience within a health care setting [59]. Research suggests that health care providers who are more informative, give more explanations, show more sensitivity to the patient's concerns, and offer more reassurance and support tend to have patients who are more satisfied with care, have a greater understanding of health issues, and are more committed to treatment recommendations [60]. Problems within the patient-provider relationship have been shown to contribute to a reduction in treatment seeking [61], engagement in health care [62], perceptions of the quality of health services received [63], as well as treatment satisfaction and emotional adjustment to illness [64]. The hypothesized mechanism for the relationship between patient-provider relationship variables and health outcomes is thought to stem from the links between positive patient-provider interactions which leads to patient satisfaction and adherence to recommended treatments [65].

In the general population, demographic characteristics have been shown to correlate with health and health care experiences. For example, Johnson et al. [66] conducted a study to examine the association between patient race/ethnicity and patient-physician communication during medical visits. The results showed that physicians behaved more verbally dominant and offered less patient-centered communication with African American patients than with White patients. Moreover, both African American patients and their physicians exhibited lower levels of positive affect than White patients and their physicians did [66]. Although racial disparities remain a significant concern, bias and discrimination in health care settings due to sexual minority status is well established [67, 68]. Other barriers for LGBT persons include physician ignorance regarding LGBT health risks and needs [69, 70], reduced access to preventive health services [71], lack of insurance coverage or access to partner benefits [72, 73] clinicians' homophobia [74] and poor access to culturally competent, preventive, and ongoing health care services [47]. Combined, the above factors may act as formidable barriers to accessing high quality health care. However, the available literature suggests that while sexual minorities may have different preferences in cancer treatments (i.e., lower rates of breast reconstruction among lesbian breast cancer patients) [75], differences in overall quality of care have not been identified.

Post-Treatment QOL and Cancer Survivorship Cancer treatments have advanced significantly in the past thirty years. Currently, about 65 % of all people with cancer can expect to live at least 5 years after their diagnosis. Nevertheless, cancer survival may be associated with short- and long-term physical and psychological morbidity secondary to the effects of cancer and related treatment. The Institute of Medicine (IOM) highlighted the importance of mental health services for cancer patients and survivors [76]. The IOM report noted that psychosocial problems are common and may include fear of cancer recurrence and death, anxiety and depression, feelings of alienation and isolation, problems with interpersonal relationships, and economic hardships related to cost of care, job loss, and employment and insurance discrimination. Given the rapidly increasing number of cancer survivors, more research looking at the impact that cancer diagnosis and treatment have on quality of life, and factors that affect the quality of cancer survivorship, is highly warranted.

Among sexual minority populations, the largest preponderance of research associated with cancer has focused on issues associated with the survivorship period and have primarily been conducted with sexual minority women with a history of breast cancer. These studies have included examinations of quality of life [75, 77], emotional adjustment [78, 79], sexual functioning [80], supportive needs and resources [81], and physical health symptoms and morbidity [82]. Results were mixed as to whether sexual orientation negatively impacts women's experiences in the survivorship period with some studies suggesting differences in adjustment and response while other studies have found no differences. Inconsistencies in results are likely due to the range of issues addressed and the relatively small number of studies that exist. As in most other areas of cancer research involving LGBT individuals, the majority of studies examining the survivorship period were unable to compare outcomes based on race/ethnicity. Further research is needed to examine the survivorship needs and experiences of LGBT people of color especially as it relates to the availability of family specific emotional and tangible support.

Conclusions

Cancer initiatives over the last 40 years have resulted in earlier detection, advanced treatment, and increased prevention efforts. Progression in the field is evidenced by a substantial decrease in overall cancer mortality rates and an increase in the 5-year survival rate in the general population. However, as the second most common cause of death in the United States, cancer remains a significant public health concern as it continues to disproportionately affect particular segments of the U.S. population [83]. Individuals at the intersections of race/ethnicity and sexual minority status may be at elevated risk for poor outcomes across the cancer care continuum due to the combined impact of poor adherence to cancer screening, barriers to adequate health care services and engagement in cancer promoting health risk behaviors. The paucity of information about the needs and experiences of sexual minorities of color suggest the need for prioritizing research that has implications for all aspects of the cancer control continuum.

References

1. Siegel R, DeSantis C, Virgo K, Stein K, Mariotto A, Smith T, et al. Cancer treatment and survivorship statistics, 2012. CA Cancer J Clin. 2012;62(4):220–41.
2. Siegel R, Naishadham D, Jemal A. Cancer statistics, 2012. CA Cancer J Clin. 2012;62(1):10–29.

3. Simard EP, Naishadham D, Saslow D, Jemal A. Age-specific trends in black–white disparities in cervical cancer incidence in the United States: 1975–2009. Gynecol Oncol. 2012;127(3):611–5.
4. Bowen DJ, Boehmer U. The lack of cancer surveillance data on sexual minorities and strategies for change. Cancer Causes Control. 2007;18(4):343–9.
5. Cochran SD, Mays VM. Risk of breast cancer mortality among women cohabiting with same sex partners: findings from the National Health Interview Survey, 1997–2003. J Womens Health (Larchmt). 2012;21(5):528–33.
6. Boehmer U, Miao X, Ozonoff A. Cancer survivorship and sexual orientation. Cancer. 2011;117(16):3796–804.
7. Machalek DA, Poynten M, Jin F, Fairley CK, Farnsworth A, Garland SM, et al. Anal human papillomavirus infection and associated neoplastic lesions in men who have sex with men: a systematic review and meta-analysis. Lancet Oncol. 2012;13(5):487–500.
8. Boehmer U, Ozonoff A, Miao X. An ecological analysis of colorectal cancer incidence and mortality: differences by sexual orientation. BMC Cancer. 2011;11:400. doi:10.1186/1471-2407-11-400.
9. Shiels MS, Pfeiffer RM, Gail MH, Hall HI, Li J, Chaturvedi AK, et al. Cancer burden in the HIV-infected population in the United States. J Natl Cancer Inst. 2011;103(9):753–62.
10. Bigby J, Holmes MD. Disparities across the breast cancer continuum. Cancer Causes Control. 2005;16(1):35–44.
11. Bouchardy C, Verkooijen HM, Fioretta G. Social class is an important and independent prognostic factor of breast cancer mortality. Int J Cancer. 2006;119(5):1145–51.
12. Bickell NA, Weidmann J, Fei K, Lin JJ, Leventhal H. Underuse of breast cancer adjuvant treatment: patient knowledge, beliefs, and medical mistrust. J Clin Oncol. 2009;27(31):5160–7.
13. Guidry JJ, Torrence W, Herbelin S. Closing the divide: diverse populations and cancer survivorship. Cancer. 2005;104(S11):2577–83.
14. Smedley BD, Stith AY, Nelson AR. Unequal treatment: confronting racial and ethnic disparities in health care (with CD). Washington, DC: National Academies Press; 2009.
15. Bowleg L. The problem with the phrase women and minorities: intersectionality—an important theoretical framework for public health. Am J Public Health. 2012;102(7):1267–73.
16. Braunstein JB, Sherber NS, Schulman SP, Ding EL, Powe NR. Race, medical researcher distrust, perceived harm, and willingness to participate in cardiovascular prevention trials. Medicine (Baltimore). 2008;87(1):1–9.
17. Chao MM, Okazaki S, Hong Y. The quest for multicultural competence: challenges and lessons learned from clinical and organizational research. Soc Personal Psychol Compass. 2011;5(5):263–74.
18. Ejiogu N, Norbeck JH, Mason MA, Cromwell BC, Zonderman AB, Evans MK. Recruitment and retention strategies for minority or poor clinical research participants: lessons from the Healthy Aging in Neighborhoods of Diversity across the Life Span study. Gerontologist. 2011;51(Suppl 1):S33–45.
19. King AC, Cao D, Southard CC, Matthews A. Racial differences in eligibility and enrollment in a smoking cessation clinical trial. Health Psychol. 2011;30(1):40.
20. McFarland W, Caceres CF. HIV surveillance among men who have sex with men. AIDS. 2001;15:S23–S32.
21. Ward E, et al. Cancer disparities by Race Socioeconomic Status. CA Cancer J Clin. 2008;52(2):78–93. doi:10.3322/canjclin.52.2.78.
22. Institute of Medicine, National Research Council. Lifestyle behaviors contributing to the burden of cancer. In: Curry S, Byers T, Hewitt M, editors. Fulfilling the potential of cancer prevention and early detection. Washington, DC: The National Academies Press; pp. 41–86.
23. Jemal A, Center MM, DeSantis C, Ward EM. Global patterns of cancer incidence and mortality rates and trends. Cancer Epidemiol Biomark Prev. 2010;19(8):1893–907.
24. Valanis BG, Bowen DJ, Bassford T, Whitlock E, Charney P, Carter RA. Sexual orientation and health: comparisons in the women's health initiative sample. Arch Fam Med. 2000;9(9):843–53.

25. Cochran SD, Mays VM, Bowen D, Gage S, Bybee D, Roberts SJ, et al. Cancer-related risk indicators and preventive screening behaviors among lesbians and bisexual women. Am J Public Health. 2001;91(4):591–7.
26. Gruskin EP, Hart S, Gordon N, Ackerson L. Patterns of cigarette smoking and alcohol use among lesbians and bisexual women enrolled in a large health maintenance organization. Am J Public Health. 2001;91(6):976–9.
27. Case P, Austin SB, Hunter DJ, Manson JE, Malspeis S, Willett WC, et al. Sexual orientation, health risk factors, and physical functioning in the Nurses' Health Study II. J Womens Health (Larchmt). 2004;13(9):1033–47.
28. Austin SB, Ziyadeh N, Kahn JA, Camargo CA, Jr, Colditz GA, Field AE. Sexual orientation, weight concerns, and eating-disordered behaviors in adolescent girls and boys. J Am Acad Child Adolesc Psychiatry. 2004;43(9):1115–23.
29. Dibble SL, Roberts SA, Nussey B. Comparing breast cancer risk between lesbians and their heterosexual sisters. Womens Health Issues. 2004;14(2):60–8.
30. Kavanaugh-Lynch MHE, White E, Daling JR, Bowen DJ. Correlates of lesbian sexual orientation and the risk of breast cancer. J Gay Lesbian Med Assoc. 2002;6(3–4):91–5.
31. Zeigler-Johnson C, Weber A, Glanz K, Spangler E, Rebbeck TR. Gender- and ethnic-specific associations with obesity: individual and neighborhood-level factors. J Natl Med Assoc. 2013(Summer);105(2):173–82.
32. Deputy NP, Boehmer U. Determinants of body weight among men of different sexual orientation. Prev Med. 2010;51(2):129–31.
33. Coulter RW, Kenst KS, Bowen DJ. Research funded by the National Institutes of health on the health of lesbian, gay, bisexual, and transgender populations. Am J Public Health. 2014;104(2):e105–12.
34. Matthews AK, Conrad M, Kuhns L, Vargas M, King AC. Project Exhale: preliminary evaluation of a tailored smoking cessation treatment for HIV-positive African American smokers. AIDS Patient Care STDS. 2013;27(1):22–32.
35. Matthews AK, Li C, Kuhns LM, Tasker TB, Cesario JA. Results from a community-based smoking cessation treatment program for LGBT smokers. J Environ Public Health. 2013;2013:984508.
36. Eliason MJ, Dibble SL, Gordon R, Soliz GB. The last drag: an evaluation of an LGBT-specific smoking intervention. J Homosex. 2012;59(6):864–78.
37. Committee on Lesbian Gay Bisexual and Transgender Health Issues and Research Gaps and Opportunities, Institute of Medicine. The health of lesbian, gay, bisexual, and transgender people: building a foundation for better understanding. Washington, DC: National Academies Press; 2011.
38. Smith RA, Brooks D, Cokkinides V, Saslow D, Brawley OW. Cancer screening in the United States, 2013. CA Cancer J Clin. 2013;63(2):87–105.
39. Ghafoor A, Jemal A, Cokkinides V, Cardinez C, Murray T, Samuels A, et al. Cancer statistics for African Americans. CA Cancer J Clin. 2002;52(6):326–41.
40. Smith ER, Adams SA, Das IP, Bottai M, Fulton J, Hebert JR. Breast cancer survival among economically disadvantaged women: the influences of delayed diagnosis and treatment on mortality. Cancer Epidemiol Biomarkers Prev. 2008;17(10):2882–90.
41. Grindel CG, McGehee LA, Patsdaughter CA, Roberts SJ. Cancer prevention and screening behaviors in lesbians. Women Health. 2007;44(2):15–39.
42. Matthews AK, Li C, Ross N, Jodi Ram B, Rebecca Ramsey M. Breast and cervical cancer screening behaviors of African American sexual minority women. J Gen Pract. 2013;1(107):2.
43. Charlton BM, Corliss HL, Missmer SA, Frazier AL, Rosario M, Kahn JA, et al. Reproductive health screening disparities and sexual orientation in a cohort study of US adolescent and young adult females. J Adolesc Health. 2011;49(5):505–10.
44. Brown JP, Tracy JK. Lesbians and cancer: an overlooked health disparity. Cancer Causes Control. 2008;19(10):1009–20.
45. Ramsey F, Hill M, Kellam C. Black lesbians matter: an examination of the unique experiences, perspectives, and priorities of the Black lesbian community. Sacramento: Zuna Institute; 2010.

46. Mays VM, Yancey AK, Cochran SD, Weber M, Fielding JE. Heterogeneity of health disparities among African American, Hispanic, and Asian American women: unrecognized influences of sexual orientation. Am J Public Health. 2002;92(4):632–9.
47. Diamant AL, Wold C, Spritzer K, Gelberg L. Health behaviors, health status, and access to and use of health care: a population-based study of lesbian, bisexual, and heterosexual women. Arch Fam Med. 2000;9(10):1043–51.
48. Kerker BD, Mostashari F, Thorpe L. Health care access and utilization among women who have sex with women: Sexual behavior and identity. J Urban Health. 2006;83(5):970–9.
49. Buchmueller T, Carpenter CS. Disparities in health insurance coverage, access, and outcomes for individuals in same-sex versus different-sex relationships, 2000–2007. Am J Public Health. 2010;100(3):489–95.
50. Tracy JK, Lydecker AD, Ireland L. Barriers to cervical cancer screening among lesbians. J Womens Health. 2010;19(2):229–37.
51. Petroll AE, Mosack KE. Physician awareness of sexual orientation and preventive health recommendations to men who have sex with men. Sex Transm Dis. 2011;38(1):63–7.
52. Sanchez DM, Pathela P, Niccolai LM, Schillinger JA. Knowledge of human papillomavirus and anal cancer among men who have sex with men attending a New York City sexually transmitted diseases clinic. Int J STD AIDS. 2012;23(1):41–3.
53. Goodall L, Clutterbuck D. Anal cytology screening in HIV-positive men who have sex with men: experience in a city centre HIV clinic. Int J STD AIDS. 2012;23(9):623–5.
54. Truesdale MD, Goldstone SE. The fear factor: drivers and barriers to follow-up screening for human papillomavirus-related anal cancer in men who have sex with men. Int J STD AIDS. 2010;21(7):482–8.
55. Tinmouth J, Raboud J, Ali M, Malloch L, Su D, Sano M, et al. The psychological impact of being screened for anal cancer in HIV-infected men who have sex with men. Dis Colon Rectum. 2011;54(3):352–9.
56. D'Souza G, Cook RL, Ostrow D, Johnson-Hill LM, Wiley D, Silvestre T. Anal cancer screening behaviors and intentions in men who have sex with men. J Gen Intern Med. 2008;23(9):1452–7.
57. LaVeist TA, Nickerson KJ, Bowie JV. Attitudes about racism, medical mistrust, and satisfaction with care among African American and white cardiac patients. Med Care Res Rev. 2000;57(4 suppl):146–61.
58. Jacobs EA, Rathouz PJ, Karavolos K, Everson-Rose SA, Janssen I, Kravitz HM, et al. Perceived discrimination is associated with reduced breast and cervical cancer screening: the Study of Women's Health Across the Nation (SWAN). J Womens Health. 2013;23(2):138–45.
59. Beach MC, Rosner M, Cooper LA, Duggan PS, Shatzer J. Can patient-centered attitudes reduce racial and ethnic disparities in care? Acad Med. 2007;82(2):193–8.
60. Suarez-Almazor ME. Patient-physician communication. Curr Opin Rheumatol. 2004;16(2):91–5.
61. Schoenthaler AM, Schwartz BS, Wood C, Stewart WF. Patient and physician factors associated with adherence to diabetes medications. Diabetes Educ. 2012;38(3):397–408.
62. Flickinger TE, Saha S, Moore RD, Beach MC. Higher quality communication and relationships are associated with improved patient engagement in HIV care. J Acquir Immune Defic Syndr. 2013;63(3):362–6.
63. Clift JB, Kirby J. Health care access and perceptions of provider care among individuals in same-sex couples: findings from the Medical Expenditure Panel Survey (MEPS). J Homosex. 2012;59(6):839–50.
64. Trevino KM, Fasciano K, Prigerson HG. Patient-oncologist alliance, psychosocial well-being, and treatment adherence among young adults with advanced cancer. J Clin Oncol. 2013;31(13):1683–9.
65. Brown JB, Stewart M, Ryan BL. Outcomes of patient-provider interaction. In: Thompson T, Dorsey A, Miller K, Parrott R, editors. Handbook of health communication. Mahwah: Lawrence Erlbaum Associates Inc.; 2003:141–61.

66. Johnson RL, Roter D, Powe NR, Cooper LA. Patient race/ethnicity and quality of patient-physician communication during medical visits. Am J Public Health. 2004;94(12):2084–90.
67. Kinsler JJ, Wong MD, Sayles JN, Davis C, Cunningham WE. The effect of perceived stigma from a health care provider on access to care among a low-income HIV-positive population. AIDS Patient Care STDS. 2007;21(8):584–92.
68. Beach MC, Saha S, Korthuis PT, Sharp V, Cohn J, Wilson IB, et al. Patient–provider communication differs for black compared to white HIV-infected patients. AIDS Behav 2011;15(4):805–11.
69. Pelletier MG, Tschurtz B. Meeting the health care needs of LGBT patients. J Nurs Care Qual. 2012;27(2):95–8.
70. Kane-Lee E, Bayer CR. Meeting the needs of LGBT patients and families. Nurs Manage. 2012;43(2):42–6.
71. Hart SL, Bowen DJ. Sexual orientation and intentions to obtain breast cancer screening. J Womens Health. 2009;18(2):177–85.
72. Gonzales G, Blewett LA. National and state-specific health insurance disparities for adults in same-sex relationships. Am J Public Health. 2014;104(2):e95–e104.
73. Ponce NA, Cochran SD, Pizer JC, Mays VM. The effects of unequal access to health insurance for same-sex couples in California. Health Aff (Millwood). 2010;29(8):1539–48.
74. Mosack KE, Brouwer AM, Petroll AE. Sexual identity, identity disclosure, and health care experiences: is there evidence for differential homophobia in primary care practice? Womens Health Issues. 2013;23(6):e341–6.
75. Matthews AK, Peterman AH, Delaney P, Menard L, Brandenburg D. A qualitative exploration of the experiences of lesbian and heterosexual patients with breast cancer. Oncol Nurs Forum. 2002;29(10):1455–62.
76. Hewitt M, Herdman R, Holland J. Meeting psychosocial needs of women with breast cancer. Washington, DC: National Academies Press; 2004.
77. Boehmer U, Glickman M, Milton J, Winter M. Health-related quality of life in breast cancer survivors of different sexual orientations. Qual Life Res. 2012;21(2):225–36.
78. Boehmer U, Glickman M, Winter M. Anxiety and depression in breast cancer survivors of different sexual orientations. J Consult Clin Psychol. 2012;80(3):382.
79. Jabson JM, Bowen DJ. Perceived stress and sexual orientation among breast cancer survivors. J Homosex. 2014;61(6):889–98 (just-accepted).
80. Boehmer U, Ozonoff A, Timm A, Winter M, Potter J. After breast cancer: sexual functioning of sexual minority survivors. J Sex Res. 2014;51(6):681–9.
81. Paul LB, Pitagora D, Brown B, Tworecke A, Rubin L. Support needs and resources of sexual minority women with breast cancer. Psychooncology. 2013;23(5):578–84.
82. Boehmer U, Glickman M, Winter M, Clark MA. Long-term breast cancer survivors' symptoms and morbidity: differences by sexual orientation? J Cancer Surviv. 2013;7(2):203–10.
83. DeSantis C, Naishadham D, Jemal A. Cancer statistics for African Americans, 2013. CA Cancer J Clin. 2013;63(3):151–66.

Part V
Healthcare Policy and LGBT Health

Chapter 17
Policy and its Impact on LGBT Cancer

Scout

Abstract Through years of public health work we now understand it is not biology but social factors that determine most of a person's lived experience of health. Thus these social factors, most especially the different manifestations of stigma, strongly determine the lived experience of health for LGBT people. The social factors represent community norms. These community norms are in turn influenced, or in cases curtailed, by public policies. This chapter will explore how public policies have an influence on the lived experience of health along the full cancer control continuum.

Through years of public health work we now understand it is not biology but social factors that determine most of a person's lived experience of health [1]. Thus these social factors, most especially the different manifestations of stigma, strongly determine the lived experience of health for LGBT people. The social factors represent community norms. These community norms are in turn influenced, or in cases curtailed, by public policies. This chapter will explore how public policies have an influence on the lived experience of health along the full cancer control continuum.

Scout (✉)
LGBT HealthLink at CenterLink: The Community of LGBT Centers, Fort Lauderdale, FL, USA
e-mail: scout@lgbtcenters.org

U. Boehmer, R. Elk (eds.), *Cancer and the LGBT Community*,
DOI 10.1007/978-3-319-15057-4_17

LGBT Policy Overview in the United States [2]

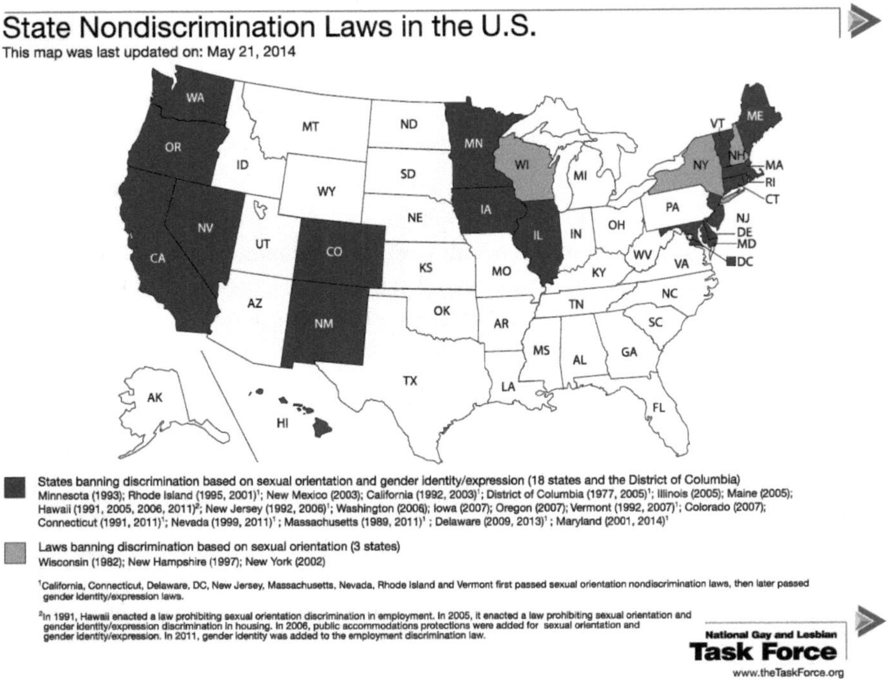

The issue map above from the National Gay and Lesbian Task Force shows the status of LGBT civil rights coverage in the United States. In each of the white regions, it is perfectly legal to fire a person for being LGBT, or refuse them housing, or access to a restaurant or hotel. In the grey regions, LGB but not T people are protected. In the black states, LGB and T people are protected. Even in the areas where nondiscrimination protections exist, this does not ensure nondiscrimination in educational environments, from elementary schools up through medical schools. To understand the experience of an LGBT person with cancer, it is important to know this information—because almost every LGBT person carries this information with them into each healthcare interaction. While it is not well understood in the mainstream population, the LGBT communities know civil rights are not guaranteed, it is too often legal for people to discriminate against LGBT people in jobs and in health.

The net effect of the lack of consistent nationwide nondiscrimination laws is that LGBT people do not have a basis of the same legal protections that provide a measure of safety and security to non-LGBT people. While community norms may have changed on some of these points, for example it is rather rare to fire someone for being gay today, they are not uniformly protected by public policy. Those who are more demonstrably different, such as trans people who cannot pass as gender normative, or effeminate gay men, or those who are also members of other stigmatized populations, such as LGBT people of color, are less likely to reap the benefits of the changing community norms.

What is Policy Inclusion for LGBT People?

Considering there are no federal nondiscrimination protections and there is a robust history of discrimination in health against LGBT people, any entity who does not go out of their way to demonstrate equitable treatment of LGBT people risks being a presumptive member of a class that discriminates against LGBT people. This is as valid for policy as it is for individual practitioners—policies that do not specify LGBT inclusion often support the historical status quo, ultimately achieving LGBT exclusion.

Crosscutting Issues: Surveillance and Research

Any discussion of policies affecting LGBT health usually starts with this topic. Health policies and services, no matter where they intersect the cancer continuum, are built on a foundation of surveillance and research. Those two foundational pieces then flow into policy-making, which then guides allocations, which in turn guide intervention programs. In this stream of health decisionmaking LGBT people are usually confounded at the very first two steps, surveillance and research.

In almost all federal surveillance systems, LGBT data are not routine demographic elements. Without data collection, there is never an evidence base of disparities from which to build explicit policy inclusion. While the first evidence of a significant smoking disparity for LGBT populations was reported in the mid-1990s [3], almost 20 years later there is still no data about LGBT cancer disparities. The piecemeal evidence that exists often does not meet the bar of proof needed for policy interventions and funding decisions. Thus the first and most widespread policy impact on LGBT cancer is the existing policy of masking LGBT health disparities by not including LGBT measures in routine surveillance or health research.

There have been several advancements in data collection over recent years. In 2012, after years of advocacy and education, the Secretary of the HHS reported they would be adding LGBT measures to the federal surveillance system which is a benchmark for more health goals than any other, the National Health Interview Survey (NHIS) [4]. Unfortunately, testing for a transgender measure was halted for more input, and has not yet resumed at the time of this writing. A newly tested "sexual identity" measure [5] was added to NHIS in Spring of 2013, and should soon yield a wave of new data to analyze.

In 2013, in an attempt to address the continued lack of progress on transgender data collection, HHS announced it was urging states to add LGB & T measures to their state surveillance systems, the Behavioral Risk Factor Surveillance System, and the associated Youth Risk Behavior System [6]. Is it is from aggregated state data from these surveys that the first clear data on risk factors are starting to emerge. For example, lesbians have a 30 % reduced odds of having an annual physical [7]. It is also these data that have already started to demonstrate that existing theories do not yet span the breadth of LGBT health disparities. For example, what theory accounts for the newly discovered fact that LGB adolescents use seat belts less often than others [8]?

Because the sample size for the BRFSS and YRBS is so high, getting tested LGBT measures on these surveys would yield a waterfall of data on LGBT cancer related behaviors. Unfortunately, even with federal urging only 17 states have now included LGBT measures [9]. In addition, not all of the measures are well-tested, so there remain concerns the resultant data, especially the trans data, might not be high value.

With the number of high quality full probability studies on LGBT smoking alone the existence of an LGBT-specific cancer disparity, has already been established. What is missing are surveillance and reporting data. Surveillance data are different from full probability studies for several reasons: first, states and the federal government rely on these data for policy decisions; second, they are considered higher standard of evidence and thus hold more weight for demonstrating need in proposals; third, since these are often the largest surveys, they are more likely to provide much needed evidence on the quality and magnitude of health gaps. Reporting data are the only way different types of cancers are tracked in different populations. Until LGBT data are included in all facets of health data collection as a routine part of a demographic battery, LGBT cancer disparities will continue to be masked by inexact science.

Crosscutting Issues: Funding

Funding mechanisms rarely state they are LGBT inclusive, which unwittingly creates ambiguity among applicants. This likely depresses the number of LGBT targeted proposals received, especially for those funding streams which are especially labor intensive, such as research proposals through National Institutes of Health (NIH). A recent analysis of NIH awards that mention LGBT by health topic area found a particular paucity of LGBT awards focused on cancer or tobacco. Of the 628 studies from 1989 through 2011 that mentioned LGBT, only 35 focused on cancer and only eight focused on tobacco [10]. The Network for LGBT Health Equity has put out a policy sheet, “LGBT Cultural Competency in Funding” [11]. In it they recommend three strategies to ensure funding announcements are welcoming to LGBT applicants:

1. When announcing funding, routinely identify LGBT people as a priority population.

2. Whenever possible, directly fund LGBT organizations.
3. Ensure the grant review process is also welcoming.

The 2011 Institute of Medicine report on LGBT health developed a series of recommendations to make NIH research more LGBT-inclusive [12]. Their seven top recommendations are listed here:

1. Create a full research agenda on LGBT health
2. Conduct consistent and routine LGBT data collection
3. Test best measures for such data collection
4. Record LGBT status in electronic health records
5. Research how to best reach our hard-to-find communities
6. Create a comprehensive training program to build the cadre of researchers
7. Set a standard whereby LGBT people are identified and routinely included in mainstream research.

As of 2015, while NIH has made significant strides on LGBT research inclusion, none of the Institute of Medicine recommendations have been implemented. The notable gaps in LGBT cancer research are poised to continue until larger scale interventions are implemented in the premier research funding institutions.

Cancer Control Continuum: Prevention

Much has been written about the effect of stigma on the health of individuals. While it remains hard to measure, stigma has a depressive effect on the health of individuals. Sometimes direct evidence of the impact of policies on individual health has been recorded, for example: LGBT people in states that pass an LGBT-unfriendly law report more mental health problems the next year [13]. Actually LGBT people in states *next to those* who have passed LGBT-unfriendly laws also report more mental health problems in the next year [13]. The national policies outlined above have a cumulative weathering effect on LGBT individuals, likely leaving them at greater risk for cancer in the first place.

Tobacco Control Policies

As is covered in the chapter on tobacco, LGBT people smoke cigarettes at rates 68 % higher than others [14]. This disparity emerges out of the stigma experienced, but is also related to policy inclusion decisions made by the tobacco industry, as compared to those made by the tobacco-control industry.

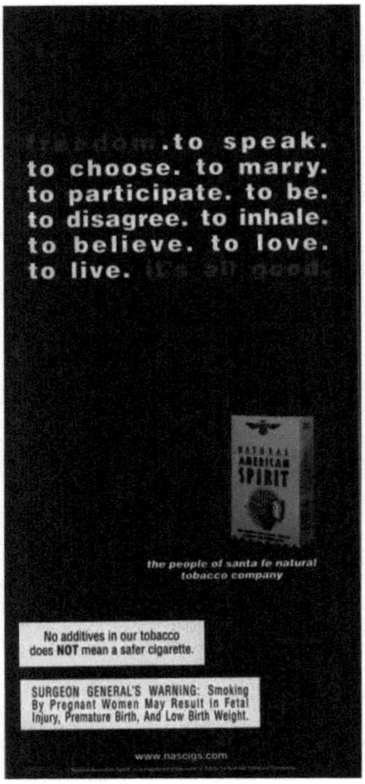

othe
er
case
es
the
toba
bacc

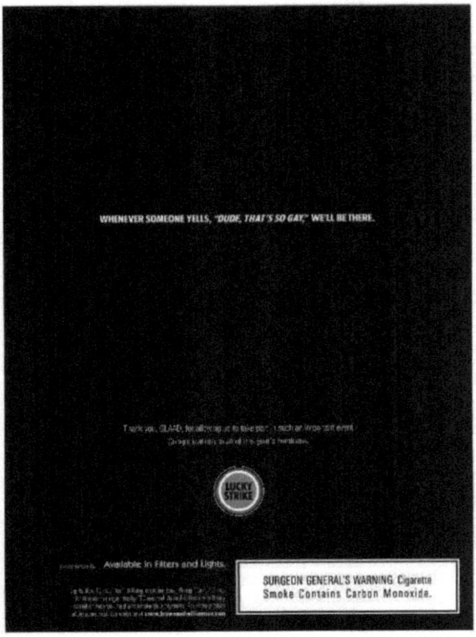

There is evidence from as early as 1993 that the tobacco industry companies were conducting market research on LGBT people [15], and tailoring outreach strategies to specifically include LGBT populations. The tobacco industry advertised early in LGBT publications, effectively setting them apart from the many companies in the 80s and 90s who were still reluctant to tailor ads for the LGBT population. Focus groups show community gratitude for this early tailoring is still a factor in LGBT opinions about the tobacco industry today [16]. The tobacco industry showed similar market savvy in tailoring the ads. Sometimes a person was added to the existing ad to make it more sexually ambiguous and therefor more LGBT tailored. In other cases the tobacco industry specifically built ads using LGBT civil rights messaging: two such examples are above.

Likewise, as early as 1993 Phillip Morris showed similar marketing savvy by heavily promoting their LGBT-welcoming philanthropic work and employment policies [15].

The tobacco control arena has been slower than the tobacco industry to use targeted marketing tactics to engage LGBT populations, but they are still ahead of many other health topic areas in LGBT inclusion. CDC's Office of Smoking and Health has funded tobacco disparity networks for many years, and has included an LGBT network among the portfolio for the last 12 years. The consistent presence of an LGBT tobacco disparity network has had a direct impact on integrating LGBT concerns into many policy decisions; much of the Network's engagement is about policy issues. The Network was instrumental in getting LGBT added to the National Partnership for Action to End Health Disparities Plan, getting a commitment of LGBT data collection from HHS Secretary Sebelius, getting LGBT added to the HHS Tobacco Control Action Plan, and to the mission statement of the new

Affordable Care Act Prevention Advisory Group. The Network advised CDC directly on data inclusion in the 2012 National Adult Tobacco Survey, leading to the first national LGBT smoking prevalence data [14]. They have advised many states on data inclusion and have had a multi-year effort to work with NIH to ensure their health research is more inclusive. In conjunction with the Network, CDC's Office of Smoking and Health has now included LGBT tailored ad in their last 3 years of mass media campaigns, the Tips Campaign from Former Smokers.

As strong as this activity is, there is still much more LGBT tailored activity from the tobacco industry as compared to the tobacco control programs. Few state level tobacco control campaigns have made it a policy to explicitly include LGBT tailored activities. Most tobacco quitlines do not train their staff on LGBT cultural competency. Some do not collect data on LGBT callers, again masking LGBT disparities. The tobacco industry has been bragging about their LGBT-inclusive employment policies since the 90s. As the employment chart earlier in this chapter shows, most of the state tobacco control programs do not have LGBT-inclusive employment non-discrimination policies. These policy gaps have a broadly depressive effect on LGBT tobacco control progress, which directly affects the prevalence of cancer among LGBT people.

Other Prevention Activities

Stimulus efforts then Affordable Care Act created a new wave of cancer prevention activities nationwide. An estimated half a billion dollars flowed into two different funding mechanisms (Communities Putting Prevention to Work and Community Transformation Grants) which in turn created local level programs focused on cancer risk reduction, specifically: physical activity, eating better, and staying smoke-free [17, 18]. As was highlighted by the LGBT HealthLink: The Network for Health Equity, despite top level LGBT inclusion in the Task Force on Prevention [19], the actual funding announcements for both of the mechanisms were at best equivocal on prioritizing LGBT inclusion [20]. Similarly, a separate funding stream focused on cancer prevention activities specifically was confined to racial and ethnic disparities. As a result, with this wave of new investment across the country, the LGBT HealthLink could identify few programs which included tailored activities for the LGBT communities. Much of this cancer prevention work is implemented by state and city health departments. Despite attempted LGBT prioritization in top-level federal policy documents, the relative lack of inclusion in federal funding announcements resulted in few tailored LGBT cancer prevention programs.

Cancer Control Continuum: Early Detection

In 1995, CDC funded The Mautner Project to launch the "Removing the Barriers" project. This project provided LGBT cultural competency training programs for healthcare providers, particularly to serve their National Breast and Cervical Cancer

Early Detection Program (NBCCEDP) sites across the country [21]. This funding showed an early willingness to welcome lesbian and bisexual women into one of the largest cancer screening programs across the country. In 2006 this funding ceased, there were no more overt LGBT activities by the CDC cancer offices until they started to co-fund the LGBT HealthLink in 2013 [21, 22].

One example related to cancer screening demonstrates both the challenges and the opportunities in the current policy environment. In October of 2013, a TV station in Colorado broke the news that a transgender woman had been denied free breast-cancer screenings at a local NBCCEDP site for not being “genetically female”. It is a credit to the growing LGBT health policy expertise at a national level that three organizations immediately sent letters to HHS and CDC asking for the rules governing who was eligible for care to be changed. Within days of the complaint the HHS LGBT liaison confirmed their HHS LGBT Issues Coordinating Committee is looking into revising the eligibility rules. By December of 2013 newly revised rules had been issued to all NBCCEDP sites across the country [23]. Their ruling was an interesting example of the policy moving forward even with a lack of data, illustrating the strategies used to create sound policies in such an environment.

> Although there are limited data regarding the risk for breast cancer among transgender women, evidence has shown that long term hormone use does increase the risk for breast cancer among women whose biological sex was female at birth. While CDC does not make any recommendation about routine screening among this population, transgender women are thus eligible under federal law to receive appropriate cancer screening. CDC recommends that grantees and providers counsel all eligible women, including transgender women, about the benefits and harms of screening and discuss individual risk factors to determine if screening is medically indicated.
> The Center of Excellence for Transgender Health and the World Professional Association for Transgender Health have developed consensus recommendations on preventive care services for the transgender population. Those recommendations include for ‘transwomen with past or current hormone use, breast-screening mammography in patients over age 50 with additional risk factors (e.g., estrogen and progestin use >5 years, positive family history, BMI>35)’. [24]

Note that CDC could not suggest any screening guidelines for the population, because as they admit, there are limited data for the risk of breast cancer in this population. But failing that, they found external guidelines, in this case developed by another organization they fund through their HIV arm, the Center for Excellence on Transgender Health. This group worked with another internationally recognized body, WPATH, to develop guidelines that could be adopted by CDC, and subsequently by the hundreds of free screening programs they fund across the country.

The example is interesting in several ways, it shows a current willingness by HHS to fix policies that are unfriendly to LGBT people and a successful if unusual pathway for moving to those fixes expediently. It highlights how policy can be created in the absence of data, often with the help of externally funded agencies. But at its core was a transgender woman who was able to take an extremely bold step; after being turned down from care she filed suit demanding such care and was willing to even go on TV to present her case. While there are many successes in this story, it takes an exceptional person to react to a healthcare barrier in such a public manner and thus this method to change policies is not easily replicable.

Fewer LGBT People with Insurance

Screening and other prophylactic health care is often a function of insurance. There is a persistent myth of LGBT affluence that would lead some to think LGBT people have higher insurance rates than others [25]. In fact, LGBT people are less likely to have insurance than their non-LGBT counterparts. An analysis of the Current Population Survey data over many years showed same sex couples were almost twice as likely to be uninsured as compared to opposite sex couples [26]. Much of this is a function of not having our relationships recognized by employers, thus not being eligible for employer-sponsored family insurance. The economists in the previous study projected that universal domestic partner coverage would reduce that insurance gap by 43 %. This insurance gap extends beyond couples as well. Over 1/3 of LGBT people with incomes under 400 % of poverty level are uninsured [27]. Trans people are significantly less likely to be insured than others.

Post-DOMA Relationship Recognition

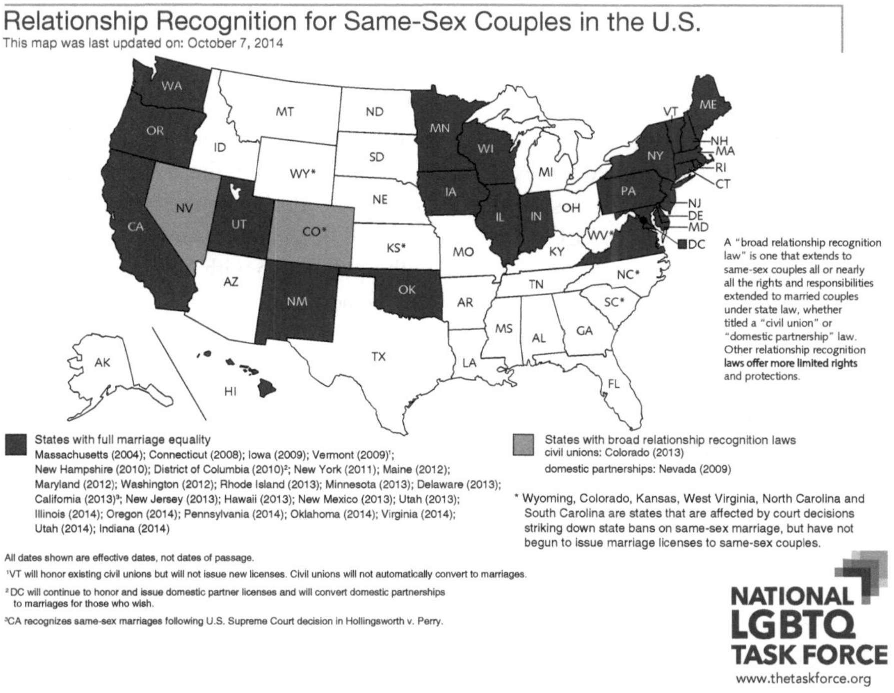

Researchers have long validated the link between marriage and better health. For people with cancer, being married usually provides a built-in advocacy and support team for the emotional and physical rigors of treatment. Until June of 2013, the Defense of Marriage Act (DOMA) had forbidden the federal government from recognizing same-sex marriage, even when performed in a state who had made such a marriage legal. The crux of the case hinged on a tax issue. Thus directly following this case the Internal Revenue Service adopted a "celebration policy", allowing same-sex marriages to be recognized by the federal government as long as they were performed in a state where they were legal [28]. The map above highlights the 25 states with full marriage equality. Many other states still ban any state equivalent of a celebration policy, although courts are increasingly ruling against these bans [29]. With this celebration policy, couples only needed to be married in a state with such recognition to get federal benefits, even if they later lived in a state without it. By early 2014 the U.S. Department of Health and Human Services announced they were also adopting the IRS celebration policy and working quickly to get it promulgated across all of their rulings [30]. This adoption of the celebration policy, and the precedent set by doing so, provides direct benefits to same-sex couples across the country. As more employers follow suit in recognizing either same-sex partners or legal marriages under employer insurance plans, a greater proportion of LGBT people will have access to cancer prevention and screening services through health insurance.

The Advent of the ACA

The advent of the Affordable Care Act is changing many different aspects of health and healthcare in the United States. As was mentioned earlier, there is a new investment in prevention across a spectrum of activities. Probably the most profound impact on the underinsured LGBT population will be via the insurance exchanges, both in simply offering insurance to those without, but also with new policy protections that will benefit the LGBT communities. In addition, section 1557 offers new anti-discrimination protections for LGBT people.

ACA: Insurance Policy Changes

Not only will the insurance exchanges cover more people, the policies enacted within them will help create an equitable base for insurance coverage. There are three levels of changes that will have the greatest impact on the LGBT population. First, insurers cannot deny or charge more individuals with a pre-existing condition like cancer [31]. Second, no one who works in the marketplaces, including insurers and employees, is allowed to discriminate against LGBT people [32]. Third, insurers cannot offer plans that discriminate based on sexual orientation or gender identity [32].

Cancer is a devastating condition in itself, to have it occur when equitable policies do not afford the same options as others can leave lasting barriers to care, some of which policy reversals still cannot rectify. In a recent public example, one lesbian was offered a job in another state, but since her new employer would not recognize her relationship her partner with cancer stayed behind to continue care in the old state [33]. Even though new ACA non-discrimination policies will prevent this from occurring among many employers in the future, this family is still left shuttling 1,000 miles each way while trying to negotiate being together for chemotherapy.

Unfortunately many of the protections of ACA are very new; they are not as widely known as would be beneficial, and they are not as widely enacted as would be beneficial. As with the case involving the trans woman and breast cancer screening, people experiencing discrimination must often be willing to engage in a public battle to get their due care. While this may be easier for someone being screened for cancer, it's harder to allot that extra energy to complaining about unfair treatment for people with a cancer diagnosis.

The trans care protections under ACA are likely to be very beneficial. Trans people have long hidden their trans status due to fear of insurance discrimination. For trans care, the levels of coverage are often divided into three tiers: mental health, hormones, and gender confirmation surgeries. Some states have interpreted these new policy protections to extend as far as to gender confirmation surgeries. Even though there is no comparable service provided to non-transgender people, states have interpreted the protections to extend to surgeries based on the principle of parity. There is less ambiguity about hormones and mental health care. Both are already offered to non-transgender people, thus the argument can be made it is discriminatory not to provide the same treatment to trans people. Likewise, it is not infrequent for a trans person to be denied coverage of a body part that does not conform with their legal sex. Thus a trans man who has a uterus cannot get routine prophylactic care, including cancer screenings. With the new policy protections this will change for all the policies which comply with federal ACA regulations. Unfortunately, there are still many policies which do discriminate, while some protections are already in place, others give insurers until 2015 to comply [34].

An example as insurance exchanges launched highlights how passing welcoming policies does not immediately change barriers to care. Before insurance exchanges opened the organizers of the new LGBT tailored interface to enrollment, Out2Enroll, sponsored focus groups to see what messaging would work with the different populations. In a presentation at the White House to launch enrollment they reviewed their results: while enrollment messaging tested successfully for LGB populations, it largely failed for trans people [27]. Fundamentally, the trans people in the focus groups did not even trust the enrollment process enough to call. They feared being treated with disrespect by the navigators, they feared not having navigators know the answers to their specific questions, and they did not think trans specific care would be covered. Here some of the most sweeping policy changes to ever protect trans health had just been built into the new insurance exchanges, but there is significant concern trans people may not have received enough tailored outreach to take advantage of the opportunity. As with many other areas in health, while the open enrollment period hit their stated goal of signing up seven million new people, there will be little information about how LGBT communities were served because those data were not collected.

ACA: Medicaid Expansion

With one in three low and middle income LGBT people reporting being uninsured [27], the expansion of Medicaid will create many more affordable insurance options for this population. Tailored outreach to the LGBT communities was included in the enrollment process, via the efforts of Out2Enroll. This website provided a community-driven interface for people interested in signing up for insurance exchanges. They also trained outreach workers in the field. Depending on the local policies of LGBT inclusion, different states included tailored outreach as well. But since LGBT data are not collected as part of the enrollment process, it will be difficult to report on the impact of these outreach efforts on reaching the low and middle-income LGBT populations.

ACA: General Policy Protections

Section 1557 of the ACA lays out nondiscrimination provisions of the Affordable Care Act; for the first time ever in healthcare, sex discrimination is explicitly banned [34]. While neither sexual orientation nor gender identity was explicitly laid out in the legislation this inclusion of sex as a category in the nondiscrimination language may now offer a pathway to achieve nondiscrimination for LGBT people.

A recent Equal Employment Opportunity Commission ruling classified trans status as a subset of sex, therefor rendering it protected by all existing rulings barring sex discrimination [35]. The HHS Office of Civil Rights has followed suit for ACA language, clarifying that gender identity is a covered category under sex discrimination [36]. EEOC goes further and is encouraging people who have experienced LGB related discrimination to file a complaint, under the idea that if it involved "sex stereotyping", it can also fall under the protection of the sex discrimination umbrella [37]. Ultimately it is likely this argument will wind its way through the court system, offering a path whereby a favorable ruling by the Supreme Court could set the stage for as much as full LGBT nondiscrimination protections anywhere sex protections are offered. If a Supreme Court decision upheld LGB and T discrimination as being protected under the current sex discrimination protections, this could impact the need for the Employment Non Discrimination Act, any educational protection act, or any other piecemeal efforts at getting civil rights. HHS's Office of Civil Rights is currently proceeding with a middle ground position, interpreting ACA protections to extend to gender identity and 'sex stereotyping' but not necessarily LGB discrimination [38]. Regulations are expected soon to clarify this position.

Cancer Control Continuum: Diagnosis and Treatment

Cancer diagnosis and treatment are quite complicated by the process of finding doctors who accept the respective insurance and are welcoming of LGBT individuals. As with civil rights, advancements are being made piecemeal, as individual agencies pass LGBT nondiscrimination policies. In 2011, this started to shift as the largest healthcare accreditation body, The Joint Commission, put out a new guidance to the hospitals they accredit to include LGBT people in their existing nondiscrimination policies [39]. Like other policy changes this change would create a large sea change in the environment, offering LGBT cancer patients redress if they are in a position to fight for it. Despite these provisions being in place, an LGBT health policy project in Missouri started to explore the policies of local hospitals and found few advertised any of the promised protections. Ultimately, despite the promise that most hospitals in the region should have adopted non-discrimination standards, patients in the region would be unable to find much evidence of non-discrimination. The Missouri project concluded that passing policies without requiring promotion of those policies was largely ineffective. If the Missouri experience is any guide, the Joint Commission's policy changes, while sweeping, may not be fully implemented nationwide.

Another area of significant new investment in care is the Patient Centered Outcomes Research Institute (PCORI) [40]. As was explained in other chapters, many of the failures in cultural competent care can be viewed as failures in patient-centered treatment, so research and intervention development in this area could be very productive for LGBT patients.

Family Medical Leave Act

The Family Medical Leave Act allows eligible spouses to take up to 12 weeks of unpaid sick leave to care for a spouse with a serious medical issue. When the Defense of Marriage Act was in force, this law did not apply to same-sex spouses, even if their state of residence recognized their marriage as legal. With the overturning of DOMA by the Supreme Court in 2013, LGBT spouses in states that recognize their marriage are now able to use the Family Medical Leave Act to care for a spouse with cancer. The Department of Labor just adopted this celebration policy for FMLA benefits in Winter of 2015. For the first time, this allows people married in states that recognize same-sex marriage to access these benefits even if they move. But the citizens that live in states which do not yet recognize same-sex marriage are not always able to move to marry. This is especially true for lower income LGBT people. For this large swath of the LGBT population, the devastation of a cancer diagnosis is still not backstopped by FMLA protections.

Cancer Control Continuum: Survivorship

Every one of the policies that affects the experience of LGBT people with cancer earlier in the continuum continues to affect them throughout the survivorship stage. If hospitals and health centers are not LGBT welcoming, that will continue to pose a barrier to getting appropriate care. If a cancer survivor cannot find welcoming doctors on their insurance plan it will be a barrier. As is discussed in Chapter 13, there are very few LGBT-tailored support groups throughout the country, leaving LGBT cancer survivors with fewer resources to stabilize emotionally after the rigors of cancer. The lack of data collection at so many levels of surveillance and reporting will continue to hinder adequate awareness of the needs of this subpopulation. Less recognition of LGBT families and general LGBT stigma will continue to exact its toll on the emotional and physical capabilities of the cancer survivor and their support team. As is covered thoroughly in the chapter 14, policy advancements and gaps continue to profoundly impact end-of-life care for this population. Since many of those policies are dependent on state-based laws, and not regulated by any uniform federal standard, progress on that front must occur state-by-state.

Policy Roadmap Towards LGBT Health Equity

Medicaid and Medicare Bully Pulpit In 2011 Obama signed an executive order directing HHS to support LGBT visitation in hospitals [41]. They approached this goal through an interesting route, by making it a condition of accepting Medicaid, which is in turn accepted by virtually every hospital in the country. As the largest payer of healthcare services in the country, the federal government has a bully pulpit to make changes to non-discrimination in health. If they were to pass a similar ruling ensuring that all Medicaid recipients promoted LGBT nondiscrimination provisions, it would create the largest single nondiscrimination change to date.

Sex Nondiscrimination That same outcome could also be achieved through court challenges under the sex discrimination protections. This has the added benefit of affecting all the non-health arenas as well, education, employment, etc. Non-discrimination protections will not be achieved by passing policies alone, as shown above, adequate promotion of these policies are needed as well as effective enforcement. When the EEOC enacted the gender identity non-discrimination ruling it created a wave of proactive human resource policy changes, because the EEOC has a long history of enforcing their rulings. Thus larger hiring institutions immediately moved to avoid any future conflicts, effectively spreading the policy widely.

Joint Commission Policy Enactment It would be devastating for any hospital or health center to lose their Joint Commission accreditation, thus performance reviews are viewed with utmost seriousness. The Joint Commission has required nondiscrimination provisions since 2012, but as advocates in Missouri discovered, they were not being implemented. There is technically an opportunity for any person treated at a hospital that claims Joint Commission accreditation to bring a complaint if they do not find LGBT nondiscrimination provisions. Once there is a basis for the Joint Commission to act on a complaint it is likely to cause a wave of preemptive changes much like with the EEOC.

HHS Disparity Population Another key move that would drive major steps towards LGBT health equity is if HHS designated LGBT communities a legal disparity population. This little-known legal option would end up adding LGBT to the list of other disparity populations wherever they are mentioned in health policies across the board. If a funding announcement already mentioned the need for receiving applications that focused on racial/ethnic minorities and low-income populations, now it would also list LGBT alongside the others. If data collection focused on disparity populations, it would now perforce include LGBT data collection as well. Likewise all the health disparity policies that echoed out towards the states would now routinely include LGBT in their listing of priority populations.

Research Integration If NIH were to adopt the recommendations of the IOM report they commissioned on LGBT health, there would be a wave of changes in research on LGBT people with cancer. Instead of a policy of exclusion, new proposals would be required to justify exclusion of LGBT people, creating a de facto policy of inclusion. Even if not a single new LGBT research study was funded, having routine LGBT integration into the existing National Cancer Institute research portfolio would be a huge boon to the field.

Data Collection The United States has a robust health surveillance and reporting system. Currently the policy standards on LGBT data collection are, as with research, set to exclude LGBT people. In a few surveys, LGBT measures are collected. Advocates continue to bring up data collection as their top priority with federal officials. If this standard is changed, and LGBT data are routinely included in all demographic measures, there would be a sea of new information about LGBT cancer. Data collection by the primary cancer outcome registry, SEER (Surveillance Epidemiology & End Results), is particularly important; there will never be any evidence of disproportionate impact of cancer on the communities until LGBT data are collected by the cancer registries.

Population Level Changes Probably the single largest move towards health equity needs to come at the population-level. As more and more people stand up like that woman in Colorado and challenge any aspect of the system that is not welcoming, more discriminatory policies will be dismantled.

References

1. Marmot M. Social determinants of health inequalities. Lancet. 2005;365(9464):1099–104.
2. National Gay and Lesbian Task Force. State nondiscrimination laws in the U.S. 2014. http://www.thetaskforce.org/reports_and_research/nondiscrimination_laws2014.
3. Stall RD, Greenwood GL, Acree M, Paul J, Coates TJ. Cigarette smoking among gay and bisexual men. Am J Public Health. 1999;89(12):1875–8.
4. Johnson C. Sebelius promises to collect LGBT data in health surveys. The Washington Blade. 2011. http://www.washingtonblade.com/2011/06/21/sebelius-promises-to-collect-lgbt-data-in-health-surveys/. Accessed 8 June 2014.
5. Miller K, Ryan JM. Design, development and testing of the NHIS sexual identity question. 2011. http://www.lgbttobacco.org/files/FinalReportSexualIdentity.pdf. Accessed 8 June 2014.
6. U.S. Department of Health and Human Services. HHS secretary Kathleen Sebelius statement on LGBT pride month. 2013. http://www.piersystem.com/go/doc/2430/1792599/. Accessed 8 June 2014.
7. Blosnich J, Foynes MM, Shipherd JC. Health disparities among sexual minority women veterans. J Womens Health (Larchmt). 2013;22(7):631–6. doi:10.1089/jwh.2012.4214.
8. Reisner SL, Van Wagenen A, Gordon A, Calzo JP. Disparities in safety belt use by sexual orientation identity among US high school students. Am J Public Health. 2014;104(2):311–8.
9. Baker K. Update of States Adopting the SO/GI Module on BRFSS/YRBS. In: Scout, editor. Update of states adopting the SO/GI module for BRFSS/YRBS; 2014.
10. Coulter RW, Kenst KS, Bowen DJ, Scout. Research funded by the National Institutes of Health on the health of lesbian, gay, bisexual, and transgender populations. Am J Public Health. 2014;104(2):e105–12.
11. Scout. LGBT cultural competency in funding. In: Scout, editor. Network for LGBT health equity. Vol 2014. Lincoln; 2011. http://blog.lgbthealthlink.org/2011/09/20/lgbt-cultural-competency-in-funding/. Accessed 11 March 2015.
12. Institute of Medicine (IOM). The health of lesbian, gay, bisexual, and transgender people building a foundation for better understanding. Washington, D.C.: The National Academies Press; 2011.
13. Hatzenbuehler ML, Keyes KM, Hasin DS. State-level policies and psychiatric morbidity in lesbian, gay and bisexual populations. Am J Public Health. 2009;99(12):2275–81.
14. King BA, Dube SR, Tynan MA. Current tobacco use among adults in the United States: findings from the National Adult Tobacco Survey. Am J Public Health. 2012;102(11):e93–e100.
15. Stevens P, Carlson LM, Hinman JM. An analysis of tobacco industry marketing to lesbian, gay, bisexual, and transgender (LGBT) populations: strategies for mainstream tobacco control and prevention. Health Promot Pract. 2004;5(3 Suppl):129S–34S.
16. Offen N, Smith EA, Malone RE. Is tobacco a gay issue? Interviews with leaders of the lesbian, gay, bisexual and transgender community. Cult Health Sex. 2008;10(2):143–57.
17. CDC. Community transformation grants. 2013. http://www.cdc.gov/nccdphp/dch/programs/communitytransformation/. Accessed 12 June 2014.
18. CDC. Communities putting prevention to work: CDC awards $ 372.8 million to 44 communities. Press release. 2010. http://www.cdc.gov/features/chronicpreventiongrants/. Accessed 12 June 2014.
19. Surgeon General. National Prevention Strategy: Strategic Directions: Eliminating Health Disparities. National prevention strategy. 2011. http://www.surgeongeneral.gov/initiatives/prevention/strategy/elimination-of-health-disparities.html. Accessed 12 June 2014.
20. Scout. The long-awaited community transformation grants? Thumbs down so far. 2011. http://blog.lgbthealthequity.org/2011/05/13/the-long-awaited-community-transform-grants-thumbs-down/. Accessed 12 June 2014.
21. Mautner Project. Mautner project. Records of the Mautner project, 1989–2010: a finding aid. 2011. 12. http://oasis.lib.harvard.edu/oasis/deliver/~sch01347. Accessed 12 June 2014.
22. Scout. Announcing: network restarts at centerlink—the community of LGBT centers. 2013. http://blog.lgbthealthequity.org/2013/10/28/announcing-network-restarts-at-national-organization-of-lgbt-community-centers/. Accessed 12 June 2014.

23. National Gay and Lesbian Task Force. Centers for Disease Control and Prevention revises guidance to include preventive screenings for transgender women. 2013. http://thetaskforceblog.org/2013/12/23/centers-for-disease-control-and-prevention-revises-guidance-to-include-preventive-screenings-for-transgender-women/. Accessed 12 June 2014.
24. Wanliss E. Do you know if Comp Cancer revised their BCCEPT guidelines to allow trans women? In: Scout, editor. Email relaying the policy change. CDC; 2014.
25. Raab B. The truth about gays and money. 2013. http://williamsinstitute.law.ucla.edu/headlines/the-truth-about-gays-and-money-2/. Accessed 12 June 2014.
26. Ash M, Badgett M. Separate and unequal: the effect of unequal access to employment based health insurance on same-sex and unmarried different-sex couples. Contemp Econ Policy. 2006;24(4):582–99.
27. Durso LE, Baker K. AC. LGBT communities and the affordable care act: findings from a national survey. Center for American progress blog. 2013. http://americanprogress.org/issues/lgbt/report/2013/10/10/76693/lgbt-communities-and-the-affordable-care-act/. Accessed 13 June 2014.
28. U.S. Department of Treasury. All legal same-sex marriages will be recognized for federal tax purpose. 2013. http://www.treasury.gov/press-center/press-releases/Pages/jl2153.aspx. Accessed 12 June 2014.
29. National Gay and Lesbian Task Force. Relationship recognition for same-sex couples in the US. map. 2014. http://www.thetaskforce.org/reports_and_research/relationship_recognition. Accessed 13 June 2014.
30. U.S. Department of Health and Human Services. HHS announces first guidance implementing Supreme Court's decision on the Defence of Marriage Act. 2013. http://www.piersystem.com/go/doc/2430/1885974/. Accessed 12 June 2014.
31. U.S. Department of Health and Human Services. How does the health care law protect me? Healthcare.gov. 2013. https://http://www.healthcare.gov/how-does-the-health-care-law-protect-me/. Accessed 14 June 2014.
32. Sellers Dorsey Foundation. Out2Enroll Q & A topics. 2013. http://out2enroll.org/topics/. Accessed 13 June 2014.
33. Scout. Out2Enroll: getting LGBT communities connected to care. Network for LGBT health equity blog. 2013. http://lgbthealthequity.wordpress.com/2013/10/14/out2enroll-getting-lgbt-communities-connected-to-care/. Accessed 11 June 2014.
34. U.S. Department of Health and Human Services. Section 1557 of the patient protection and affordable care act. Health and Human Services website. 2013. http://www.hhs.gov/ocr/civilrights/understanding/Section1557/. Accessed 11 June 2014.
35. McGovern AE. Macy v. Holder: Title VII and workplace justice for transgender employees. J Law Public Policy. 2012.
36. U.S. Department of Health and Human Services. Corrective actions taken in sex discrimination cases Enforcement of "Section 1557" of the ACA. 2013. http://www.hhs.gov/ocr/office/1557_bulletin.pdf. Accessed 8 June 2014.
37. Scout. It was legal to fire me for being LGBT—last year. Video interview of EEOC Commissioner Chai Feldblum explaining how LGB people are encourated to file comlaints under Macy v. Holder ruling. 2012. https://http://www.youtube.com/watch?v=HLChaY8r8xE. Accessed 8 June 2014.
38. Prachniak C. Health and human services attorney: new regulations won't cover LGB discrimination. Network for LGBT health equity blog. 2014. http://blog.lgbthealthequity.org/2014/04/05/hhs-discrimination/. Accessed 13 June 2014.
39. The Joint Commission. Patient-centered communication standards for hospitals (Issue 1). R3 report: requirement, rationale, reference. 2011. http://www.jointcommission.org/assets/1/18/r3 report issue120111.pdf. Accessed 8 June 2014.
40. Patient-Centered Outcomes Research Institute. How we're funded. PCORI blog. http://www.pcori.org/about-us/how-were-funded/. Accessed 8 June 2014.
41. Office of Public Engagement. Hospital visitation regulations go into effect today. White House blog. 2011. http://www.whitehouse.gov/blog/2011/01/18/hospital-visitation-regulations-go-effect-today. Accessed 10 June 2014.

Chapter 18
Current Policy and Research on Cancer in LGBT Communities Internationally

I Mary Poynten

Abstract This chapter focuses on cancer policy and research from a number of countries around the world. It endeavours to determine if cancer rates in LGBT communities in these countries differ when compared with the general population. There are few countries with national LGBT-specific policies for screening and managing cancers. No country could be identified where demographic data on sexual identity/orientation were collected in population-based cancer registries. Thus the current knowledge of cancer risk, incidence and mortality in LGBT communities in these countries is gleaned from population-based surveys, results from studies of infection-related cancers, in particular HIV, and from clinical, behavioural and epidemiological research.

As population-based demographic data on sexual identity are unavailable in relation to cancer diagnoses, risk factors as surrogates for cancer risk, such as smoking, excess alcohol consumption and human papillomavirus (HPV) infection are explored. The prevalences of these factors are compared between lesbian, gay, bisexual, transgender and heterosexual populations where possible. General health data are also examined by sexual identity.

The main conclusions of the study are the higher incidence of some risk factors in the LGBT community in many but not all countries, the strong link between HIV and an increased incidence of infection-related cancers, and the issue that unless sexual identity can be documented in census and cancer registry data, population-based data on cancer incidence in LGBT people will remain rare. A "combination prevention" approach to cancer in LGBT communities, similar to that of HIV prevention is proposed.

I. M. Poynten (✉)
The Kirby Institute, The University of New South Wales, Sydney, Australia
e-mail: Mpoynten@kirby.unsw.edu.au

U. Boehmer, R. Elk (eds.), *Cancer and the LGBT Community*,
DOI 10.1007/978-3-319-15057-4_18

Introduction

Though there has been an increased focus on LGBT health in recent years, the incidence and risk factors for cancer among LGBT people remain insufficiently studied in countries other than the United States[1]. In most countries, there is scarce high quality statistical information available on LGBT people, as medical systems such as national health and cancer registries do not routinely record diagnoses by sexual orientation. Thus it is not possible to develop estimates that link cancer incidence or mortality to sexual orientation. Consequently, efforts to address cancer disparities associated with sexual orientation are greatly impeded [2, 3]. Other factors contribute to this lack of data. Many LGBT people grew up with legal sanctions on their sexual behaviour and may be reluctant to disclose sexuality in health-related settings, even after homosexuality has been legalised in their country [4]. In a large number of countries, identifying as LGBT remains criminalised and highly stigmatised. Collection of health-related data is close to impossible and as a result there are no data on cancer among LGBT populations available. Due to perceived and actual homophobia, biphobia or transphobia, many LGBT patients do not disclose their sexual orientation to health care providers [5]. Often the issue of sexual orientation is never raised in cancer settings, and the person is presumed to be heterosexual. The current knowledge of cancer risk, incidence and mortality in LGBT communities arises from population based surveys, results from studies of infection-related cancers, in particular HIV, and from clinical, behavioural and epidemiological research. Many studies are small and prone to sampling bias, which limits the generalisability of findings [6]. Obtaining a representative sample of LGBT people is difficult as there is usually no well-defined sampling frame. The recent availability of same-sex marriage registers may offer a new and promising avenue by which a reasonably representative sample may be drawn [7]. As in settings where health care is provided, there may be reluctance to disclose sexual identity in research settings [8, 9]. The LGBT population, like all other populations, is a very heterogeneous group.

Published Policies and Legislation

It is beyond the scope of this chapter to review all global health policies and legislations as they relate to LGBT communities. An on-line search of policies from Canada, Australia and the United Kingdom, limited to English language documents was undertaken. Search terms included “health”, “policy” “health act” “LGBT”, “lesbian”, “gay”, “government” and “federal”. Examples of policies and legislations in these three countries are discussed below. No national cancer-specific LGBT policies could be identified.

a. Australia

The Australian National LGBTI Health Alliance has estimated that the number of LGBT Australians aged over 65 years will reach 500,000 by 2051 [4]. The Australian Federal Government's Commonwealth Department of Health and Ageing's 2012 National Ageing and Aged Care strategy clearly states that LGBT people are a group requiring particular attention due to the past and continuing experience of discrimination. It highlights the limited recognition of LGBT people's needs by service providers and in policy frameworks and accreditation processes [10]. In the Australian National Women's Health Policy of 2010, being a lesbian or a bisexual woman is recognised as a social determinant of health. More broadly sexuality, sex and gender identity are also considered to be important determinants of health. The policy declares that for same-sex attracted women, "the fear or experience of insensitive treatment or of blatant discrimination can be a major barrier to accessing appropriate and acceptable health care". The policy emphasises that in order to minimise the hurdles that same-sex attracted women face when accessing services, it is important to first understand the needs of these groups of women [11].

b. United Kingdom (UK)

There are an estimated 3.6 million LGBT people living in UK, approximately 5% of the population. The UK Health Equality Act (2006) prohibits discrimination on the grounds of sexual orientation in the provision of goods and services, including health care [1]. The 2007 Equality Act (Sexual Orientation) Regulations state there should be equal treatment in all public services, including in the National Health Service [12]. A number of non-governmental organisations have released policies and strategies on health issues, including cancer diagnosis and treatment, affecting LGBT communities in the UK. These documents highlight the need to improve the evidence base on cancer in LGBT communities by conducting more research and the need to eliminate obstacles to healthcare access for LGBT people [1, 13].

a. Canada

In 1996, the Canadian Human Rights Act was amended to explicitly include sexual orientation as one of the prohibited grounds of discrimination [14]. Canada has promoted the equality of same-sex partners, including the legalisation of same-sex marriage in 2005. A question on sexual identity was added to the Canadian Community Health Survey (CCHS) in 2003, which has been very valuable in describing the health and social needs of the Canadian LGBT community. In 2009, 1.1% of Canadians aged 18–59 reported that they considered themselves to be homosexual (gay or lesbian) and 0.9% considered themselves to be bisexual [15, 16]. Commentators on the Canadian health system have made observations on the exclusion of LGBT populations from mainstream health promotion research, policy and practice [17]. However, community organisations funded through government sources have worked to develop health promotion programs and policies to increase the visibility of and the services provided to LGBT people [18]. Province-wide guidelines on screening for transgender people for breast, cervical, ovarian, uterine and prostate cancers have been published for British Columbia [19].

Population-Based Studies and Surveys

In 1989, Denmark became the first country to establish marriage-like partnerships with legal implications for same-sex couples. The largest population-based study of cancer among the LGBT community is a Danish cohort study which linked information from the Danish Civil Registration System on men and women in registered same-sex partnerships with the Danish cancer registry and the Danish AIDS registry. Data were linked for the time period between 1989–1997 and results were compared with the general Danish population. 1614 women and 3391 men in same-sex partnerships were included, with an average follow-up of 4.1 years and 4.6 years respectively. Among women, the overall cancer incidence differed little between women in same-sex partnerships and women in the general population, albeit based on wide confidence intervals (relative risk (RR) 0.9 (95 % CI 0.4–1.9). Men in same-sex partnerships were twice as likely to develop cancer compared with men in the general population. However, this was almost entirely a result of extremely high incidence rates of Kaposi's sarcoma (KS) (RR 136.0, 96–186), non-Hodgkin's lymphoma (NHL) (RR 15.1, 10.4–21.4) and anal cancer (RR 31.2, 8.4–79.8). The overall cancer incidence rate was not significantly different when these cancers were excluded from the analysis. Though the findings are pivotal, the study does have a number of limitations. No information was available on sociodemographic factors such as education and income, and the study's authors caution on how representative participants are of all LGB men and women in Denmark [7]. The sample size was relatively small. Further data from these linked registries from 1982 to 2011 were published in 2013. In this updated study, 0.1 % of all partnerships were same-sex marriages and 1.0 % comprised women and 1.9 % men registering same-sex cohabitation. Cohabitation status was a variable created by determining the number and gender of adults sharing the same address as cohort members. Of concern, all-cause mortality was markedly increased in all age groups in same-sex married women (hazard ratio (HR) 1.89, 95 % CI 1.60–2.23) compared with opposite-sex married women, with the greatest differences seen in cancer (HR 1.62, 95 % CI 1.28–2.05) and suicide related mortality (HR 6.4). The mortality rates of men in same-sex marriages had declined since the 1990s. Though still raised when compared with opposite-sex married men, the mortality rates were similar to those among unmarried, widowed or divorced men [20].

Other population-based surveys include the national Canadian Community Health Survey (CCHS). Since 2003, respondents have been asked if they are heterosexual, homosexual (lesbian or gay) or bisexual. In cross-sectional analyses of results for women (60937 heterosexual, 354 lesbian and 424 bisexual), lesbian and bisexual women were more likely to smoke than heterosexual women (odds ratio (OR) 1.77, 95 % CI 1.22–2.57 and 2.04, 95 % CI 1.47–2.83 respectively). Lesbian and bisexual women were twice as likely to report excess alcohol consumption compared with heterosexual women (OR 2.67 (95 % CI 1.67–4.28) and 2.00 (95 % CI 1.30–3.09) respectively) [15]. Gay and bisexual men in the 2003 CCHS had similar rates of daily smoking or excess alcohol consumption as heterosexual men [16].

A national Dutch survey of patients attending general practices was conducted in 2001.19685 people were approached and 65% participated. Sexuality was reported by 98.2% of 9684 participants, with 0.6% identifying as bisexual men, 1.5% as gay men, 1.2% as bisexual women and 1.5% as lesbian women. The SF36 questionnaire, a standardised measure of functional health and wellbeing, was administered and results demonstrated lower acute and general mental health status in LGB people. Cancer rates were not reported. In this study, sexual orientation was not linked to current cigarette smoking in men or women. A lower proportion of LGB people were currently using alcohol, but those who currently used alcohol were more likely to report recent excess consumption (adjusted OR 1.72, 95% CI 1.17–2.99) [21]. Private Lives 2 is the second national Australian on-line survey of health and well-being of LGBT Australians. It was administered in 2011, with 3835 respondents completing the survey. According to results from the SF36 questionnaire, the general health of male respondents was lower than the national average. The general health of female respondents was lower still, and transgender men and women reported the lowest levels of general health. Only a small numbers of cancers were reported (2.1% of respondents in total; 2.4% men, 1.8% women, 2.5% transgender women, 0% transgender men). The most common cancers were skin (19 cases), prostate (16 cases) and breast cancer (12 cases). Of note, breast cancer screening rates did not appear to be lower, with 56.2% of women aged 50–69 years reporting having a mammogram in past 2 years compared with 55.2% of similar-aged women in the general population [22].

Risk Factors for Cancer

Much of the existing research and proposed evidence for cancer disparities among LGBT communities is based on differing rates of risk factors for cancer. Behavioural factors such as cigarette smoking and excess alcohol consumption have been associated with a number of cancer types. Nulliparity and being overweight or obese have been associated with breast cancer. Chronic HPV infection has been causally linked with cervical and other ano-genital cancers and cancers of the head and neck (particularly the oropharynx and tonsil). A number of these risk factors, including behaviours and infectious agents, are discussed here.

Cigarette Smoking and Alcohol Consumption

Surveys in Australia show varying rates of smoking among LGBT populations. The National Drug Strategy Household Survey in 2010 showed current smoking rates for the general population at 17.5%, while the smoking rate for those identifying as homosexual/bisexual was 34.2% [23]. Descriptive and small studies of transgender health also suggest high rates of smoking. Forty four percent of transgender men and 35.4 % of transgender women in the Private Lives survey smoked on more than five occasions in the preceding month [24]. Among Australian people living with HIV, the HIV Futures study reported a decrease in smoking rates from 54.6 % in 2002 to 30.2 % in 2013 [25]. While rates of smoking have fallen among gay and bisexual men and people with HIV, the Sydney Women and Sexual Health survey shows that the reported high rates of smoking among lesbians and other same-sex attracted women have remained constant between 2006 and 2012 [26]. In the Private Lives survey, 60 % of respondents considered themselves non-smokers, 13.7 % identify as ex-smokers which is comparable with national data where 57.8 % have never smoked and 24.1 % ex-smokers. Reported alcohol use was lower than national averages [22, 23]. Results from a 2007 online survey of 6178 lesbian and bisexual women (LBW) in the UK showed that two thirds of respondents (4118 women) reported a smoking history and 40 % drank at least three times a week [27].

Tobacco has been identified as the most important risk factor for cancer in the UK, with its use linked to 19.4 % of all cancer cases newly diagnosed in 2010. In contrast, infectious agents only accounted for 3.1 % of cancer cases in the UK [28]. In order to address the perceived increase in cigarette smoking among gay men, a UK pilot smoking cessation study was developed. The study aimed to design, recruit and deliver smoking cessation group interventions to gay men in London in consultation with community groups. The intervention was adapted to meet the specific needs of gay men. Of the 98 gay men recruited, 76 attended at least the first session. After 7 weeks, 76 % confirmed they had ceased smoking [29].

Human Papillomavirus Infection

Human papillomavirus (HPV) has been classified by the International Agency for Research on Cancer as a human carcinogen for several cancer types, including anal, cervical, penile, vulval, vaginal and oropharyngeal cancers (in particular tonsillar and base of tongue cancers) [30]. Approximately 85 % of anal cancer is caused by high risk types of HPV, and the high risk type HPV16 is by far the most common cause (90 % of all HPV-related anal cancer) [31].

There have been increasing numbers of studies of prevalence and incidence of ano-genital HPV among men who have sex with men (MSM) in recent years. MSM are consistently more likely than heterosexual men to have anal HPV detected. A systematic review and meta-analysis of studies in MSM that reported prevalence and incidence of anal HPV detection, anal cancer precursor lesions (high grade squamous intraepithelial lesions, HSIL) and anal cancer showed that anal HPV and anal cancer precursors were very common in MSM. In HIV-positive men, the pooled prevalences of anal HPV16 and HSIL were 35·4 % (95 % CI 32·9–37·9) and 29·1 % (95 % CI 22·8–35·4) respectively. In HIV-negative men, the pooled prevalences of anal HPV16 and HSIL were 12·5 % (95 % CI 9·8–15·4) and 21·5 % (95 % CI 13·7–29·3) respectively [32].

Though the great majority of studies identified in this systematic review were from North America, a number of studies on anal HPV from other countries have recently been published. In a cross-sectional Irish study of 113 MSM with detectable HPV DNA, 68 men (42 %) had at least one high risk HPV type detected [33]. A Netherlands cross-sectional study recruited HIV positive (317, 41 %) and HIV negative (461) MSM. Both anal and penile high risk HPV infection were significantly more prevalent in HIV positive MSM (65 % vs 45 %, $p < 0.001$ and 32 % vs 16 %, $p = 0.001$ respectively) [34]. The Study for the Prevention of Anal Cancer (SPANC) is a 3-year prospective study of HIV negative and positive gay men aged ≥35 years in Sydney, Australia. By March 2013, 342 participants (median age 49 years; 28.7 % HIV positive) had attended a baseline visit. The vast majority of men (85.8 %) had one or more HPV types detected. Almost two thirds had at least one high risk HPV type (64.4 %) and almost a third had HPV16 (30.3 %) detected. Similar to other published studies, the SPANC study found that anal high risk HPV detection was significantly associated with positive HIV status ($p = 0.010$) [35]. A multi-centre cohort study of 551 HIV positive MSM conducted in Spain between 2007 and 2011 detected anal high risk HPV in 82 % of men [36]. In a cross-sectional study of 445 men with HIV attending public clinics in urban Brazil, men who had sex with women and men (MSWM) and MSM were much more likely than heterosexual men to have anal high risk HPV detected (OR 7.33 and 7.92 respectively) [37].

In-depth interviews and focus groups were conducted in Peru to explore knowledge, attitudes and experiences regarding HPV and genital warts among Peruvian male to female transgender and MSM populations. The study found that knowledge of HPV was limited. Unfortunately, it did not examine knowledge of the association between HPV and cancer [38]. An Italian cross-sectional study assessed knowledge and attitudes towards HPV and HPV vaccination among a random sample of 1000 LGB people. Less than two thirds of participants (60.6 %) had heard of HPV. Knowledge was higher among women and those with higher involvement with LGB community organisations. Though willingness to be vaccinated against HPV was high (73.3 %), only 1.7 % reported being vaccinated [39]. Of 1041 MSM recruited between 2008 and 2009 from community venues in Vancouver, Canada, 71.3 % had heard of HPV and 67.0 % said they were willing to receive HPV vaccine. Interestingly, for MSM aged less than 26 years old, the median time from first sexual contact with males to disclosure of sexual identity to a health care provider was 3.0 years (IQR 1–8 years). Thus many young MSM would already be infected with HPV by the time they self-reported as gay or bisexual. This highlights the limitations associated with delivering vaccination programs for young MSM through health care providers [40].

The incidence of HPV-associated oropharyngeal cancers is rapidly increasing. In 2007, oral HPV detection was measured in 500 MSM (50 % HIV-positive) attending Melbourne Sexual Health Centre, Australia. Oral HPV was found to be significantly associated with HIV infection. One in five HIV positive MSM (19 %) had at least one HPV type detected compared with less than one in ten HIV negative men (7 %, $p < 0.001$). HPV16 was detected in 4.4 % of HIV positive men compared with 0.8 % of HIV negative men. Other risk factors for oral HPV included smoking, recent tooth-brushing and more lifetime tongue-kissing and oral sex partners [41].

The quadrivalent HPV vaccination provides protection against the two HPV types that are responsible for most ano-genital cancers (HPV16 and HPV18) and the two types that are responsible for most ano-genital warts (HPV6 and HPV11). The vaccine has been proven to be safe and effective in both males and females. An ongoing national school-based, government-funded, HPV vaccination program for females aged 12–13 years commenced in Australia in 2007. The impact of this program has been evaluated in different populations. Among 112 083 new patients attending sexual health services, a decline in number of diagnoses of genital warts was noted for young female residents (p trend<0·0001) after the HPV vaccination program was implemented. There was also a statistically significant decline in genital warts among young heterosexual men (p <0·0001) which was interpreted as being due to herd protection. There was no change in the number of diagnoses in gay men [42], demonstrating that gay men will gain little if any herd protection from the vaccination of women. The Australian government approved a subsided male HPV vaccination program which commenced in February 2013 and is targeted at high school males aged 12–13 years with a catch up only to the age of 15 [43]. This will clearly benefit very young MSM in Australia. Though HPV-related cancers will be prevented in the decades to come, today's generation of adult MSM remain unprotected.

HIV-Related Cancers

It is evident that information and data on cancer rates and mortality are far more extensive for gay men with HIV than for LGBT people in general [44]. This is due primarily to the presence of HIV and AIDS registries, which often capture information on sexual behaviours, at least among men diagnosed with HIV. Though an exhaustive review of published literature in this area is beyond the scope of this chapter, the studies discussed here consistently demonstrate the increased risk of cancer among gay and bisexual men living with HIV. In a Scottish study of data linkage from cancer and HIV registries from 1981 to 1996, the incidence of cancer among people living with HIV was 11 times higher than the general population. Among gay and bisexual men, the incidence of cancer was 21 times higher than men in the general population (standardised incidence ratio (SIR) 21.4, 95% CI 17.4–26.1) [45]. In a Spanish study linking AIDS and cancer registry data, compared with other people living with HIV, MSM and MSWM had the highest rates of Kaposi's sarcoma (SIR 3003.23) and any invasive cancer (SIR 53.94) and the second highest rates of non-Hodgkin's lymphoma (after heterosexual men living with HIV, SIR 240.66) [46]. Combined data from 1997 to 1998 on cancer rates among 8385 men (25.8% homosexual) from two hospital HIV cohorts and a cohort of HIV seroconverters in Italy and France were studied. Observed cancer rates among MSM were compared with expected rates (derived from rates in men in the general population). There were markedly increased observed rates of cancer at any site (SIR 44.2), Kaposi's sarcoma (SIR 2055), cancer of the salivary glands (SIR 65.5), non-Hodgkin's lymphoma (SIR 124) and Hodgkin's disease (SIR 11.2) [47].

Breast Cancer

It is important to emphasise that being a LBW is not in itself a risk factor for breast cancer. The fundamental issue is whether LBW are at greater risk of breast cancer because the risk factors for breast cancer are more prevalent among LBW [5, 48]. These risks include behavioural factors such as excess alcohol consumption and smoking (potentially) [49, 50], reproductive factors such as higher rates of nulliparity and delayed childbirth [51]. There is no consensus on whether these risk factors are indeed more common among LBW.

A threefold increase in fatal breast cancer among LBW has been found in studies from the United States. A recently published systematic review of breast cancer in LBW by UK-based researchers was undertaken in 2009. No published incidence rates of breast cancer could be identified. The review included nine studies of breast cancer prevalence among LBW, mostly small studies of varying methodological quality. Of note, only two were from countries other than the United States (Denmark and UK). These two studies are discussed in this chapter. The authors emphasise that these sparse results validate the call for sexual orientation data to be collected within routine statistics [52]. The UK data included in the systematic review above was an online survey of LBW conducted in 2007. No details of the study methodology are available. Of the 6178 responses, 8 % of LBW reported a diagnosis of breast cancer between ages 50 and 79 [27].

The national UK Lesbians and Health Care Survey was undertaken between 1997 and 1998. 1066 lesbians responded and three quarters of respondents reported that they believed that LW had the same risk of breast cancer as heterosexual women. Twenty one percent of women reported that they never practised breast self-examination; the same proportion as among the general population. However, only 16 % of LBW performed regular monthly breast self-examination, compared with 41 % of women in the general population. Interestingly, 19 % believed their risk of breast cancer was higher than that of heterosexual women [8]. Findings from a national Australian survey showed that Australian LBW aged between 50–69 had similar mammogram rates to the national rates in this age group (56.1 vs 55.2 %), which suggests that Australian LBW are not under-screened for breast cancer [22].

Cervical Cancer

Studies from the United States have found significant differences in prevalence of cervical cancer by sexual orientation. In pooled data from California Health Interview surveys from 2001 to 2005, bisexual women had more than double the prevalence of cervical cancer compared with other women surveyed [2]. However, in the Danish same-sex partnership cohort study described above, invasive cervical cancer rates among women in same-sex relationships were similar to those in opposite-sex relationships. Of note, there was statistically significantly less in situ cervical disease reported in women in same-sex relationships. Although the numbers were small and thus definitive conclusions difficult to make, the authors suggest that this may represent inadequate attendance at screening programs by lesbian women [7].

Disparities exist in recommendations for cervical cancer screening for LBW. Additionally, confusion persists among health care providers and among LBW themselves over the need for screening and the frequency of screening [8, 53, 54]. The British Columbia Cervical Screening Program in Canada recommends that all women who have ever been sexually active (touching and intercourse) should be regularly screened [55]. In Australia, each state's guidelines state that LBW should be screened routinely, similar to heterosexual women [56]. It has been noted that historically, the UK National Health Service Cervical Screening Programme (NHSCSP) policy did not provide consistent advice for lesbians, which may have led to non-attendance for screening [6].

It has been observed that lesbian women, in particular those who have never had sexual contact with a man, have been considered a low risk group for cervical cancer [12], despite published studies finding similar prevalences of cervical atypia between LBW and heterosexual women [57]. In Sydney Australia, a large cross-sectional study of women who have sex with women (WSW) was conducted between 1995 and 1998. Among 356 WSW (9.6 % of all new female presentations) there was no difference in the prevalence of abnormal cytology (CIN1, CIN2-3) when compared with 286 heterosexual women [54].

A Lesbians and Health Care mail-out survey enrolled 1066 lesbians in the UK over a 12 month period in 1997–1998. The survey found that 55 % of women attended regularly for a pap test, 12 % of those eligible had never had a pap test and 15 % reported they no longer attended. Of those women who had been screened, 15 % reported abnormal smears. One in two women perceived that lesbian women had a lower risk of cervical cancer than heterosexual women [8]. In the UK online survey of LBW discussed previously, 15 % of LBW aged over 25 had never had a pap test. Of these women, 20 % had been told they were not at risk, providing further evidence of the misperceptions surrounding the need for cervical cancer screening among LBW [27].

A UK study enrolled 606 women with cervical cytology results, from specialised lesbian sexual health clinics. One in four women had a history of sex with a man. Of those eligible, 17 % had never had a pap test and 25 % had not had a pap test for over 4 years. Ten women (1.7 %), including a woman who reported she was exclusively lesbian, had cervical abnormalities (5 Cervical Intraepithelial Neoplasia (CIN)1, 1 CIN2 and 4 CIN3). One in five (22 %) lesbian women said lesbian women have less need for screening than heterosexual women [53]. In Victoria, Australia, 409 lesbian women at a GLBT community event completed a self-report survey. The survey found that two thirds of women were appropriately screened, one quarter of women were under-screened and one in ten had never had a pap test. Women aged 40 or more and interestingly, those who had disclosed their sexual orientation to their health care provider, were more likely to be appropriately screened [51]. In the national Australian on-line survey of health and well-being of LGBT Australians administered in 2011, 56 % of women reported a pap test in past 2 years, similar to the 59 % of women who participated in the national cervical screening program between 2008 and 2009. Thirty-nine percent of transgender men reported a pap test in the past 2 years [22].

The findings from these studies demonstrate there is a pressing need for education of LBW and health service providers as to the risk of cervical cancer and the necessity of routine screening among LBW [12, 53]. Further research into barriers to cervical screening for LBW needs to be undertaken [12].

Anal Cancer

Among men, anal cancer has consistently been associated with a history of sex with other men, thought to be due to anal exposure to HPV [7, 58]. Much of the data on anal cancer among MSM comes from HIV registries. A nested case control study in the Swiss HIV cohort study found a 30 fold higher rate of anal cancer compared with the general population. Of the 59 anal cancer cases that were reported, 73 % were diagnosed in MSM. Risk factors included current smoking (OR 2.59), exposure to HPV (OR 4.52) and low CD4 count. A CD4 count less than 200 cells/μL 6 or 7 years prior to diagnosis was most highly associated (OR for < 200 vs ≥ 500 cells/μL = 14.0, 95 % CI 3.85–50.90) [59]. The French HIV and HPV cohort study followed 247 HIV positive MSM with anal HPV detection, anal cytology and high resolution anoscopy (HRA) for anal cancer precursor HSIL every 6 months for 3 years between 2002 and 2005. Over half of the men (132, 53 %) had anal HSIL detected. Risk of anal HSIL increased with increasing age, a CD4 count less than 50 cells/μL when starting cART and infection with HPV16 and/or HPV18 [60]. In the French Hospital Database on HIV there were 124 cases of anal cancer diagnosed among men between 1992 and 2004. Three quarters of the men had a history of sex with another man. The prevalence of anal cancer was higher among MSM with HIV than women or heterosexual men with HIV and increased over time, despite the introduction of combined antiretroviral therapy (cART) [61]. In a follow-up study using the same database in the years from 2005 to 2008, HIV positive MSM had an extraordinarily increased standardised incidence ratio of 109.8 (95 % CI 84.6–140.3) compared with the general population [44].

The incidence of anal cancer in the Netherlands has doubled in the last few decades. Part of this increase can be temporally linked to an increase in the HIV positive MSM population in the Netherlands over this time [62]. From 1995 to 2012 the overall incidence of anal cancer in MSM in the Dutch HIV Observational cohort database was 116 per 100,000PY. Low nadir CD4 (HR 2.41, 95 % CI1.5–3.89), excess alcohol consumption (HR 2.23, 95 % CI 1.28–3.89) and smoking (HR 1.60, 95 % CI 1.07–2.41) were all associated with anal cancer in MSM [63]. In Denmark, 36 anal cancer cases were reported in the Danish HIV Cohort Study from 1995 to 2009. Not only did HIV positive MSM have over 100 fold risk of anal cancer (IRR 101.4, 95 % CI 39.3–261.5), they had a three-fold increase in mortality rate compared with HIV negative anal cancer controls [64].

The causal link between anal HPV infection and anal cancer is well established. However, the natural history of anal HPV infection is still being investigated, particularly as it relates to rates of progression and regression of anal HSIL. Furthermore, the safety and efficacy of available treatment options for HSIL is yet to be proven in randomised controlled trials [65] and more research on preventive and therapeutic strategies against HSIL is underway [66]. There is ongoing assessment and discussion around the performance of anal cytology and HRA for screening for anal cancer and little is known of the psychosocial and quality of life impacts of anal cancer screening. The SPANC study, discussed above is a prospective study of HIV negative and positive gay men aged 35 years and over in Sydney, Australia. 420 men have been recruited by March 2014, with a target sample size of 600 men. The study aims to provide data on anal HPV natural history and to inform the development of anal cancer screening guidelines for gay men in Australia [9].

Anal cancer is the most common non-AIDS defining malignancy in those living with HIV in Australia [67]. The prognosis of anal cancer is closely related to tumour size. Studies from the US have shown that 5 year survival for tumours equal or less than 2 cm is 80 %, whereas the 5 year survival for tumour larger than 5 cm is only 45 % [68]. A French study including 69 people with anal cancers less than one cm found a 100 % cancer specific survival and 89 % disease free survival at 5 years [69]. As the results from research such as the SPANC study may not be available for a number of years, and there is no consensus on screening approaches for anal cancer, digital ano-rectal examination (DARE) for early detection of anal cancer is being advocated as a simple, inexpensive method of screening. It is unknown how many clinicians screen using DARE. A questionnaire was distributed to HIV physicians in Melbourne Australia. Thirty six physicians (86 %) responded and although 86 % said it was important or very important to screen, only 22 % were screening their HIV positive gay patients via DARE [70]. The acceptability of DARE among HIV positive gay men was examined in the same city. Of 142 men offered enrolment, 102 (72 %) participated. Four men were referred to surgeons, with one subsequently diagnosed with anal cancer. The examinations were found to be almost universally acceptable, with 98 % of men stating they would probably have the examination again [71].

Prostate Cancer

In many countries, the notion of an inequality in healthcare for prostate cancer between heterosexual and non-heterosexual men has caused concern. To explore this issue, 460 heterosexual men and 96 MSM completed an anonymous online survey between December 2010 and April 2011. These men resided in 17 countries, including the US (63 %), Australia (18 %), Canada (9 %) and the UK (6 %). Of note, non-heterosexual men had significantly lower grade disease when diagnosed than heterosexual men ($p=0.02$) and treatment outcomes were similar between groups. Therefore, there was no evidence for disparities in treatment found in this survey and indeed, non-heterosexual men appeared to be more likely to be screened [72]. This is similar to findings in California, where other men had three times higher risk of prostate cancer than MSM [2]. In the 2011 national on-line survey of health and well-being of LGBT Australians, 27 % of males and 21.5 % of transgender females had been screened in the past 2 years with either serum prostate specific antigen or digital rectal examination. Among men aged 65–75 years of age, screening was almost universal (86.3 %) [22].

Though treatments for prostate cancer potentially will have a significant impact on subsequent sexual function, there has been very little research in this area among MSM. One such study was a qualitative pilot study of MSM treated for prostate cancer in Ontario, Canada. Between July 2011 and March 2012, 15 participants (seven treated with surgery, eight with radiotherapy) were interviewed. Men treated with surgery experienced more erectile dysfunction during anal intercourse and decreased sexual activity post-treatment, suggesting that radiotherapy has less impact on sexual function [73]. These finding need to be further explored in larger studies.

Head and Neck Cancer

Only a small number of published studies on head and neck cancer and sexual orientation were available from countries other than the United States. In the Danish same-sex partnership cohort study described above, men in same-sex partnerships had over five times the risk of tonsillar cancer compared with other men (RR 5.6, 95 % CI 0.60–20.2) [7]. The International Head and Neck Cancer Epidemiology Consortium performed a pooled analysis of 5,642 head and neck cancer cases and 6,069 controls from four population-based and four hospital-based case controlled studies. Data was sourced from 12 countries, including the US. The number of women reporting same-sex sexual activity was very small and thus data on women having sex with women were not presented in the report. Men reporting a history of same-sex contact had a markedly increased risk (OR 8.89, 95 % CI 2.14–36.8) of cancer of the base of tongue compared with controls and also compared with other higher risk groups, such as women reporting oral sex contact ever (OR 4.32). These men did not have a raised risk of tonsillar cancer (OR 1.28, 95 % CI 0.25–6.64) [74].

Conclusions

A number of countries other than the United States have recognised the need for a national approach to improvements in health in the LGBT community and thus instituted policy and legislative change. However, the majority of countries around the world have at best neglected or all too frequently, marginalised and criminalised LGBT communities, with no consideration of their health and well-being. Thus globally, there are vast possibilities for developing and implementing national

LGBT-specific policies for screening and managing cancer. Only a limited number of published population-based surveys provided data on cancer risk, prevalence, incidence and mortality in LGBT communities. No country could be identified where demographic data on sexual identity/orientation were collected in national cancer registries. In Australia, a large scale population-based survey showed low rates of refusal to complete a question on sexual orientation, demonstrating the feasibility of asking such questions in large scale research [75].

Of all cancer types, the most extensively researched and published is anal cancer among MSM. Numerous studies reported on cancer among MSM living with HIV. Indeed the amount of data on cancer in MSM with HIV was disproportionally high compared with that available for MSM in the general population. Few studies were available of risks of cancer among lesbian and bisexual women. Importantly, apart from case reports, only one study was identified in the published literature among transgender people, where rates of cancer were reported to be similar between transgender people and control groups in Belgium [76]. It is critical that the alarming paucity of research in cancer in transgender populations is addressed without delay.

The largest of studies, the Danish cohort study, showed a worrying trend in increases in cancer-related mortality among all age groups of same-sex married women compared with opposite-sex married women, after no difference was found a decade ago. In 2003, men in same-sex partnerships were twice as likely to have cancer compared with men in the general population. However, this was almost entirely a result of extremely high rates of KS, NHL and anal cancer [7]. The mortality rates of men in same-sex marriages had declined since the 1990s. Though still raised when compared with opposite-sex married men, the rates were similar to mortality rates among unmarried, widowed or divorced men [20].

The studies presented here provide further evidence that MSM regardless of HIV status have a markedly increased risk of anal cancer, while HIV positive MSM have a 100 fold increased risk of anal cancer [44, 63]. Tonsillar and base of tongue (HPV-related) cancers also are more prevalent among MSM. Conversely, prostate cancer risk appears to be either the same or decreased compared with heterosexual men. Though papers on cervical cancer rates among LBW were not identified, similar rates of cervical cancer precursor lesions were found among women having sex with women compared with heterosexual women [54].

Differing findings as to risk factors are reported between countries and within countries. These differences in reported rates of smoking and alcohol consumption may reflect differences in sampling frames. In Canada, LBW were twice as likely to smoke as heterosexual women [15]. There was no difference among men by sexual orientation [16]. In the Netherlands, sexual orientation was not linked to current cigarette smoking in men or women [21]. In Australia, some studies showed smoking rates in the LGBT community double those of the general population [26], whereas other studies found smoking rates in the LGBT community were comparable to national data [22]. Descriptive and small studies of transgender health also suggest high rates of smoking among transgender people. In Canada, LBW were twice as likely to report excess alcohol consumption compared with heterosexual women [15]. There was no difference among men by sexual orientation [16]. In a UK study, 40 % of LBW consumed alcohol at least three times a week [27]. In the Netherlands, LGB people were more likely to report excess alcohol consumption [21], whereas in Australia, reported alcohol use in the LGBT community was lower than national averages [22]. It is unclear whether sampling differences or true international differences are responsible for the disparities in these findings.

When reviewing the infectious causes of cancer, MSM are consistently more likely than heterosexual men to have anal HPV detected. The studies discussed here demonstrate the increased risk of cancer among gay and bisexual men living with HIV. The incidence of any cancer among gay and bisexual men living with HIV was 21 fold higher in Scotland, 54 fold in Spain and 44 fold higher in Italy and France, compared with men in the general population [45–47].

Patterns of health-care utilisation are influenced by the often negative attitudes and experiences within the healthcare system [77]. For instance, LBW are less likely to have a regular family doctor [15]. These in turn may influence cancer outcomes. There is a lack of training for health care professionals providing cancer and palliative care services to LGBT people [78], and health promotion strategies such as tobacco control programs consistently omit LGBT-specific programs and messaging. It is beyond the scope of this chapter to examine ways to address the impact that stigma and discrimination have on health-related behaviours and outcomes, but an approach to cancer in LGBT communities that may be explored is "combination prevention", similar to that of HIV prevention. The UNAIDS definition of combination prevention programs for HIV is "rights-based, evidence-informed, and community-owned programmes that use a mix of biomedical, behavioural, and structural interventions, prioritized to meet the HIV prevention needs of particular individuals and communities …. Well-designed combination prevention programmes are carefully tailored to national and local needs and conditions …. They mobilize community, private sector, government, and global resources in a collective undertaking. They require and benefit from enhanced partnership and coordination. "[79, 80]. This evidence-informed approach may include biomedical strategies (for instance screening and vaccination), behavioural strategies (for instance health promotion targeting smoking and alcohol use among certain groups) and structural interventions. These structural interventions need to address the social, cultural, political and economic environment that affects individual and collective vulnerability and risk. For cancer and the LGBT community, these interventions may be legislation, programmatic and policy changes. They could be standardised and compulsory training of health care providers in LGBT health, planning by public health and healthcare agencies for the specific demands of LGBT cancer survivors and their family members [2] and inclusion of GLBT people in all population-based government health and well-being policies [22]. These changes combined with sensitive documentation of sexual orientation and gender identity in census and cancer registry data [2, 18] and indeed any government funded research [4], would ideally improve our knowledge of the impact of cancer among LGBT people.

References

1. Cancer Research UK. Policy statement: health inequalities in cancer and LGBT communities. 2008. 1st Feb 2014.
2. Boehmer U, Miao X, Ozonoff A. Cancer survivorship and sexual orientation. Cancer. 2011;117:3796–84.
3. Boehmer U, Cooley T, Clark M. Cancer and men who have sex with men: a systematic review. Lancet Oncol. 2012;13:e545–53.
4. National LGBTI Health Alliance. LGBTI Health 2013: people, profiles and perspectives. LGBTI Health Update [Internet]. 2013; 3.
5. Dhami K, Breast Cancer Care. Lesbian and bisexual women and breast cancer: a policy briefing. London; 2011 1907001484, 9781907001482.
6. Henderson H. Why lesbians should be encouraged to have regular cervical screening. J Fam Plann Reprod Health Care. 2009;35:49–52.
7. Frisch M, Smith E, Grulich A, Johansen C. Cancer in a population-based cohort of men and women in registered homosexual partnerships. Am J Epidemiol. 2003;157:966–72.
8. Fish J, Anthony D. UK national lesbians and health care survey. Women Health. 2005;41:27–45.
9. Machalek D, Grulich A, Hillman R, Jin F, Templeton D, Tabrizi S, et al. The study of the prevention of anal cancer (SPANC): design and methods of a three-year prospective cohort study. BMC Public Health. 2013;13:946. doi:10.1186/1471-2458-13-946.
10. Australian Government Department of Health. National Lesbian, Gay, Bisexual, Transgender and Intersex (LGBTI) ageing and aged care strategy. 2012. http://www.health.gov.au/lgbtistrategy. Accessed 1 March 2014.
11. Department of Health and Ageing, Australian Government. National women's health policy 2010. p. 92–101. Commonwealth of Australia 2010. National Circuit, Barton ACT 2600 ISBN: 978-1-74241-363-1 Online ISBN: 978-1-74241-364-8 Publications Number: D0102.
12. Fish J. Cervical screening in lesbian and bisexual women: a review of the worldwide literature using systematic methods. Leicester: De Montfort University; 2009.
13. Musingarimi P. Health issues affecting older gay, lesbian and bisexual people in the UK. UK: The International Longevity Centre [Internet]; 2008. 1st February 2014.
14. Government of Canada. Canadian Human Rights Act (R.S.C., 1985, c. H-6). Justice laws website, [Internet]. 1996. http://laws-lois.justice.gc.ca/eng/acts/H-6/. Accessed 1 March 2014.
15. Steele L, Ross L, Dobinson C, Veldhuizen S, Tinmouth J. Women's sexual orientation and health: results from a Canadian population-based survey. Women Health. 2009;49:353–67.
16. Brennan D, Ross L, Dobinson C, Veldhuizen S, Steele L. Men's sexual orientation and health in Canada. Can J Public Health. 2010;101:255–8.
17. Mulé N, Ross L, Deeprose B, Jackson B, Daley A, Travers A, et al. Promoting LGBT health and wellbeing through inclusive policy development. Int J Health Equity. 2009;8. doi:10.1186/1475-9276-8-18.
18. Rainbow Health Ontario. LGBT Health and Public Policy. Ontario, Canada. 2014. http://www.rainbowhealthontario.ca/research/policy.cfm. Accessed 1 March 2014.
19. Trans Care Project. Trans care medical issues: trans people and cancer. Vancouver: Vancouver Coastal Health; 2006.
20. Frisch M, Simonsen J. Marriage, cohabitation and mortality in Denmark: national cohort study of 6.5 million persons followed for up to three decades (1982-2011). Int J Epidemiol. 2013;42:559–78.
21. Sandfort T, Bakker F, Schellevis F, Vanwesenbeeck I. Sexual orientation and mental and physical health status: findings from a Dutch population survey. Am J Public Health. 2006;96: 1119–25.
22. Leonard W, Pitts M, Mitchell A, Lyons A, Smith A, Patel S, et al. Private lives 2: the second national survey of the health and wellbeing of gay, lesbian, bisexual and transgender (GLBT) Australians (Monograph Series number 86). Melbourne. The Australian Research Centre in Sex, Health and Society, La Trobe University; 2012.

23. Australian Institute for Health and Welfare. Australia's welfare 2011. Canberra: AIHW; 2011.
24. Pitts M, Smith A, Mitchell A, Patel S. Private lives: a report on the health and wellbeing of GLBTI Australians. (Monograph series no 57, the Australian Research Centre in Sex, Health and Society). Melbourne: La Trobe University, Gay and Lesbian Health Victoria; 2006.
25. Grierson J, Pitts M, Koelmeyer R. HIV futures seven: the health and wellbeing of HIV positive people in Australia (Monograph series no 88, the Australian Research Centre in Sex, Health and Society). Melbourne: La Trobe University; 2013.
26. Mooney-Somers J, Deacon R, Comfort J, Richters J, Parkhill N. Women in contact with the Sydney gay and lesbian cmmunity: report of the Sydney women and sexual health (SWASH) survey 2006, 2008, 2010 and 2012. Sydney: ACON & Centre for Values, Ethics and the Law in Medicine (VELiM), University of Sydney; 2013.
27. Hunt R, Fish J. Prescription for change: lesbian and bisexual women's health check. London: Stonewall, de Montfort University; 2008.
28. Parkin D, Boyd L, Walker L. The fraction of cancer attributable to lifestyle and environmental factors in the UK in 2010. Br J Cancer. 2011;105:s77–s81.
29. Harding R, Bensley J, Corrigan N. Targeting smoking cessation to high prevalence communities: outcomes from a pilot intervention for gay men. BMC Public Health. 2004;4:43. doi:10.1186/1471-2458-4-43.
30. Bouvard V, Baan R, Straif K, Grosse Y, Secretan B, El Ghissassi F. A review of human carcinogens—part B: biological agents. Lancet Oncol. 2009;10:321–2.
31. De Vuyst H, Clifford G, Nascimento M, Madeleine M, Franceschi S. Prevalence and type distribution of human papillomavirus in carcinoma and intraepithelial neoplasia of the vulva, vagina and anus: a meta-analysis. Int J Cancer. 2009;124:1626–36.
32. Machalek D, Poynten I, Jin F, Fairley C, Farnsworth A, Garland S, et al. Anal human papillomavirus infection and associated neoplastic lesions in men who have sex with men: a systematic review and meta-analysis. Lancet Oncol. 2012;13:487–500.
33. Sadlier C, Rowley D, Morley D, Surah S, O'Dea S, Delamere S, et al. Prevalence of human papillomavirus in men who have sex with men in the era of an effective vaccine; a call to act. HIV Med. 2014;15(8):499–504.
34. Van Aar F, Mooij S, Van Der Sande M, Speksnijder A, Stolte I, Meijer C, et al. Anal and penile high-risk human papillomavirus prevalence in HIV-negative and HIV-infected MSM. AIDS. 2013;27:2921–31.
35. Poynten I, Tabrizi S, Jin F, Cornall A, Phillips S, Templeton D, et al. High-risk anal human papillomavirus (HPV) types in Australian homosexual men—predictors, prevalence and patterns of infection. Eurogin; 3rd–6th November; Florence, Italy 2013.
36. González C, Torres M, Benito A, Del Romero J, Rodríguez C, Fontillón M, et al. Anal squamous intraepithelial lesions are frequent among young HIV-infected men who have sex with men followed up at the Spanish AIDS Research Network Cohort (CoRIS-HPV). Int J Cancer. 2013;133:1164–73.
37. Guimarães M, Grinsztejn B, Melo V, Rocha G, Campos L, Pilotto J, et al. Anal HPV prevalence and associated factors among HIV-seropositive men under antiretroviral treatment in Brazil. J Acquir Immune Defic Syndr. 2011;57(Supplement 3):3S217–S24..
38. Nureña C, Brown B, Galea J, Sánchez H, Blas M. HPV and genital warts among Peruvian men who have sex with men and transgender people: knowledge, attitudes and treatment experiences. PLoS One. 2013;8(3):e58684.
39. Pelullo C, Di Giuseppe G, Angelillo I. Human papillomavirus infection: knowledge, attitudes, and behaviors among lesbian, gay men, and bisexual in Italy. PLoS One. 2012;7(8):e42856.
40. Rank C, Gilbert M, Ogilvie G, Jayaraman G, Marchand R, Trussler T, et al. Acceptability of human papillomavirus vaccination and sexual experience prior to disclosure to health care providers among men who have sex with men in Vancouver, Canada: implications for targeted vaccination programs. Vaccine. 2012;30:5755–60.
41. Read T, Hocking J, Vodstrcil L, Tabrizi S, McCullough M, Grulich A, et al. Oral human papillomavirus in men having sex with men: risk-factors and sampling. PLoS One. 2012;7(11):e49324.

42. Donovan B, Franklin N, Guy R, Grulich A, Regan D, Ali H, et al. Quadrivalent human papillomavirus vaccination and trends in genital warts in Australia: analysis of national sentinel surveillance data. Lancet Oncol. 2011;11:39–44.
43. Garland S. The Australian experience with the Human Papillomavirus vaccine. Clin Ther. 2014;36:17–23.
44. Piketty C, Selinger-Leneman H, Bouvier A, Belot A, Mary-Krause M, Duvivier C, et al. Incidence of HIV-related anal cancer remains increased despite long-term combined antiretroviral treatment: results from the french hospital database on HIV. J Clin Oncol. 2012;30:4360–6.
45. Allardice G, Hole D, Brewster D, Boyd J, Goldberg D. Incidence of malignant neoplasms among HIV-infected persons in Scotland. Br J Cancer. 2003;89:505–7.
46. Galceran J, Marcos-Gragera R, Soler M, Romaguera A, Ameijide A, Izquierdo A, et al. Cancer incidence in AIDS patients in Catalonia, Spain. Eur J Cancer. 2007;43:1085–91.
47. Serraino D, Boschini A, Carrieri P, Pradier C, Dorrucci M, Dal Maso L, et al. Cancer risk among men with, or at risk of, HIV infection in southern Europe. AIDS. 2000;14:553–9.
48. All Party Parliamentary Group on Cancer. Report of the all party parliamentary group's inquiry into inequalities in cancer London; 2009.
49. Gaudet M, Gapstur S, Sun J, Diver W, Hannan L, Thun M. Active smoking and breast cancer risk: original cohort data and meta-analysis. J Natl Cancer Inst. 2013;105:515–25.
50. Nyante S, Gierach G, Dallal C, Freedman N, Park Y, Danforth K, et al. Cigarette smoking and postmenopausal breast cancer risk in a prospective cohort. Br J Cancer. 2014;110(9):2339–47.
51. Brown A, Hassard J, M F, Szabo E, Wakefield M. Lesbian's experience of cervical screening. Health Promotoion J Australia. 2003;14:128–32.
52. Meads C, Moore D. Breast cancer in lesbians and bisexual women: systematic review of incidence, prevalence and risk studies. BMC Public Health. 2013;13:1127-.
53. Bailey J, Kavanagh J, Owen C, McClean K, Skinner C. Lesbians and cervical screening. Br J Gen Pract. 2000;50:481–2.
54. Fethers K, Marks C, Mindel A, Estcourt C. Sexually transmitted infections and risk behaviours in women who have sex with women. Sex Transm Infect. 2000;76:345–9.
55. BC Cancer Agency. About cancer screening: cervix; 2012 [1st March 2014].
56. Australian Government Department of Health. National Cervical Screening Program 2013; http://www.cancerscreening.gov.au/internet/screening/publishing.nsf/Content/cervical. Accessed 1 March 2014.
57. Marrazzo J, Koutsky L, Stine K, Kuypers J, Grubert T, Galloway D, et al. Genital human papillomavirus infection in women who have sex with women. J Infect Dis. 1998;178:1604–9.
58. Daling J, Weiss N, Hislop T, Maden C, Coates R, Sherman K, et al. Sexual practices, sexually transmitted diseases, and the incidence of anal cancer. N Engl J Med. 1987;317:973–7.
59. Bertisch B, Franceschi S, Lise M, Vernazza P, Keiser O, Schöni-Affolter F, et al. Risk factors for anal cancer in persons infected with HIV: a nested case-control study in the Swiss HIV Cohort Study. Am J Epidemiol. 2013;178:877–84.
60. de Pokomandy A, Rouleau D, Ghattas G, Trottier H, Vézina S, Coté P, et al. HAART and progression to high-grade anal intraepithelial neoplasia in men who have sex with men and are infected with HIV. Clin Infect Dis. 2011;52:1174–81.
61. Piketty C, Selinger-Leneman H, Grabar S, Duvivier C, Bonmarchand M, Abramowitz L, et al. Marked increase in the incidence of invasive anal cancer among HIV-infected patients despite treatment with combination antiretroviral therapy. AIDS. 2008;22:1203–11.
62. van der Zee R, Richel O, de Vries H, Prins J. The increasing incidence of anal cancer: can it be explained by trends in risk groups? NethJ Med. 2013;71:401–11.
63. Richel O, Van der Zee R, Smith A, De Vries H, Prins J. Gradually decreasing anal cancer incidence in the HIV + population in the Netherlands after a decade of cART. Sex Health. 2013;10:586.
64. Legarth R, Helleberg M, Kronborg G, Larsen C, Pedersen G, Pedersen C, et al. Anal carcinoma in HIV-infected patients in the period 1995-2009: a Danish nationwide cohort study. Scand J Infect Dis. 2013;45:453–9.
65. Macaya A, Muñoz-Santos C, Balaguer A, Barberà M. Interventions for anal canal intraepithelial neoplasia. Cochrane Database Syst Rev. 2012;12:CD009244.

66. Coutlée F, de Pokomandy A, Franco E. Epidemiology, natural history and risk factors for anal intraepithelial neoplasia. Sex Health. 2012;9:547–55.
67. van Leeuwen M, Vajdic C, Middleton M, McDonald A, Law M, Kaldor J, et al. Continuing declines in some but not all HIV-associated cancers in Australia after widespread use of antiretroviral therapy. AIDS. 2009;23:2183–90.
68. Madeleine M, Newcomer L. Chaper 5 cancer of the anus. SEER survival monograph: cancer survival among adults. In: Ries L, Young J, Keel G, Eisner M, Lin Y, Horner M-J, editors. US SEER program, 1988-2001, patient and tumor characteristics Bethesda: National Cancer Institute, SEER Program; 2007. p. 43–7.
69. Ortholan C, Ramaioli A, Peiffert D, Lusinchi A, Romestaing P, Chauveinc L, et al. Anal canal carcinoma: early-stage tumors<or= 10 mm (T1 or Tis): therapeutic options and original pattern of local failure after radiotherapy. Int J Radiat Oncol Biol Phys. 2005;62:479–85.
70. Ong J, Chen M, Temple-Smith M, Walker S, Hoy J, Woolley I, et al. The inside story. Physicians' views on digital ano-rectal examination for anal cancer screening of HIV positive men who have sex with men. J Med Screen. 2013;20:188–91.
71. Read T, Vodstrcil L, Grulich A, Farmer C, Bradshaw C, Chen M, et al. Acceptability of digital anal cancer screening examinations in HIV-positive homosexual men. HIV Med. 2013;14:491–6.
72. Wassersug R, Lyons A, Duncan D, Dowsett G, Pitts M. Diagnostic and outcome differences between heterosexual and nonheterosexual men treated for prostate cancer. Urology. 2013;82:565–71.
73. Lee T, Breau R, Eapen L. Pilot study on quality of life and sexual function in men-who-have-sex-with-men treated for prostate cancer. J Sex Med. 2013;10:2094–100.
74. Heck J, Berthiller J, Vaccarella S, Winn D, Smith E, Shan'gina O, et al. Sexual behaviours and the risk of head and neck cancers: a pooled analysis in the International Head and Neck Cancer Epidemiology (INHANCE) consortium. Int J Epidemiol. 2010;39:166–81.
75. Byles J, Forder P, Grulich A, Prestage G. It's okay to ask. Inclusion of sexual orientation questions is feasible in population health surveys. Australia New Zealand. J Public Health. 2013;37:390–1.
76. Wierckx K, Elaut E, Declercq E, Heylens G, De Cuypere G, Taes Y, et al. Prevalence of cardiovascular disease and cancer during cross-sex hormone therapy in a large cohort of trans persons: a case-control study. Eur J Endocrinol. 2013;169:471–8.
77. McNair R. Lesbian health inequalities: a cultural minority issue for health professionals. Med J Aust. 2003;178:643–5.
78. Reygan F, D'Alton P. A pilot training programme for health and social care professionals providing oncological and palliative care to lesbian, gay and bisexual patients in Ireland. Psycho-Oncology. 2013;22:1050–4.
79. UNAIDS. Combination prevention: strategic HIV prevention programmes founded on good practice. A background paper for the UNAIDS Prevention Reference Group Meeting. Geneva; 2009 3–5 December 2009. Report No.
80. UNAIDS. Combination prevention HIV: tailoring and coordinating biomedical, behavioural and structural strategies to reduce new HIV infections: a UNAIDS discussion paper In: Joint United Nations Programme on HIV/AIDS, editor Geneva; 2010.

Chapter 19
The Challenges Remain: Needed Next Steps in Alleviating the Burden of Cancer in the LGBT Community

Ronit Elk and Ulrike Boehmer

Abstract Recently, there have been significant improvements in federal policy that have positively impacted many aspects of healthcare for LGBT patients and their families. Despite this, significant challenges remain. In order to improve outcome and survival in the LGBT community, as well as to reduce suffering in LGBT patients and families, there are steps that we as a community and society need to take. In this chapter we focus on these obstacles and the necessary action steps.

Despite the recent and very significant improvements in federal policy, and notwithstanding the valiant efforts of dedicated researchers, some of whose work is profiled in this book, significant ongoing challenges remain, hurdles that continue to impede our ability to reduce the risk of cancer in the LGBT community, of detecting cancer early, and thus improving outcome and survival, and equally important, of reducing suffering in both the LGBT person and their loved ones. There are several important steps that we as a community and as a society have to take if we are to overcome these. It is these obstacles, as well as the steps necessary to overcome them that we focus on in this chapter.

There are two reasons for focusing on these; the first is to raise awareness about the ongoing obstacles, which are hurdles that can in fact be overcome, but which require sustained and coordinated effort and persistence. Our second goal is to both inspire and challenge the reader into taking action– in either working to remove the obstacles, or in tackling one or more of the many remaining gaps in knowledge. We know that change can happen, as we are living in its midst. If the priority action areas identified in this chapter are tackled, consider in how many thousands of LGBT lives we can re-

R. Elk (✉)
College of Nursing, University of South Carolina, Columbia, SC, USA
e-mail: ELK@mailbox.sc.edu

U. Boehmer
Department of Community Health Sciences, Boston University School of Public Health, Boston, MA, USA
e-mail: boehmer@bu.edu

U. Boehmer, R. Elk (eds.), *Cancer and the LGBT Community*,
DOI 10.1007/978-3-319-15057-4_19

duce cancer risk, for how many hundreds of thousand lives we can improve outcome and survival, and how much suffering we can prevent in the LGBT community.

Gaps in Research Across the Cancer Continuum

Notwithstanding the remarkable accomplishments of some dedicated researchers, many of whom contributed to this book, there remains an *enormous gap* in knowledge of cancer in the LGBT community, *across the entire cancer continuum*. Some, but certainly not all, of these gaps are listed here for two purposes. The first is to demonstrate the broad range of research in cancer in the LGBT community that remains unaddressed. The second is so that future researchers or students with an interest in any of these areas can find a wealth of research opportunities. These issues must be investigated further if we are to reduce the burden of cancer in the LGBT community.

Gaps in Research in Reducing the Risk of Cancer

Pathways by which health outcomes influence risk factors: In Chap. 4, Fredrikson-Goldsen et al. highlight the need for research that delineates pathways by which health outcomes can be influenced by risk factors that result from a sexual or gender minority status. They recommend studying the interplay of factors such as social exclusion and discrimination, in combination with the presence/absence of personal/social resources that may result in adverse health behaviors, such as smoking, some of which have been linked to the etiology of cancer. Fredrikson-Goldsen et al. also suggest assessing the protective factor of marriage as an influence on health behaviors, only recently granted to the LGBT community in more than two thirds of US states. Although it has been shown that smoking is more prevalent among LGB adolescents and at a younger age, in Chap. 5, Burkhalter stresses the need for studies focusing on the etiology of smoking disparities among sexual and gender minorities. Also unstudied to date are tobacco prevention and cessation interventions specifically targeted to the LGBT community.

Gaps in Research in Screening for and Early Detection of Cancer

In Chap. 6, Clark et al. point out the wide range of studies to determine the prevalence of screening, identify those subgroups less likely to be screened, and study interventions appropriate to those subgroups that would enhance screening. Lacking are population-based studies to determine the barriers to and facilitators of screening. Also missing are studies of subgroups within the LGBT community, including racial and ethnic minorities, and intervention studies to test methods of reducing barriers. Research is also needed on cancer screening recommendations made by providers to LGBT individuals, the outcome on screening adherence of LGBT-sensitivity training programs for healthcare staff, such as the one provided by the National LGBT Cancer Network or the Human Rights Campaign Health Equality Index. In Chap. 7, Blank et al. highlight the need for more research on effective screening, screening intervals, relative benefits and risks of screening, and screening training, especially how to direct appropriate screening messages to gay and bisexual (GB) men, men who have sex with men (MSM), and transgender people.

Gaps in Research in Cancer Survivorship

As documented by Amiel et al. (Chap. 10) and Haigentz (Chap. 11), cancer in sexual minority men is under-researched, including associated psychosocial issues, despite strong epidemiological data of increasing cancer rates among sexual minority men with HIV-infection. Focusing on women with breast cancer in Chap. 9, Boehmer highlights the many gaps that remain in terms of our knowledge of sexual minority women undergoing or who have undergone treatment. There is a need for research on understanding sexual minority women's experiences with disclosure to their provider and their experience within the health care system. Lacking are studies about sexual minority women's perceptions of treatments and their outcomes, treatment preferences, decision-making and adherence to treatments. Boehmer points out that it is key that we conduct such studies in order to ensure that sexual minority women achieve their desired role in decision making, are fully informed about treatments and side effects, and are supported in coping with late and long-term effects. Boehmer highlights several other areas of missing research. Little is known on health care providers' perceptions and attitudes towards sexual minorities, knowledge of and skills in caring for sexual minorities. We know almost nothing about sexual minority women diagnosed with Stage IV cancers, or those with a recurrence or secondary cancers. The experiences of sexual minority women undergoing treatment at these stages, and their unique needs and preferences need to be explored. Survivorship Care Plans are designed to achieve coordinated care with the overall goal of enhancing quality of care for cancer survivors. However, there are no studies that have determined whether survivorship plans for sexual minority women are tailored to address their unique needs. Research is needed to understand the experiences of caregivers to the sexual minority cancer patient. There is a dire need for intervention studies. The economic burden of cancer on sexual minority women's lives, families, and relationships has been unexplored to date. Studies of subgroups of sexual minority women, including those from an ethnic or racial minority, rural areas, those who are older, and others are missing from the literature and are necessary to provide us with an understanding of the needs and challenges facing each of these unique groups. In their introduction to Chap. 13 on Cancer Survivorship, Margolies and Kamen begin by referring to a review by Boehmer [1], pointing out that despite the large number of LGBT cancer survivors, they have for the most part remained invisible in research. There is limited information on the support-seeking behavior of LGBT cancer survivors. In Chap. 14, Elk highlights the paucity of research that focuses specifically on understanding the needs, preferences, and perspectives of LGBT people at end of life, and how their preferences and those of their partners influence their end of life care decisions. Other than the literature focusing on those with HIV and AIDS, there have only been a handful of studies focusing on the experiences of LGBTs at end of life and a few focusing on their anticipated future. Large-scale research in this area remains a priority, for it is only through this process that we can build the necessary evidence to design evidence-based programs tailored to the unique needs of LGBT patients who are facing a life-limiting illness.

Gaps in Research on Cross-Cutting Issues

The Diversity of the LGBT Community Because much of what is known about the LGBT community and cancer has been painstakingly researched, at times overcoming tremendous obstacles to identify LGBT individuals that fit the respective study criteria, insufficient attention has been paid to the diversity of the LGBT community. Along the cancer continuum, there is a need to consider the intersectionality of LGBT people, examining LGBTs' multiple identities and the ways in which they interact [2]. For example, in Chap. 9 Boehmer indicates although racial and ethnic minorities are included in studies of sexual minority cancer survivors, the number of sexual minority women who are racial and ethnic minorities is too small to be able to come to any reliable conclusions. Other intersections, such as LGBT individuals who are poor or foreign-born need to be examined as well. In Chap. 16, Matthews et al. point out the paucity of information on the needs and experiences of sexual minorities of color with cancer *across the cancer continuum.* A similar vacuum in research exists across the cancer continuum among the transgender population. As Lombardi and Banik point out in Chap. 15, the IOM report [2] has identified the lack of any cancer-focused research among transgender individuals other than a small number of case studies focusing on hormone therapy and hormone sensitive cancers. Furthermore, the IOM report identified the need for more research in the health disparities of transgender people and pointed out that research among these population groups remains a high priority [2].

Healthcare Settings The healthcare setting remains unwelcoming to LGBT individuals. Healthcare staff may be prejudiced, are often untrained in understanding the LGBT community, and there is a serious shortage of tailored programs for LGBTs with cancer. While it is no longer socially acceptable to engage in overtly discriminatory behaviors in healthcare settings, Eliason and Dibble (Chap. 12) explain that some healthcare providers harbor overtly negative attitudes, resulting in refusal of care or receipt of inappropriate care. Although this is a minority, most LGBT patients will unfortunately continue to experience a more subtle form of discrimination during visits to a health care setting, including micro-insults such as condescension or insensitivity, resulting in the patient's hyper vigilance and often not coming out. Fredriksen-Goldsen et al. (Chap. 4), Eliason and Dibble (Chap. 12), Elk (Chap. 14), Lombardi and Banik (Chap. 15), and Scout (Chap. 17), all describe research that clearly indicates LGBT people continue to experience various forms of discrimination in healthcare settings, which may result in concealing their sexual and gender identities, which in turn may impact the quality and timeliness of care LGBT patients receive. Lack of cultural competence training and lack of familiarity with LGBT patients' circumstances (for example, LGBT individuals are significantly less likely than heterosexuals to list biological family members as support sources, instead listing members of family of choice) and unique needs are primary causes and ones that we can target for change.

The Next Wave of Research on LGBT and Cancer: Guiding Frameworks

Up to now, the groundbreaking studies discussed throughout this book were predominantly framed from the perspective of health disparities or health inequities, (e.g., lower rates of screening, more cancer risk behaviors), comparing LGBT individuals to heterosexual individuals. This remains a compelling approach, which needs to be continued to fully explore all aspects of cancer for LGBT individuals and to reveal all aspects of structural discrimination and deprivation that hinder LGBT people from living long healthy lives. Researchers also frequently assess the unique aspects of LGBTs that are not mirrored by heterosexuals (e.g., disclosure of sexual identity, experiences stemming from living as a minority).

Many of the frameworks that guide other health research or the research of other health issues that affect LGBT patients need to be applied to cancer more fully in the future. Moving forward it is important to make use of these additional frameworks to deepen the understanding of the LGBT communities in the context of cancer. Consistent with the recommendations of the IOM report [2], the *life-course framework* can be applied to an understanding of cancer, prevention, and cancer risk factors, acknowledging that events at each stage of life influence subsequent stages and recognizing that experiences are shaped by one's age cohort and historical context. Similarly, the *minority stress model,* which posits that sexual and gender minorities experience chronic stress as a result of their stigmatization [2] will need be fully explored in the context of cancer, including studies that examine the neurophysiological responses to the stress experienced by LGBT people, including studies that explore biomedical pathways of minority stress on immune function. Another framework, *syndemic theory,* which has been used for understanding HIV risk in the LGBT population, is likely suitable and beneficial for understanding LGBT patients and cancer as well. *Syndemic theory* refers to the understanding that two or more conditions are interconnected and interacting synergistically, thereby contributing to an excess burden of disease in the LGBT population, as has been shown for the HIV epidemic in the US [3]. Yet another approach, the Health Equity Model [4], is described in detail by Fredriksen-Goldsen et al. (Chap. 4). These authors explain that the health equity approach aims not only to reduce disparities but also to fully maximize efforts embedded within social contexts so that all people can attain their full health potential. Other models for deepening the understanding of LGBT health in the context of cancer are the resilience of LGBT individuals and the LGBT community. Resilience has also been utilized as a framework for understanding prevention of HIV among gay and bisexual men [5]. These frameworks are not intended as an exhaustive list of approaching LGBT populations and cancer, but as examples of approaches to apply in future cancer-related studies.

Lack of Tailored Programs for LGBT Patients and Lack of Training of Healthcare Professionals

An immediate and significant outcome of the limited state of research on cancer and LGBT communities is the lack of evidence-based programs that address this population specifically.

Lack of Risk-Reduction Programs

Although there are many studies indicating the need for culturally sensitive, tailored interventions to reduce behavioral risk among LGBT people, see Fredriksen-Goldsen et al. (Chap. 4), the reality is that there is a dearth of programs designed to address specific behavioral risks in modifying cancer-related risk behaviors. For example, of the 14,000 substance abuse treatment centers in the US, Fredriksen-Goldsen et al. explain that only 6 % of these target lesbian or gay clients. In Chap. 3, Tracy provides another example: the lack of an evidence-base for health promotion materials developed for sexual minority women on safe sex practices. In Chap. 5, Burkhalter discusses data that indicate a high prevalence of smoking among LGB youth and LGBT adults, higher than their heterosexual counterparts, pointing to a strong need to find effective culturally-tailored programs. Thanks to the effort of the Network for Health Equity (now called LGBT HealthLink) headed by Dr. Scout, there has been progress in the field of smoking, such as advising the CDC on data inclusion in the 2012 National Adult Tobacco Survey, which led to the first national LGBT smoking prevalence data. Also, the CDC's Office of Smoking and Health now has several LGBT tailored ads in their mass media campaigns. There remains much work to be done, however; few state-level tobacco control campaigns include LGBT tailored activities, and most tobacco quit line staff are not trained in LGBT cultural competency. In Chap. 17, Scout describes how the Affordable Care Act (described below) created a new wave of cancer prevention activities nationwide, with half a billion dollars flowing into community grants that created local level programs focused on several cancer risk reduction strategies. However, despite top-level LGBT inclusion in the Task Force on Prevention, the actual funding announcements for these mechanisms did not result in prioritization for LGBT inclusion. Despite the prioritization of inclusion of LGBT people in federal documents, other funding sources that were earmarked for city and state cancer prevention efforts resulted in only a few tailored LGBT cancer prevention programs.

Lack of Screening Programs

To date, as Clark et al. (Chap. 6) tell us, no recommendations for cancer screening specific to lesbian and bisexual women have been developed or recommended by the agencies that develop such guidelines, like the Centers of Disease Control and Prevention (CDC) and the American Cancer Society. Dibble and her colleagues (referred to in Clark et al.'s chapter) developed and tested an intervention that was found to enhance some forms of cancer screening, but this intervention has not been implemented in other settings despite its proven efficacy. Interestingly, Scout (Chap. 17) explains that in the absence of guidelines for screening of transgender men and women, the CDC adopted the guidelines for transgender women created by the Center for Excellence on Transgender Health in December 2013, following national pressure after a transgender woman filed suit. The result is that all uninsured transgender women are eligible for free screening under the National Breast and Cervical Cancer Screening program.

Lack of Evidence-Based Survivorship Programs

As indicated earlier, there is an absence of evidence-based interventions and programs for sexual minority individuals with cancer, including survivorship care plans tailored to this population. Margolies and Kamen (Chap. 13) state that the most requested service by cancer survivors is targeted support groups for LGBT survivors. Yet, although support systems can have a profound impact on recovery and health outcomes, there are very few LGBT-tailored support groups in the US, and very few that are tailored to the needs of same-sex partners supporting the person with cancer. In addition, Margolies and Kamen explain that most cancer support groups operate under the one-size- fits-all model, which is often not appropriate for LGBT cancer patients in so many regards (e.g., pink paraphernalia may not be viewed as healing by lesbians and gender nonconforming patients.)

In order to provide patient-centered palliative and end of life care and services to LGBT patients and their families, which are currently unavailable, Elk (Chap. 14) stresses that it is essential that the physical, psychological, social, cultural and spiritual needs of these patients are recognized, understood, and to the fullest extent possible, met. This includes recognition and acceptance of sexual and gender minorities and all that is entailed, including acceptance and full recognition of the partner, who should be fully involved in the care and decision-making process. Care must also be delivered in an environment that is nonjudgmental and understanding. Similar recommendations are provided by Amiel et al. in Chap. 10, for urologists and other cancer treatment providers to address the unique needs of gay and bisexual men for survivorship services and techniques for providers to make their practice more welcoming for gay and bisexual men facing cancer.

Recommendations A particularly useful framework for thinking about the programmatic and policy needs of LGBT populations is the *social ecological perspective*, which recognizes that an individual's health is affected by community and social circumstances [2]. Therefore, LGBT health programs should consider LGBT individuals in their various contexts, including their interpersonal relationships, and strive for broad policy changes.

Access to Screening Although mandates in the Affordable Care Act and the repeal of the Defense of Marriage Act (DOMA) may reduce the number of LGBT people without insurance, some LGBT people will nonetheless be denied access to cancer screening, either because of lack of insurance or not being in a married or committed relationship to obtain partner benefits. Clark et al. (Chap. 6) make several recommendations to enhance these, including increased marketing of the National Breast and Cervical Cancer Early Detection Program to underserved lesbian and bisexual women. The use of electronic medical records, in which patient identifying information is retained, may be of value, as is education to health care providers on high-quality ways of enhancing screening in sexual and gender minorities.

Tailored Programming Margolies and Kamen (Chap. 13) speak of the need for tailoring that should be applied to survivorship programs for LGBT patients, for example, supportive care for patients with anal cancer among gay and bisexual men may need to address the sexual side effects of this type of cancer. Other suggestions include the use of patient navigators, matching patients with others in their peer network.

Nondiscrimination Policy Prior to 2011, it was up to individual healthcare organizations whether to have a nondiscrimination policy. As Scout (Chap. 17) explains, this changed when the Joint Commission, the largest healthcare accreditation body, issued a new guidance to all healthcare organizations, indicating that in order to receive accreditation LGBT people had to be included in the organization's nondiscrimination policies.

Training in Cultural Competence and Accreditation of Healthcare Agencies Training in LGBT cultural competence at the professional level, including medical and nursing schools and schools of allied health and public health, currently not an integral part of study, is an essential first step. The AAMC (Association of American Medical Colleges) Advisory Committee on Sexual Orientation, Gender Identity, and Sex Development has recently created a publication with a set of competency guidelines as a resource for medical educators [6]. This publication represents a major step forward in giving medical schools, academic medical centers, and other health organizations a roadmap for improving care for LGBT people.

The provision of LGBT cultural training competence to all health care providers will go a long way to promote better understanding and care of LGBT patients. Such national training programs are now available, and healthcare agencies that provide such training receive certification as a Leader in LGBT Healthcare from the Human Rights Campaign Health Equality Index (HEI). If the Joint Commission were to make this a mandatory training for all health care facilities to receive accreditation, this would result in substantial improvements in care of LGBT patients.

Safe Space Active welcoming of LGBT patients including the Safe Space symbol, to indicate that the clinic and its healthcare staff openly support the LGBT community is one of the methods of enhancing inclusiveness and acceptance of LGBT patients described by Margolies and Kamen (Chap. 13).

Monumental Recent Developments

In the sections above, we have described the dearth of LGBT-focused research and of LGBT-tailored programs, and have made recommendations for how to remedy these. However, we are living in a time of change, and we would be remiss if we were not to provide a perspective into the significant developments that have taken place over the last few years, advances that have the potential to significantly improve the healthcare of LGBT people. In addition to the HEI certifications and the Joint Commission accreditation guidelines described above, these include (1) the Affordable Care Act, (2) the repeal of the Defense of Marriage Act (DOMA) DOMA, (3) actions by the Department of Health and Human Services (HHS) and (4) the Presidential Memorandum.

Affordable Care Act (ACA)

This landmark Act will change the face of healthcare in the US. According to Scout (Chap. 17), the most profound impact on the underinsured LGBT population will be via the insurance exchanges, both in offering insurance to those without it, but also with new policy protections that will benefit the communities. With one in three low and middle income LGBT persons reporting being uninsured, the expansion of Medicaid will create many more affordable insurance options for this population. In addition, Sect. 1557 offers new anti-discrimination protections for LGBT people. There are three levels of changes that will have the greatest impact on the LGBT population: Insurers cannot deny a person or charge them more if they have a preexisting condition, such as cancer. Second, no one in the health care market, including insurers and employers, is allowed to discriminate against LGBT people and third, insurers cannot offer plans that discriminate based on sexual orientation or gender identity [7]. Protection for transgender people is also likely to be extremely beneficial; coverage now is being interpreted to include mental health and hormones but this is a moving target and not consistently interpreted. Since this is a new law, many of the protections stated in it are not as widely known as they need to be.

Repeal of DOMA

In a turning point decision in June 2013, the US Supreme Court struck down sections of the discriminatory DOMA, which was followed in 2014 by the Supreme Court's rejection to decide on appeals of same-sex marriage laws, setting into motion a rapid expansion of legal same-sex marriage to many more US states and the equal legal treatment of same-sex marriages from the federal government. Scout (Chap. 17) highlights the direct benefits to same-sex couples across the country. As more employers follow suit in recognizing either same-sex relationships or their marriages under employer insurance plans, a greater proportion of LGBT people will have access to cancer prevention and screening services through health insurance. Elk (Chap. 14) explains, however, that although this ruling is for same-sex married couples, it does not change any of the discriminatory state laws that still exclude same sex couples from state-conferred marriage rights in approximately 15 remaining states. This aspect has direct implications for the end of life care of a partner of an LGBT person. For example, receipt of a same-sex spouse's Medicare benefits (health benefits provided to someone over the age of 65) is *only* possible if she/he is married under the law of the state where he/she is living at the time of filing for benefits. Less well known are the changes that took place in the nation's largest health care system, the Department of Veterans Affairs (VA). Following the repeal of the discriminatory US military "Don't ask, don't tell" policy in 2010, increased protection and access to VA care became possible for LGBT veterans. Specifically, the VHA Directive 2011-024 regulated the provision of health care for transgender and intersex veterans, ensuring that transgender individuals eligible for VA care may now use the VA for hormonal therapy, mental healthcare, preoperative evaluation, and medically necessary post-operative and long-term care following sex reassignment surgery [8].

Presidential Memorandum 20511 of 2010

In 2010, President Obama signed an executive order directing HHS to support LGBT visitation in hospitals. As Elk (Chap. 14) explains, prior to this landmark mandate, partners of LGBT patients who were unconscious or not coherent could have been challenged by the hospital from both visiting their partners in hospitals, or acting as health care surrogates for partners who were incapacitated, including at end of life. The President directed the Department of Health and Human Services (HHS) to address these issues and in response, the Centers for Medicare and Medicaid (CMS), an HHS agency, amended its rules. Hospitals that accept Medicaid and Medicare must respect patients' advance directives and are prohibited from denying visitation priveleges based on, inter alia, sexual orientation. This means that in all hospitals that accept Medicaid and Medicare, the LGBT patient has the legal right for his/her loved one to visit in the hospital. However, Elk cautions that unlike in visitation of LGBT partners where federal law governs, in the case of an advance care directive, state law governs. This means that if an LGBT patient has not executed an advance directive granting rights to their same-sex partner, state health care surrogacy laws take over i.e., abiological family member can take over decision-making such as whether to continue treatment or whether to remove a loved one from a ventilator or other healthcare decisions so critical to end of life care, and they can do so regardless of the wishes of the same-sex partner. Whether this happens or not is determined by the state's legal perspective towards same-sex marriage (http://www.hrc.org/resources/entry/health-care-proxy). LGBT individuals who live in the states that still resist same-sex marriage are at risk of the state health care surrogacy laws taking over [9]. Scout (Chap. 17) points out that the federal policy about visitations was achieved by making it a condition of accepting Medicare, and comments that as the largest payer of healthcare services in the country, the federal government has a bully pulpit to make changes to non-discrimination in health. If they were to pass a similar ruling ensuring that all Medicaid recipients promoted LGBT nondiscrimination provisions, it would create the largest single nondiscrimination change to date. This is a lofty goal, but certainly a worthy target to work towards.

Major Obstacles and Recommendations for Action

A number of ongoing challenges are preventing the rapid expansion of knowledge through research and the development of evidence-based programs for LGBT populations and cancer.

Lack of National and State Surveillance Data Collection

The first step in identifying cancer prevalence, incidence, and mortality rates in any population group includes the examination of cancer registry data. These data are either collected at the state-level in partnership with the CDC's National Program of Cancer Registries, or by the SEER (Surveillance, Epidemiology and End Results) Program of the NCI. *Yet, to date cancer registries in the US do not include information on sexual orientation and gender identity* [2, 10, 11]. As addressed in over half of this book's chapters, this lack of systematic data collection acts as a significant barrier to understanding cancer incidence, treatment, and survival of LGBT people. This lack of information has prevented the identification of disparities in cancer incidence and mortality among LGBT people compared with heterosexual and cisgender persons, resulting in insufficient information suitable for the development of LGBT-specific screening guidelines. Unfortunately, as described by Dr. Poyten (Chap. 18), the lack of systematic data collection remains equally abysmal in other countries,.

There have been improvements in recent years, in that an increasing number of government and state-sponsored surveys include measures of sexual orientation. For example, many state-sponsored surveys e.g., CHIS (California Health Interview Survey)) ascertain sexual orientation, as do other government-sponsored surveys, e.g., National Health Interview Survey, National Survey of Family Growth, etc. However, even here there is still a need for considerable improvements, in that to date questions that ascertain gender identity are still mostly missing with few exceptions, such as the Behavioral Risk Factor Surveillance System (BRFSS), to which a number of states added questions about gender identity. Furthermore, while an increasing number of states opted to include sexual orientation above and beyond the mandatory BRFSS modules, only a consistent inclusion of both sexual orientation and gender identity questions in all US states will provide for a comprehensive national assessment of the health of LGBT communities in the US.

Recommendations for Action Scout (Chap. 17) explains why surveillance data are different from full probability studies. "First, states and the federal government rely on it for policy decisions; second, it is considered higher standard of evidence and thus holds more weight for demonstrating need in proposals; third, since these are often the largest surveys, it is more likely to provide much needed evidence on the quality and magnitude of health gaps. Reporting data are the only way different types of cancers are tracked in different populations. Until LGBT data are included in all facets of health data collection as a routine part of a demographic battery, LGBT cancer disparities will continue to be masked by inexact science (Scout p. 5.)" Sell and Dunn [12] and Boehmer et al. [13] have made compelling arguments for the inclusion of sexual orientation and gender identity as critical demographic variables that should be included in all surveillance and epidemiological research systems. Until this is the case, we will never be able to adequately address the needs of the LGBT population across the cancer continuum. Advocating for these data to be collected as part of all national and state surveillance and epidemiologic research systems must remain our first priority.

Lack of Research Funding

The key method of advancing knowledge is through conducting research; the National Cancer Institute (NCI) of the National Institutes of Health (NIH) is by far the largest funder of cancer research. In FY 2013 (the latest year for which data are available) their budget was $ 4.79 billion, of which 41.8 % were allotted to Research Project grants (total number funded in 2013 are 4816) (see: http://obf.cancer.gov/financial/factbook.htm). Yet, a recent analysis of grants funded by the entire NIH found only 628 studies from 1989 to 2011 that mentioned LGBT [14]. Of these, only 5.6 % focused on cancer and only 1.4 % on tobacco [14]. The gap of funding by the NIH on LGBT research is vast.

The American Cancer Society is the largest not-for-profit funder of cancer research. Over a 15-year period, only six grants focusing on LGBT populations were funded, all six during a 7-year period when one of the chapter authors (R.E.) served as Director of Cancer Control and Prevention Research, none before and none since.

This limited funding of LGBT cancer research by both the NIH and ACS occurred despite both organizations' embrace of an inclusive definition of health disparities, each acknowledging sexual orientation and the greater burden of cancer in LGBT communities. Further within the ACS, this inclusive approach relied heavily on a knowledgeable LGBT-research-friendly and out Program Director, who encouraged applicants to apply for funding of their LGBT focused applications. Positive changes took place in terms of research focusing on LGBT health at the NIH in 2012; a cross-institutional Funding Opportunity Announcement (in effect until 2015) was released that focuses specifically on the health of LGBTI groups. The extent to which this Funding Opportunity resulted in funded LGBT research studies has yet to be evaluated.

In order to be funded, peer review committees have to review LGBT application and deem them worthy of funding. For the ACS, it is clear that the programmatic strategies of including LGBT health disparities within the definition of cancer health disparities, the appointment of peer reviewers with LGBT expertise, and the knowledge of an LGBT-research-friendly and out Program Director, encouraged applicants to apply for funding. Although this is but a small example of making change possible, think of how much change we can achieve if at the NIH, each Institute had a Program Officer knowledgeable and welcoming of LGBT applications and each review committee included reviewers with LGBT expertise.

Recommendations for Action In 2011, the Institute of Medicine report on LGBT health [2] outlined a set of recommendations that would advance the knowledge and understanding of LGBT health, such as routinely collecting data on sexual and gender minorities in all federal surveys and in electronic health records [15]. Other key IOM recommendations focus on the NIH; suggesting a full research agenda on LGBT health, the training of LGBT researchers, and the routine collection of data on LGBT; i.e., for every grant submitted, researchers would have to justify why LGBT people were excluded if they were not automatically included in the study. Another often-mentioned change that researchers in particular wish to see is for the Director of NIH to explicitly recognize LGBTI individuals as minorities, "through the guidelines established … define the terms 'minority group' and 'subpopulation'" (492B(g)[2] http://grants.nih.gov/grants/funding/women_min/guidelines_amended_10_2001.htm).

There have been several key positive changes at the NIH in terms of research focusing on LGBT health; for example, the issuing of a cross-institution Funding Opportunity Announcement in 2012 that is still in effect, that focuses specifically on the health of LGBTI groups. In 2013 the NIH Director outlined a three-pronged plan for increasing the portfolio of grants that focus on LGBT populations, including the creation of a LGBTI Research Coordinating Committee (RCC) under the National Institute on Minority Health and Health Disparities which is a trans-NIH committee that facilitates and coordinates activities related to LGBT issues across the NIH and the Department of Health and Human Services. In 2014 the NIH LGBTI RCC, in conjunction with the NIH Office of Equity, Diversity and Inclusion, developed a website containing information about the committee and its activities, as well as programs at NIH and other LGBT-focused material (see: http://edi.nih.gov/people/portfolios/about). A report just released by the Department of Health and Human Services, indicates that the NIH will take additional steps to advance research in LGBT health. One new example is the launch Health Inequity Exploration Research Supplements for existing research grants. These changes are both necessary and laudable, but are only the tip of the iceberg; more importantly, at the time of writing, none of the IOM recommendations have been implemented. Only with the implementation of all the IOM recommendations will we see the beginning of the needed movement towards building a research knowledge base of cancer in the LGBT community, and only with that knowledge can we begin to implement necessary programmatic and legislative changes. It is possible that this will in fact be implemented in the next few years; the recently released report states that the NIH will release a strategic plan for sexual and gender minority health research that aligns with the recommendations issued by the IOM (see: http://www.hhs.gov/lgbt/resources/reports/dhhs-lgbt2014annualreport.pdf).

The Academic Obstacle

In addition to the two major research obstacles described above, there is another barrier not often discussed. The majority of health related research is conducted within the context of academia; where promotion and tenure are very tightly controlled, and where senior faculty input plays a key role in a "yay" or "nay" vote for either promotion or tenure. Unfortunately, until recently, faculty who built their careers around research focusing on LGBT groups (other than HIV research), by virtue of their research focus, often hampered their career, facing homophobia and discrimination by their academic institution and the academic community. Many faculty members have been advised not to conduct research in the LGBT field, and those who do are susceptible to having their work marginalized or described as 'biased' and 'lacking rigor' [16]. While HIV and AIDS-related research, which after initial tremendous struggles has been consistently funded [1, 14], there are comparably fewer grant-funded academic cancer researchers with a focus on cancer in LGBT populations, given the significant obstacles they face. Despite the many hurdles within academia and the dire funding, a National Summit on Cancer in LGBT Communities was held in NY in 2014, the first such summit on cancer in the community ever held. We owe a debt of gratitude to each of these courageous and inspiring leaders who have led the way.

Recommendations for Action It is imperative that academic institutions develop a climate where institutional discrimination is diminished, tokenism is not accepted and departments do all to create a climate of inclusivity and cultural competency

[16]. Within that context, bias against LGBT-focused research conducted by faculty must be highlighted and addressed. In many ways, academic institutions will likely follow suit and reward LGBT-focused research, once gender and sexual minorities will be part of minority definitions and protections via federal policies and guidelines, similar to changes that occurred within academia with respect to racial and ethnic minorities. There are some organizations that can serve as role models for future LGBT Centers that focus on cancer and LGBT health in academia. For example, The Center for LGBTQ Studies (CLAGS) is the first University based center (at CUNY) with the specific goal of nurturing academic excellence in scholarship focused on the LGBT community. They have recently launched LGBT Scholars of Color Conference in which the goal is for LGBT Scholars of Color to network with other scholars, receive mentoring by senior scholars in academic skills including research, navigate the tenure process and help build the pipeline for the future. Twenty years ago this would not have been thought possible; however, this is just the beginning. For now these Centers are a precious rarity. Think what the future of academia and the future for LGBT health focused research would be if many more similar organizations proliferated across the US. One strategy for such proliferation would be for NIH to fund Centers of Excellence in LGBT health. This was a strategy used to jumpstart the field of disability research and HIV research; it would be a welcome addition to the field of LGBT health research. With adequate funding and institutional support, Cancer Research Centers that focus on LGBT populations could and should be established around the country, becoming leaders in cancer research and collaborating with LGBT community organizations. Until then, individual researchers will continue to focus on their areas of interest and passion and continue to write grants, conduct studies and publish their results. The results of these studies are essential to gain deeper understanding into our knowledge of cancer prevention, early detection and survivorship strategies for LGBT populations, which are so necessary to develop evidence-based programs.

Conclusion

In this chapter we have highlighted the major obstacles LGBT health and cancer research continues to face, and the resultant lack of much needed research and programs. We have also made several significant recommendations, that if (when) implemented will bring about significant improvements in the provision of prevention, early detection, quality care, and support to our LGBT brothers and sisters. We invite all our readers to become involved in whatever manner suits your wishes and skill sets best. Remember, there is absolutely no *logical* reason why the Cancer Registries do not include information on gender identity and sexual orientation, why the NIH and other funders of cancer research like the American Cancer Society do not implement the IOM Report guidelines. There is no logical reason why all healthcare settings don't openly embrace LGBT patients, and there is no logical reason why targeted cancer prevention, screening and survivorship research is not conducted and funded, and evidence-based programs developed and implemented. The recent monumental developments are indeed that, monumental, and bring in their wake huge improvements. However, we cannot, and must not rest until these substantial obstacles are overcome and we are able to conduct the necessary research and provide the services that the LGBT community needs and deserves.

References

1. Boehmer U. Twenty years of public health research: inclusion of lesbian, gay, bisexual, and transgender populations. Am J Public Health. 2002;92(7):1125–30.
2. Institute of Medicine. The health of lesbian, gay, bisexual, and transgender people: building a foundation for better understanding. Washington, DC: The National Academies Press; 2011.
3. Herrick AL, Lim SH, Plankey MW, Chmiel JS, Guadamuz TT, Kao U, et al. Adversity and syndemic production among men participating in the Multicenter AIDS cohort study: a life-course approach. Am J Public Health. 2013;103(1):79–85.
4. Fredriksen-Goldsen K, Simoni J, Walters K, Kim H-J, Lehavot K, Yang J. Reconceptualization of health disparities by sexual orientation and gender identity: LGBTQ Health Equity Model. Am J Orthopsychiatr. 2014;84(6):653–63.
5. Herrick AL, Stall R, Goldhammer H, Egan JE, Mayer KH. Resilience as a research framework and as a cornerstone of prevention research for gay and bisexual men: theory and evidence. AIDS Behav. [Research Support, N.I.H., Extramural]. 2014;18(1):1–9.
6. Hollenbach AD, Eckstrand KL, Dreger A, Edited for the AAMC, Editors. Implementing curricular and institutional climate changes to improve health care for individuals who are LGBT, gender nonconforming, or born with DSD. A resource for medical educators. Washington, DC: Association of American Medical Colleges (AAMC); 2014.
7. Sellers Dorsey Foundation. Out2Enroll Q & A Topics. 2013. http://out2enroll.org/topics/. Accessed: 13 June. 2013.
8. Alenkin N. The transgender veteran experience: policy impacts on treatment. Los Angeles: USC Center for Innovation and Research on Veterans & Military Families; 2012.
9. Hernandez JO. Gay rights one baby-step at a time: protecting hospital visitation rights for same-sex partners while the lack of surrogacy rights lingers: comment on "Ethical challenges in end-of-life care for GLBTI individuals" by Colleen Cartwright. J Bioeth Inq. [Comment]. 2012;9(3):361–3.
10. Bowen DJ, Boehmer U. The lack of cancer surveillance data on sexual minorities and strategies for change. Cancer Causes Control. 2007;18(4):343–9.
11. Brown JP, Tracy JK. Lesbians and cancer: an overlooked health disparity. Cancer Causes Control. 2008;19(10):1009–20.
12. Sell RL, Dunn PM. Inclusion of lesbian, gay, bisexual and transgender people in tobacco use-related surveillance and epidemiological research. J LGBT Health Res. [Article]. 2008;4(1):27–42.
13. Boehmer U, Miao X, Ozonoff A. Cancer survivorship and sexual orientation. Cancer (0008543X) [Article]. 2011;117(16):3796–804.
14. Coulter RWS, Kenst KS, Bowen DJ, Scout. Research funded by the National Institutes of Health on the health of lesbian, gay, bisexual, and transgender populations. Am J Public Health. 2014;104(2):e105–12.
15. NIH LGBT Research Coordinating Committee. Consideration of the Institute of Medicine (IOM) Report on the health of lesbian, gay, bisexual, and transgender (LGBT) individuals. Washington DC: National Institutes of Health; 2013.
16. LaSala MC, Jenkins DA, Wheeler DP, Fredriksen-Goldsen K. LGBT faculty, research and researchers: risks and rewards. J Gay Lesbian Soc Serv. 2008;20:253–67.

Index

U. Boehmer, R. Elk (eds.), *Cancer and the LGBT Community*,
DOI 10.1007/978-3-319-15057-4

MIX
Papier aus verantwortungsvollen Quellen
Paper from responsible sources
FSC® C105338

If you have any concerns about our products,
you can contact us on
ProductSafety@springernature.com

In case Publisher is established outside the EU,
the EU authorized representative is:
Springer Nature Customer Service Center GmbH
Europaplatz 3, 69115 Heidelberg, Germany

Printed by Libri Plureos GmbH
in Hamburg, Germany